PRESCRIPTION ALTERNATIVES

PRESCRIPTION ALTERNATIVES

Earl Mindell, R.Ph., Ph.D.
and Virginia Hopkins, M.A.

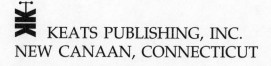
KEATS PUBLISHING, INC.
NEW CANAAN, CONNECTICUT

Prescription Alternatives is not intended as medical advice. Please consult a health professional should the need for one be indicated.

Printed in the United States of America

Library of Congress Cataloging-in-Publication Data

Mindell, Earl.
   Prescription alternatives / Earl Mindell and Virginia Hopkins.
      p.   cm.
   Includes bibliographical references and index.
   ISBN 0-87983-790-X
   1. Naturopathy.   2. Drugs, Nonprescription—Utilization.   3. Alternative medicine—Popular works.   4. Consumer education.   I. Hopkins, Virginia.
II. Title
  RZ999.M54   1998
   615.5'35—dc21   98-16266
                                                      CIP

10 9 8 7 6 5 4 3 2

Keats Publishing, Inc.
27 Pine Street (Box 876)
New Canaan, Connecticut 06840-0876

Website address: www.keats.com

CONTENTS

Introduction   vii

PART I
LAYING THE FOUNDATION FOR GOOD HEALTH

1. Changing the Pill-Popping Mindset   3
2. How to Avoid Prescription Drug Abuse   19
3. How Your Body Processes Drugs   32
4. How Drugs Interact with Food, Drink and
   Supplements   43
5. How Drugs Interact with Other Drugs   50
6. Surgery, Drugs and Nutrition: Minimizing the Damage
   and Maximizing Your Recovery   54
7. How to Read Drug Labels and Information Inserts   59

PART II
PRESCRIPTION DRUGS AND THEIR NATURAL ALTERNATIVES

8. The Six Core Principles for Optimal Health   71
9. Drugs for Heart Disease and Their Natural Alternatives   87

10. Drugs for the Digestive Tract and Their Natural
    Alternatives   184
11. Cold, Cough, Asthma and Allergy Drugs
    and Their Natural Alternatives   224
12. Drugs for Pain Relief and Their Natural Alternatives   284
13. Antibiotics, Antifungals and Their Natural Alternatives 327
14. Drugs for Insomnia, Anxiety and Depression and
    Their Natural Alternatives   363
15. Diabetes Drugs and Their Natural Alternatives   400
16. Drugs for Eye Diseases and Their Natural Alternatives   421
17. Drugs for the Prostate and Their Natural Alternatives   447
18. Synthetic Hormones and Their Natural Alternatives   454
19. Drugs for Osteoporosis and Their Natural Alternatives   485
20. Drugs for Herpes and Their Natural Alternatives   502
Resources   507
Recommended Reading   508
References   510
Index   529

INTRODUCTION

IF YOU HAVE THIS book, you're probably taking at least two prescription drugs, or you know somebody who is. If you or someone you love is taking any type of medication, from an allergy medicine to a beta-blocker, you'll want to know how the medicine affects the body and how to stay healthy while on it. We'll give you that information in this book, but we're also going to tell you how you can solve your health problems without the drugs. Ultimately we hope that this book inspires you to get off your prescription drugs and keep yourself healthy primarily through lifestyle, diet and nutrition. We have found that almost everyone taking a long-term prescription drug can wean themselves off drugs and create good health—and often vibrant, radiant good health—using simple, safe, natural remedies with no side effects.

As a general rule, prescription drugs cause imbalances in the body ranging from depletion of vitamins and minerals, to constipation and lowered immune function. *Prescription Alternatives* gives you a tool for easily and immediately accessing information about how the drugs you are taking affect your body, the steps you can take to counteract these imbalances and what alternative treatments are available.

There is no possible way we could cover every drug available, or every interaction or problem with every drug. We have tried to cover the most commonly used drugs in detail, but ultimately we urge you to take responsibility for any drug use by consulting with your pharmacist and reading the drug insert. Knowledge of the side effects and interactions of drugs is changing every day. It is our goal to teach you how to be a knowledgeable and conservative drug user, who knows how to ask the right questions and get the necessary information to stay healthy.

The United States is currently the only country in the world that allows drug companies to advertise prescription drugs directly to the consumer. It used to be that prescription drugs could only be touted to physicians. But now consumer ads on TV tantalize you with great promises of health and well-being, skim through the side effects as quickly as possible and then suggest you contact your physician or a drug company hotline for more information. The drug companies are also responsible for the expensive, slick, four-color ads you now see in consumer magazines and newspapers. You are bombarded with $3 billion worth of advertising for prescription and over-the-counter drugs every year. That should give you an idea of how valuable you are as a drug consumer and of the staggering profits the drug companies rake in every year.

Drugs have powerful effects on the body, so please don't abruptly stop taking any prescription medication. It's best to work with a health-care professional to monitor your health as you switch from drugs to natural health.

I

Laying the Foundation for Good Health

CHAPTER 1

Changing the Pill-Popping Mindset

WHAT DO YOU WANT when you go to an M.D.? Most of us, if we're being honest, would say we want the doctor to give us a name for our disease and a pill to make it go away. We call this the pill-popping mindset and it has become a deadly habit.

We have been convinced, through *multibillion* dollar advertising and marketing campaigns on TV and in popular magazines and newspapers, that everything "wrong" with us is a result of genetics or our biochemistry and that we should look for a pill that will fix the mistake that nature made. But only a fraction of a percent of what is wrong with us is attributable to genetics and biochemistry. For most of us what's wrong is a consequence of an unhealthy lifestyle: poor nutrition, overeating, lack of exercise, chronic stress, not enough sleep and exposure to toxins such as pesticides. These are all choices we make that we can do something about. Taking drugs to solve health problems caused by an unhealthy lifestyle is not a good strategy for a high quality life, or even for a long and healthy life.

In an article published in the *Journal of the American Medical Association* (JAMA), researchers studying "adverse drug events" or ADEs in people admitted to a big city hospital estimated that 140,000 Americans die every year from ADEs. An earlier study from the University of Arizona estimated that 28 percent of hospitalizations were attributable to prescription drug-related problems. We haven't even counted the hundreds of thousands of elderly people who die at home or in nursing homes and are never autopsied.

If a disease were killing that many people every year we would have millions of dollars mobilized to study it and we would be wearing ribbons on our lapels to increase awareness of the problem. To put this in some perspective, breast cancer kills about 46,000 American women each year and according to the Centers for Disease Control, about 40,000 Americans are dying from AIDS every year.

An FDA research group recently estimated that mistakes made in the prescription and dispensation of medications result in 938,000 "injuries" a year. That's close to a million people injured by drugs. Do you think that the drug companies, the hospitals or the physicians responsible for manufacturing and dispensing the drugs are paying for the staggering cost of these injuries? Of course not. We all pay for it through sky high insurance rates and taxes.

As you'll read later, at least 11 million people are abusing prescription drugs, resulting in not only a drop in quality of life, but a huge cost to the taxpayer in the form of increased accidents, workmen's compensation claims, an increase in days of work missed, hospitalizations due to drug overdoses and drug treatment centers.

If we look at the problem in dollars, according to studies published in JAMA, mistakes in prescribing drugs and the treatment of drug side effects cost about $76 billion every year. Other studies put the number as high as $136 billion. That $76 billion comes out of the high insurance rates you're paying, the taxes that go to Medicare (which is collapsing under the weight of its economic burden), and straight out of your pocket. That means you're spending hundreds of dollars a year to keep the drug companies in business, while they keep peddling dangerous and improperly studied drugs.

According to a study published in the *Western Journal of Medicine*, some $20 billion could be saved each year in hospital costs simply by supplementing folic acid and vitamin E. This is based on the well-studied fact that folic acid deficiencies contribute to neural tube birth defects and low birth weight premature babies, and that just 100 IU of vitamin E daily dramatically reduces the risk of heart disease. Imagine the billions that could be saved both in drug sales and overall health costs if everyone took a good multivitamin!

Tragically, avoiding prescription drugs isn't quite as easy as asking your M.D. for alternatives. The powerful international drug companies have wormed their way into the very heart of medicine like an insidious parasite, controlling what's taught in medical school, the continuing medical education courses M.D.s take to keep their medical license, how insurance pays for drugs and now they are even going so far as to "align with" or buy HMOs (health maintenance organizations) so they can more directly control your drug intake.

BIG DRUG BROTHER IS WATCHING YOU

A couple of years ago in *Forbes* magazine, a spokesman for a major drug company proudly boasted about how profitable his company was going to be in the next decade because they were aligning themselves with HMOs and would work with them to ensure "greater patient compliance" in taking drugs. This is a stunningly insensitive point of view. Obviously the man had considered the financial implications of what he was saying, but not the effect on the people involved. These people don't want greater "patient compliance" so that you'll get better, they want it so that you'll take more drugs. If their drugs were working, they wouldn't have to be so concerned about patient compliance.

Every year the big drug companies take a stronger and stronger stranglehold on the health of America and the alternative health community becomes more like David fighting Goliath. It's important that you be aware of how your health is being controlled (and ruined) by the greed of a medical system that is designed not to heal but to push drugs.

Here's a typical scenario of how this unholy drug company/HMO alliance is already playing out across America. Let's take a typical 63-year-old woman named Ann, who goes to her HMO for an annual checkup, carrying a bag full of her pills, as instructed. Ann is already on the drug treadmill, taking an ACE inhibitor to lower her blood pressure which is marginally high, a cough suppressant to treat the nagging cough caused by the ACE inhibitor, sleeping pills to help her sleep because her cough keeps waking her up, the estrogen Premarin for hormone replacement therapy, the synthetic progesterone Provera to offset the cancer-promoting effects of the estrogen (which along with the sleeping pills makes her feel tired and mentally foggy), the antiosteoporosis drug Fosamax which is giving her heartburn, Tagamet to treat the heartburn and Metamucil to treat the constipation and indigestion caused because the Tagamet is suppressing her stomach acid, which was low to begin with.

Ann isn't feeling too great, but she's been reading more about natural health and has decided she wants to go off all her drugs, replacing them with changes in lifestyle. She's hoping her physician will help her with a weight loss program to lower her blood pressure and a natural progesterone cream for her osteoporosis and hormone replacement therapy. She also plans to use psyllium instead of Metamucil until her constipation goes away and plans to use melatonin if her increased exercise doesn't always help her sleep. She has a list of what she wants to do and eagerly brings it in to her physician. He tells her that he doesn't "know about that hocus-pocus natural stuff," and that if she wants to continue being treated by her HMO she needs to cooperate and take the drugs he prescribes. "But doctor," she pleads, "since I started on all these drugs life is hardly worth living! I'm tired all the time, I'm coughing all the time and I'm depressed. I want to get off these drugs." Her doctor brushes her off, saying everything in her bag is approved by the HMO and the insurance company and if she has health complications caused by doing something different than he prescribes her insurance might not cover it or her rates could go up.

This really scares Ann. What if she needs surgery and her physician, angry because she hasn't toed the HMO line, claims it was caused because she didn't follow instructions? "Okay," says Ann, "I'll take the drugs. But I looked up this ACE inhibitor I'm taking and it says one of its common side effects is a nagging cough. Couldn't you put me on a different drug to lower my blood pressure?" Her physician impatiently pulls out her chart, quickly scans it and says, "This is the drug approved by this HMO for your problem. I'm afraid you'll have to live with it."

Ann meekly takes her bag of drugs and leaves, obediently filling a new prescription for Prozac on her way out. She never takes it, but the records show that she filled the prescription, so her physican and HMO will be happy. She realizes she's on her own, unless she decides to work with an M.D. who uses alternative medicine who's not in her HMO.

Why does Ann have to take a drug that is causing side effects? Because that's the one made by the drug company her HMO is in cahoots with. And why might her insurance company not cover future procedures or even raise her rates? Because the drug companies and HMOs are also in cahoots with the insurance companies (this isn't strictly legal, so it's not being openly boasted about). The effect is that the insurance companies, instead of the physician, get to decide which drugs may be prescribed for which health problems and Ann's health and well-being are pushed aside for the health of corporate profits.

The picture of a patient in effect being forced to take drugs or suffer the consequences is frightening. It begins to put the drug company/HMO/insurance company alliance on the level of drug pushers on the street. This is nothing less than extortion. Believe me, the future looks even more like Big Drug Brother will be watching over your shoulder and telling you how to live your life when all medical records are on a nationally computerized system and refusal to take a drug could mean cancellation of HMO services or health insurance.

What you can do to fight this practice is write to the politicians you've voted into office and object; try to give your health insurance business to a company that covers preventive and alternative health care (they're springing up all over the country; check your Yellow Pages); raise a fuss at your HMO and demand they cover alternative medical practices; and above all, stay healthy so you don't have to use them!

TAKING BACK THE POWER TO STAY HEALTHY

Too many of us have put our health in the hands of our physician. We have a philosophy that says, "I should be able to eat as much sugar and fat as I want, drink as much coffee, soda pop and alcohol as I want, overwork, undersleep, underexercise and not suffer any consequences." After all, with the miracle of modern medicine, you can just go to the physician and you will receive a pill or surgery to fix your problem and insurance will pay for 80 percent of it. Such a deal.

The truth is that we begin suffering from our bad habits in our forties, and for too many people, life from about age 50 on is one round after another of physicians, surgeries and drug side effects. We may be kept alive, but what is our quality of life?

This is not to suggest that you need to eat nothing but brown rice and tofu and run five miles a day, but it is to suggest that if you're hooked on sugar or fat you scale back, and that if you're a couch potato you get up and move your body. (You'll get more specifics in the next chapter.) When your physician offers you a drug, don't unquestioningly take it, but ask questions first.

THE MYTH OF THE FDA AS OUR PROTECTOR

Not long ago there was a television news program about a controversial new fake fat recently approved by the FDA. A woman in a grocery store was asked by the TV commentator what she thought about the new product. Her response was, "Well, if the FDA has approved it, it must be safe."

Nothing could be further from reality. Although the FDA is supposed to be an impartial government watchdog organization protecting us consumers from greedy corporations looking to make a buck at the expense of our health, in truth it is a politically driven machine largely controlled by food and drug manufacturers. FDA drug approval has much more to do with political maneuvering and who's throwing around the most money and power, and very little to do with how safe and effective a food or drug is. You absolutely cannot assume that just because a food or drug carries the label "FDA Approved," that means you can take it without concern.

Remember, those FDA-approved drugs are killing at least 140,000 people a year. That's an epidemic! Meanwhile, the FDA is wasting millions of dollars harassing people who sell natural supplements. There are bizarre tales of FDA "troops" flying in through alternative health practitioners' doors with guns drawn, confiscating their files and taking them to court, all because they were selling a vitamin in the way the FDA hasn't approved.

How many people have been killed by nutritional supplements and herbs prescribed by alternative practitioners? Zero. That's right. Zero. Now let's look again at the minimum number of people who have died because they took FDA-approved drugs—about 384 *every day* just in the U.S. Next time you're about to walk out of your physician's office with a prescription in your hand, remember that number and think again about whether FDA approval should give you confidence.

If that isn't enough, think about the thousands of women whose children have reproductive cancers because they took the drug DES when they were pregnant. How about all the children with missing limbs whose mothers took thalidomide? Or all the women who took estrogen in the '50s and '60s, thinking they would be forever young, when in truth the Grim Reaper was about to knock on the door with reproductive cancers.

A more recent example of the FDA's level of concern for your health is the drug combination known as fen-phen (dexfenfluramine/Redux or fenfluramine/Pondimin and phentermine), prescribed to millions for weight loss in spite of the fact that it was not a combination approved by the FDA. Phentermine is an amphetamine-like drug (amphetamines are known on the street as speed), while dexfenfluramine and fenfluramine are Prozac-like drugs that raise serotonin levels, offsetting the jitteriness caused by the phentermine.

The FDA knew perfectly well that this unstudied drug combination was being handed out like candy to anyone who wanted to lose a few pounds, and chose to look the other way. Even when evidence came out of Europe, which had been using the combination for a longer period of time, that fen-phen could cause pulmonary hypertension (almost always a fatal disease) in a small percentage of women, they still chose to look the other way. The FDA and the media did stage press conferences with reassuring sound bites about how the risk of dying from heart disease due to obesity was so high that it was preferable for some women to take the chance of getting pulmonary hypertension. What they forgot to mention is that in no study have women ever kept the weight off after they stopped taking fen-phen, nor did they mention that the FDA themselves had never approved either drug for long-term use.

Then the Mayo Clinic found that a population of women with odd and potentially deadly heart valve damage had all been taking fen-phen, yet it still took the FDA months to ask the manufacturer to pull the fenfluramine and dexfenfluramine off the market. We don't even know that these drugs by themselves cause the problem; it is most likely the combination of the drugs that causes the problem. The latest numbers are that as many as 30 percent of the people who have taken this combination long term may have heart valve damage. This amounts to hundreds of thousands of people (mostly women) with possibly permanent damage to their hearts!

But the saga is not yet over. Now the combination of Prozac and phentermine, called Pro-phen or phen-Pro, is being substituted. The makers of Prozac are loudly protesting the use of this new combination (to avoid future lawsuits), but they are doing it so loudly that millions of women are sure to hear about it and in their desperation to lose weight, they are likely to try it anyway. And their physicians will most likely prescribe it to them, telling themselves that if they don't prescribe it, the patient will just go elsewhere to get it.

Since it's likely that it is the combination of higher serotonin and an amphetamine-like drug that is causing the heart damage, Pro-phen could harm thousands of people who are, in effect, being guinea pigs for drug experimentation.

One of the saddest parts of this latest tragedy with prescription drugs is that when dexfenfluramine was under consideration for approval by the FDA, it was very nearly not approved because in high doses it causes cause brain damage in laboratory animals, and they knew that it could cause pulmonary hypertension. The FDA's advisory committee of scientists actually voted against approving the drug, but it was approved anyway, with the condition that further studies be done on brain damage and long-term use. A year later those studies had not even begun.

Most likely, the FDA will continue its shameful behavior of protecting the drug companies and it will look the other way while hundreds of thousands of people experiment with the combination of Prozac and phentermine. The drug manufacturers will rake in millions of dollars worldwide and the physicians and weight loss clinics who push these drugs will also rake in millions. The only losers will be the women and men who become ill from using the drugs, and their families who suffer along with them.

THE PRESSURES OF BEING AN M.D.

If you have a typical M.D. he has probably scared you half to death with threats and warnings about what will happen if you go off your drugs, but that's only because he doesn't know any other way. He has been taught that it's too difficult to help a patient make lifestyle and diet changes, and is at risk of losing his medical license if he doesn't conform.

Helping the whole patient, not just a set of symptoms, takes time and thoughtfulness. Physicians are not trained to help you as a whole person. They are trained to diagnose a disease and find a pill to treat it with. If they take more than 10 or 15 minutes with a patient they start to lose money because their malpractice insurance is so high or their HMO is dictating the amount of time they are allowed to spend with a patient.

Being an M.D. at this time in history is fraught with problems. In medical school and during residency, M.D.s-in-training are given an inhuman workload, putting them in a state of chronic stress and sleep deprivation which makes them particularly susceptible to brainwashing. This is not to say that medical students are consciously being brainwashed, but that is the effect. What they are taught in medical school becomes a mindset, a sort of gospel; they are taught that deviating from the gospel can mean the death of a patient, a lawsuit or loss of a medical license. This is a very compelling set of circumstances for toeing the party line, even if it's clearly not working.

The drug companies have a powerful presence from the beginning of the medical student's education. Did you know that drug companies court medical students with free meals and medical supplies and that they often "sponsor" talks in medical school? Why do medical schools allow this clearly unethical practice? Who do you think is funding the majority of their research and studies? Right, the drug companies. The effect is that drug companies are dictating what is taught in our medical schools.

Once an M.D. has a practice he is courted by drug companies with free samples and if he prescribes enough of their product, offers of free vacations or other perks. Drug companies also sponsor CME (continuing medical education) courses, which are required for keeping a medical license. The ultimate drug company "bribery" is sending an M.D. on an exotic vacation and including CME courses along with it. The physician spends a few hours a day listening to lectures on how to prescribe the company's drugs and the rest of his time on the beach or golf course.

Pressure to conform also comes from the physician's state medical board which has the power to take away his license. Physicians are subject to having their medical license taken away if they fail to conform to the "standard of care" dictated by the board. Thus, a physician who fails to prescribe the "right" class of drugs for a common problem such as high blood pressure can be threatened with the loss of his license.

The typical physician leaves medical school half a million dollars in debt and is eager to begin a lucrative practice to pay off loans. He or she may be starting a family and paying a mortgage. The last thing in the world he or she needs is any type of threat to their medical license. The pressure to conform and go along with the status quo is tremendous.

Now physicians have another force operating against them: the unholy alliance of drug companies and HMOs/insurance companies. If the insurance company and drug company make a back room deal stipulating that only certain drugs are to be prescribed for certain problems (i.e., the insurance company can tell the physician which drugs can be prescribed for which disease), that takes prescribing out of the hands of the physician. Insurance company involvement in drug prescribing has been justified under the guise of saving money by approving cheaper generic drugs, but in truth there are plenty of expensive patent drugs being prescribed because the drug company agreed to supply them at a reduced price in exchange for exclusive prescription of their drug. The effect of this practice is that your physician cannot always prescribe the drug he or she feels would be best for you.

Now the physician's job has been reduced to seeing a patient for 10 to 15 minutes, making a diagnosis and finding out which drug his HMO requires him to prescribe for that disease. How long has it been since you have met a physician who is happy with the job? It's easy to see why there is such widespread dissatisfaction in the profession. Being a physician no longer has much to do with healing.

Intelligent, well-intentioned and courageous M.D.s who genuinely want to heal their patients must struggle to break free of the "diagnose and prescribe a pill" mindset. It takes time, perseverance and a willingness to venture into the brand new territory of preventive, natural and holistic approaches to healing. It takes a willingness to be challenged by the state medical board and to be fired by an HMO. Be sympathetic to the pressures brought to bear on your physician, but don't ever be pressured or bullied yourself into taking drugs you don't need.

PORTRAIT OF A CONVENTIONAL MEDICINE APPROACH

What's the difference between a conventional medical approach and an alternative approach to a health problem? Let's say a woman in her fifties named Pam goes to her physician for an annual checkup and he finds that her blood sugar levels are high. In spite of the fact that she is at least 50 pounds overweight he never questions her eating habits, but tells her she is "prediabetic" and prescribes oral diabetes drugs to "control" the problem.

Pam dutifully and unquestioningly takes the drug, while continuing her habit of eating pastries for breakfast along with three or four cups of sugar-laden coffee, drinking soda pop all day long, snacking on candy bars and chips in the afternoon, and having pudding or pie for dessert. Her idea of a vegetable is ketchup or peas from a can and her carbohydrates are all refined white rice, white bread and pasta. She gets virtually no exercise aside from cleaning the house and never drinks any water.

The drug Pam is taking for her prediabetic condition gives her chronic indigestion, so she starts taking a drug called Tagamet, which reduces her digestive symptoms, but now her stomach acid, which was low to begin with, is practically nonexistent so she's not digesting her food and is not getting any nutrients from her food. The drug is also putting stress on her kidneys and it happens her estrogen is low too, so she starts getting chronic urinary tract infections.

Pam is put on antibiotics for her urinary tract infection, but that lowers her immune system defenses and kills all the beneficial bacteria in her colon, so she gets a bad case of the flu that just won't go away and she has constant gas from the colon imbalance.

She starts taking antihistamines for the chronic sinus infection she's developed and her physician tells her he thinks a hysterectomy will solve her urinary tract problems. She gets the hysterectomy and is put on synthetic hormones, which make her feel depressed and weepy, so the physician gives her some Prozac.

Do you get the picture? This is an extremely common scenario. We'll bet you nearly every family physician in America has been through either this exact scenario or a variation on the theme.

The woman is now taking a diabetes drug, an H2 blocker (Tagamet), antihistamines, synthetic hormones and Prozac. She's exhausted all the time, she's mentally flaky and emotionally withdrawn and is just waiting for her next health problem to hit, which it will. She's on the royal road to heart disease or a stroke and is likely to begin losing her eyesight soon. She's got arthritis and chronic headaches.

What is the future of someone like this? Her quality of life is horrible, she's no fun to be around anymore, she'll cost the medical system and taxpayers hundreds of thousands of dollars before she dies and she feels helpless. She's doing everything the physician tells her to do, like a good girl, and she's still sick and getting sicker by the day. Her future? More drugs, more drug side effects, more disease, more surgeries and more pain. This is no way to live and yet this is how millions of Americans, caught in the insidious web of an unhealthy lifestyle, conventional medicine and drugs, will live out their so-called golden years.

Now let's take a look at a different scenario.

PORTRAIT OF AN ALTERNATIVE APPROACH

Now let's say Pam is wary of taking pills and goes to a naturopathic doctor referred to her by a friend. This doctor looks at her blood and urine tests and talks to her about her eating and exercise habits. He asks her if she's willing to make some changes in her diet and to start getting some exercise and she agrees to do that if it's not too hard. She's tried diets before she says, and they never work. The doctor tells her that he's asking for a permanent lifestyle change, not a temporary diet, and she agrees to try it out for six months.

The doctor asks her to make an appointment with his staff nutritionist to create a diet and supplement program that's manageable for her, gives her the phone number of a support group of other people in a similar position, and recommends an exercise program especially designed for older women at the local YMCA.

The staff nutritionist asks Pam to restrict her sugar to one small treat a day, encourages her to substitute fruit when she gets serious sugar cravings, recommends some cookbooks that will teach her how to prepare whole grains and fresh vegetables, and asks her to drink eight glasses of water every day. She gives Pam some sample meal plans and encourages her to ask the women in her support group for ideas about shopping and preparing these new foods.

The nutritionist also gives Pam a prescription for a multivitamin, as well as a vitamin and mineral formula for stabilizing blood sugar that contains chromium, zinc, vanadyl sulfate and some herbs.

The doctor asks Pam to come back in a month to have her blood sugar checked again and encourages her to call if she's having problems with any part of the new lifestyle.

A month later Pam returns, delighted to report that she's lost 10 pounds, has much more energy and has made wonderful new friends both in her support group and in her exercise group. Her blood sugar test comes out normal and her blood pressure has dropped a few points. She's complaining about indigestion on the new diet, so the doctor asks her to try taking betaine hydrochloride before meals to supplement what may be low stomach acid and to notice whether any particular food is bothering her. The nutritionist asks her to keep taking the formula for blood sugar for another two months and asks her to now cut her sugar treats down to three times a week.

Pam returns in three months and her blood sugar is still normal, she's lost 15 more pounds, her digestion is fine and she's joined a synchronized swimming group. She reports that she hasn't felt better in years and she loves her new lifestyle.

What is the future of someone like this? She's happy, she's healthy, she's physically fit, she's emotionally and mentally stable, she's not taking any drugs and her golden years are likely to be truly golden. Her medical costs are minimal and her enjoyment of life is maximal.

This scenario is just as real as the one before it. What a dramatic difference!

Modern medicine is wonderful if you have a life-threatening infection that requires antibiotics, if you need surgery, if you have a broken bone or need a diagnosis for a disease, but for nearly all other health problems you're better off working with alternative medicine. By now there are many thousands of M.D.s who are combining safe, effective alternative medicine with what they learned in medical school and giving excellent health care. Unfortunately you are unlikely to find them at your HMO.

If you're confused about how to choose a health care professional who will truly be a partner in your health care, I'd like to recommend an excellent book that can guide you and also gives many resources and references to use in your search. It's called *Five Steps to Selecting the Best Alternative Medicine: A Guide to Complementary and Integrative Health Care*, by Mary and Michael Morton (New World Library, Novato, Calif., 1996).

HOW TO STAY ALIVE AND WELL IN THE HOSPITAL

Stan was a cardiologist for 35 years in a major American city. He was in and out of a large hospital every day looking after his patients, and of course was intimately familiar with all the goings-on in his medical community. After he retired, Stan was told by his physician that he needed to be hospitalized for some surgery. This normally calm, cool and collected professional went into a panic. He was terrified at the prospect of being hospitalized. He made his wife promise that either she or his sister would be by his side at all times during his hospital stay, day and night. He conferred with his physician ahead of time about what drugs he would be getting, how often, and in what dosages, and wrote this all down for his wife and sister. He instructed them to double and triple check any medication he was given against what he had written, and told them that under no circumstances was he to be given anything else unless he or his physician, in person, specifically approved it.

It may sound like Stan was being paranoid, but in reality he was just being smart. After decades of working in a hospital, he was all too aware of how easy it is for patients to be injured and even killed by improper medication. According to a Harvard study done a few years ago, these types of errors result in 200,000 injuries to hospital patients every year.

Have an Advocate

Don't panic if you need to be hospitalized, but do have a friend or relative be your advocate to make sure you're getting the proper care and medication. Stan's concerns were confirmed in a study published in JAMA in which 4,000 patients admitted to two Boston hospitals over a six-month period were tracked by Harvard researchers. They found 247 "adverse drug events," meaning medication errors that injured the patient in some way. Of these, 70 or 28 percent were considered preventable. Of the 70, 56 percent were caused by physician error and 34 percent by improper administration by a nurse.

Watch for Errors Like a Hawk: This Is Your Life

You can protect yourself by keeping track of what medications you are being given. *Before* you go into the hospital, ask your physician what medications you will be given; the exact brand name and generic name; what they are prescribed for; the dosage, i.e., how many milligrams (mg) per pill, and how many pills you take each time; how many times in a 24-hour period you will be given them; in what form (i.e., oral, intravenous, etc.); and for how many days. Make your own daily chart with these details, and each time you are given a medication by a nurse, double check what the physician told you against what the nurse is giving you. If anything changes, ask why, and if you don't receive a satisfactory answer, refuse the medication until you can personally check with your physician or with the hospital pharmacist. If you are not able to function to do this, have a friend or relative do it for you. This may sound like a lot of trouble to go to, and you may get some resistance from the hospital staff, including your physician, but on the other hand, it could save your life.

The most frequent types of medication mistakes are:

- Prescribing the wrong drug, i.e., mixing up the names of drugs that sound alike or giving inappropriate drugs to seniors and children.
- Giving the wrong dosage of a drug, i.e., too much or not enough, or too frequently or not frequently enough.

- Mixing drugs without being aware of adverse drug interactions.
- Giving a drug via the wrong route, i.e., orally instead of intravenously.
- More than one physician prescribing drugs without paying attention to what the others are ordering.
- The side effects from a drug not being monitored.
- Stopping a drug too soon or not continuing it long enough.

CHAPTER 2

How to Avoid Prescription Drug Abuse

WHEN YOU THINK of a person who abuses drugs you probably have in mind a gang member in the inner city, a troubled teen or a Hollywood celebrity who let fame and riches get out of hand. But our educated guess is that there are probably more people abusing prescription drugs than street drugs, at an equal cost in lives ruined and ended, and at a far greater cost to the taxpayer.

Those most at risk for prescription drug abuse are the elderly, people with a history of drug abuse such as alcoholics and, believe it or not, those in the medical profession with access to the drugs.

Elderly people tend to be much more sensitive to the effects of a drug, and a slight overdose or negative side effect has a much greater potential to cause illness and even death. A recent report by the General Accounting Office, an investigative branch of Congress, found that more than 17 percent of elderly Americans not in an institution were receiving at least one of 20 drugs considered inappropriate for the elderly.

The rapidly increasing aging population represents a huge financial feedbag for the drug companies. If you are over the age of 50 and your blood pressure or cholesterol reading are even slightly above the so-called "normal" levels for your age, you will automatically be put on a drug to make those numbers seem more normal. Most of the time they will only cause ill health and side effects for which your physician will prescribe more drugs, which will cause more side effects, and so forth and so on until you're so sick you wind up in a nursing home. Please read the sections in this book on drugs for high blood pressure and cholesterol and their natural alternatives very carefully before agreeing to take a blood pressure or cholesterol medication.

But you don't have to be elderly or an alcoholic to become hooked on prescription drugs. Anybody can become hooked on prescription drugs. People who have never used street drugs, tobacco or alcohol are just as susceptible to prescription drug abuse as those who have. Those who abuse prescription drugs usually start out rationalizing their problem as okay because a physician wrote out the prescription. This is a dangerous assumption.

A tragic prescription drug-abuse scenario is the recovering alcoholic who breaks a bone or has surgery and is given a potent narcotic pain reliever such as Vicodin or Demerol by a physician who never asks whether the person has a drug abuse problem. The patient trustingly takes the drug, supposedly for a week or two, and gets hooked into another downward spiral of addiction and dependence.

In case you think prescription drug abuse is uncommon, according to the U.S. Department of Health and Human Service Administration's 1993 National Household Survey on Drug Abuse, 138 million Americans are abusing alcohol, nearly 19 million are abusing marijuana, over 10 million are abusing illicit drugs such as cocaine, crack and heroin and over 11 million people are abusing prescription drugs. Other surveys estimate that as many as 50 percent of the drug overdoses treated in the hospital are a result of prescription drug abuse. On the Drug Enforcement Agency's (DEA) list of the top 20 most-abused controlled substances, 12 or more than half are prescription drugs.

The drugs most likely to be abused are painkillers (especially opioids and narcotic analgesics), sedatives, tranquilizers and stimulants. Of the top 10 prescribed drugs in the U.S., three are narcotic painkillers. We obviously have a huge problem in the U.S. with addiction to narcotic painkillers. Shouldn't somebody at the FDA, our government watchdog agency that we pay for with our taxes, be taking a hint from this statistic and taking some action?

THE 20 MOST ABUSED DRUGS

Legalized drug abuse is common in America, mostly in the form of physicians writing out prescriptions for medications that are addictive or consciousness altering. And of course the pharmaceutical companies are making a bundle. Are the physicians who write out these prescriptions and the companies that sell them any better than the drug lords and street pushers we despise so much?

The DEA has a list of the 20 most-abused drugs in America, which is enlightening for those of us who think of drug abuse as only happening in the inner cities.

All the boldface drug names on this list are prescription drugs. The drugs with an * after them are in the benzodiazepine family. Codeine (8) and hydrocodone (13) are addictive narcotics used as painkillers and cough suppressants. Propoxyphene (9) is another addictive narcotic used for pain, but there is no evidence it is any more effective than a placebo for pain, and aspirin works as well. Oxycodone (17) is combined with acetaminophen (Tylenol) in the widely used drugs Percocet and Tylox or with aspirin in Percodan. Oxycodone is similar to a narcotic and is addictive. Try acetaminophen or aspirin alone first, and use these drugs only as a last resort. Methadone (20) is a synthetic narcotic used to replace heroin. Reportedly, addicts who use methadone don't get the same high as on heroin, but avoid the withdrawal. Nevertheless, this is a highly addictive substance with a wide range of side effects.

1. Cocaine
2. Heroin
3. Marijuana
4. **Alprazolam*** (Xanax)
5. **Diazepam*** (Valium)
6. **Clonazepam*** (Klonopin)
7. **Lorazepam*** (Ativan)
8. **Codeine**
9. **D-propoxyphene** (Darvon)
10. Methamphetamine
11. **Misc. benzodiazepines***
12. PCP
13. **Hydrocodone** (Tussionex)
14. Amphetamine
15. Hashish
16. **Chlordiazepoxide*** (Librium)
17. **Oxycodone**
18. **Temazepam*** (Restoril)
19. LSD
20. **Methadone**

THE PAINKILLERS

People who are addicted to painkilling drugs is not the same as people with cancer or other illnesses who take painkillers for legitimate pain. If anything, legitimate pain is undertreated in the U.S. because of the stigma and fear of drug addiction. This type of pain is what the drugs are made for in the first place and they should be used accordingly! Nobody should have to suffer pain unnecessarily. There is no gain or heroism in this type of preventable suffering.

If you have a legitimate need for painkilling drugs and have to take them for more than a week or two, you will eventually have to go through physical withdrawal from them. If this is done very gradually it doesn't need to be traumatic or painful. Those who get in trouble with these drugs are the ones who *deny* they're physically dependent on them. This is generally a sign that they've become physically *and* emotionally dependent.

Painkillers are the most-abused prescription drugs. For most abusers, the first introduction to painkillers is after surgery, a broken bone, a back injury or treatment for headaches. If the drugs are taken for more than a week or two, physical dependence will begin and withdrawing from the drug becomes increasingly difficult as each day passes. Every time the person tries to stop taking the drug, the discomfort of withdrawal becomes confused with the original pain. Complicating the picture even more, the painkiller will dull emotional pain long after the physical pain has worn off. People will convince themselves, their families and their physicians that the physical pain is still present, but it is withdrawal symptoms and emotional pain that are really being treated.

Painkillers with Potential for Abuse

Butalbital
Butorphanol (Stadol)
Buprenorphine (Buprenex)
Codeine (often mixed with other painkillers such as acetaminophen)
Darvon
Darvocet
Demerol
Dezocine (Dalgan)
Dilaudid
Ergotamine
Fioricet

Fiorinal
Hydrocodone
Levorfanol
Meperidine
Methadone
Methotrimeprazine (Levoprome)
Morphine
Nalbuphine (Nubain)
Oxycodone
Pentazocine (Talwin)
Percocet
Percodan
Propoxyphene
Roxicet
Roxiprin
Sumatriptan (Imitrex)
Talwin
Tramadol (Ultram)
Tussionex
Tylox
Vicodin

THE STIMULANTS

Stimulant drugs prescribed under the guise of antidepressants or appetite suppressants are the next most commonly abused prescription drugs. These are sold on the street as "uppers;" most of the so-called legitimate drugs are variations of the street drug called speed or methamphetamine. These drugs create a false sense of confidence and energy, speed up the metabolism, increase the heart rate and raise blood pressure. They can also cause irritability. Typically the abuser of these drugs is a woman who goes to the physician for anxiety, depression or some other emotional problem. If she is overweight, lethargic and depressed, a stimulant will be her physician's drug of choice. What she really needs is someone to talk to, but she gets drugged instead and having nowhere else to turn, she'll keep turning to the drugs. What goes up must come down and withdrawing from stimulant

PRESCRIPTION ALTERNATIVES

drugs can be extremely difficult, with severe rebound depression and weight gain.

The latest fad in antidepressants are the SSRIs (selective serotonin re-uptake inhibitors) such as Prozac and Zoloft. These "uppers" raise levels of the feel-good brain chemical serotonin and they also create a false sense of emotional detachment. As might be expected, drug manufacturers claim that these drugs are not addictive, but hundreds of thousands of people who have had to withdraw from them would disagree. We also have no idea what the long-term effect is of fiddling around with the brain chemistry this way, and there is mounting evidence that these drugs may be causing permanent changes in the brain.

In a particularly horrifying turn of events, drug companies selling SSRIs now see children as a potential new market for their antidepressants, and the FDA has given them the go-ahead to test the drugs on children. While the market for SSRIs for adults has finally begun to drop, for children it more than doubled between 1994 and 1996. In our "pill for every ill" culture, will children be taught to take drugs instead of learning to ride out the normal ups and downs of life? What will the long-term effects be on the growing, changing, evolving brain chemistry of a child? We don't know and we may never know. What we do know is that antidepressants are no substitute for love, affection, a supportive and communicative family atmosphere, good diet and exercise.

Stimulants with Potential for Abuse

Amphetamines
Antidepressants
Caffeine
Cylert
Dexedrines
Diethylpropion
Fenfluramine (can cause depression, drowsiness, impotence)
Mazindol
Methylphenidate (Ritalin)
Phenmetrazine
Phentermine
Phenylpropanolamine (nonprescription, i.e., Dexatrim, Acutrim)

THE BENZODIAZEPINES

The benzodiazepines are a class of drugs widely used to treat anxiety, depression related to anxiety, insomnia and generally as tranquilizers. Most nonbarbiturate sleeping pills are benzodiazepines. There are other sedatives and tranquilizers not in this class, all of which are addictive, but for the most part they have been replaced by the benzodiazepines. You can pretty much assume that if you're taking a drug for anxiety, to ease tension, nervousness or stress, or to help you sleep, that it has the potential for abuse. The barbiturates are another story, which will be covered next.

During the 1970s hundreds of thousands of women became hooked on the trendy anti-anxiety drug Valium, which is a benzodiazepine. Their physicians reassured them that the drug wasn't addictive, because the medical literature claimed it was only habit-forming in some people who were "prone to addiction." Physicians also reassured women that the drugs only created a physical dependence if they were taken in very high doses for a long period of time. Nothing could be farther from the truth, but it sold millions of dollars worth of drugs to unsuspecting women who thought they were temporarily being helped through a hard time.

Let's talk about the phrase "prone to addiction." Although some people do tend to have a more "addictive" personality than others, nearly any human being who is going through a hard time physically, emotionally, mentally or spiritually is "prone" to addiction. It is human nature to try to correct an imbalance in the body or the psyche and if a drug gives the illusion that balance has been achieved, it has the potential for abuse. What is most insidious is the physician in the white coat, that authority figure whom we have been trained not to question, who tells us the pill will be good for us and solve our problem.

Drug addiction can begin as innocently as taking something to help you sleep or to help you through a difficult time in your life. Insomnia is a very common symptom of stress and anxiety. Physicians tend to regard the benzodiazepines as harmless temporary aids for people who are stressed, anxious and not sleeping, but they are quite addictive, interact dangerously with alcohol and many other drugs and have lists of side effects as long as your arm. Please don't ever be fooled into thinking these are benign, harmless drugs. There may be a time in your life when you need to take them for some reason, but be vigilant and be aware that you will need to go through withdrawal.

All of the so-called anti-anxiety drugs have the potential for abuse. When the short-acting benzodiazepines such as lorazepam (Ativan) came out, they were applauded for their diminished potential for abuse. Experience has shown us that the short-acting versions simply created physical dependence and withdrawal symptoms right away!

Possible Withdrawal Symptoms from Anti-Anxiety Drugs

Anxiety
Confusion
Fatigue
Fear
Hallucinations
Headache
Insomnia
Loss of appetite
Mental fogginess
Seizures
Shakiness
Sweatiness

Anti-Anxiety Drugs with Potential for Abuse

Alprazolam (Xanax)
Chlorazepate (Tranxene)
Chlordiazepoxide (Librium, Mitran)
Diazepam (Valium, Zetran, Dizac)
Flurazepam (Dalmane)
Halzepam (Paxipam)
Lorazepam (Ativan)
Meprobamate (not a benzodiazepine) (Equanil, Miltown)
Oxazepam (Serax)

Prazepam
Quazepam (Doral)
Temazepam (Restoril)
Triazolam (Halcion)

THE BARBITURATES

The barbiturates are a class of drugs widely acknowledged to be addictive, but still occasionally prescribed. They were much more widely prescribed before the benzodiazepines came along. Their withdrawal symptoms can be severe enough to be fatal. There is really no reason these days to be taking a barbiturate drug. Some of the names of the barbiturates are phenobarbital (Solfoton, Bellergal), mephobarbital (Mebaral), amobarbital (Amytal), butabarbital (Butisol), secobarbital (Seconal), pentobarbital (Nembutal). The barbiturates also deplete folic acid. A folic acid deficiency can cause birth defects and high homocysteine levels, a risk factor for heart disease.

I DON'T KNOW HOW TO HEAL YOU SO TAKE THIS DRUG . . .

Ironically the prescription drugs most likely to be abused are those most likely to be prescribed when your physician *doesn't know how* to treat your problem.

For example, conventional medicine is notoriously unable to help back pain. If you go to your physician with back pain chances are you'll be given pain-killing drugs or surgery, neither of which will heal the back. But since your physician doesn't know what else to do and you are in terrible pain, he'll keep prescribing the drugs for you. Every year thousands of people become hooked on painkillers they first took for back pain. (If you have chronic back pain, before you do anything else, read the book *Healing Back Pain* by John Sarno, M.D., Warner Books, 1991.)

Chronic headaches are another source of pain that conventional medicine is often unable to heal effectively. The medical solution tends to be a potent painkiller, when the cause is usually a hormonal imbalance, a food sensitivity or chronic stress and tension.

Women who visit a physician's office complaining of nervousness, lethargy or depression are likely to be drugged. Most of these women only need someone to talk to.

When your physician prescribes a drug for an illness he doesn't know how to treat, see an alternative health care professional such as a naturopathic doctor, an acupuncturist or a chiropractor.

WHEN ARE YOU ADDICTED?

If the physician prescribed it, the drug must be okay, right? When your physician prescribes drugs for a real medical need, such as for pain after surgery, that's okay. But if you're still taking the drug every day six weeks or six months or six years later, you have a problem. In spite of their extensive training in prescribing drugs, physicians are ill-equipped to recognize the symptoms of drug addiction and even less well equipped to help a patient withdraw from drugs. Your physician is just as afraid of the stigma of having a drug-addicted patient as you are of being one. It's much easier to write you another prescription than to take the time and trouble to help you through drug withdrawal—a painful, complicated and emotionally wrenching process. To help you withdraw from a drug, find a different physician from the one who has been prescribing you drugs. Beware of physicians who insist that addictive drugs won't hurt you; that's their own form of denial and it's no help to you.

Keep in mind that two of the primary symptoms of addiction versus a purely physical dependence are denial that there is a problem and repeated attempts to stop taking the drug, followed by a relapse. One of the requirements for getting unhooked from a drug is having the personal honesty to admit there's a problem and the courage to follow through and take action.

In our culture of instant gratification, we tend to forget that qualities such as contentedness, inner calm, inner peace and emotional balance are won through the accumulation of wisdom, experience and introspection. The truth is that the vast majority of people prescribed a benzodiazepine, an antidepressant or some other type of drug that affects the mind and emotions, simply need some help making it over a rough spot in their lives. They need a sympathetic ear; somebody to listen objectively and caringly.

The distinctions made by drug manufacturers and the medical profession between drugs that are "habit-forming" and "addictive" are strictly academic and seem to have been created largely to justify prescribing dangerous drugs. If you are hooked on a drug, the difference between one that is addictive and one that is habit-forming is academic. Our definition of an addictive drug is one that creates a dependence that falls outside of a legitimate medical need. If you have been using a drug for so long that you find you can't stop, you are addicted, regardless of what the drug is.

How you answer the following questions may give you some indication of whether you are inappropriately dependent on your medication:

1. Do I need to take my medicine more often than it was prescribed?
2. Do I become tense, nervous, anxious if I don't take the medicine for more than one day?
3. Can I sleep without it?
4. Do I have to have extra supplies because I am afraid I will run out?
5. Do I have two M.D.s writing prescriptions for the same drug, in case one cuts me off?
6. Do I feel in a fog mentally when I take the drug?
7. Do I feel more alert when I take the drug?
8. Do I talk about the drug a lot to my friends and family?
9. If a pill breaks do I save up the bits and pieces?
10. Have I tried to stop taking the drug without success?
11. Do I want to stop taking the drug?
12. Have I tried to stop taking the drug and experienced such bad withdrawal symptoms that I went back on it?

If you answered "yes" to any of these questions, please consider the possibility that you are abusing the drug or drugs you are taking and get some help. Resources for prevention and recovery are listed in the back of the book.

CAN YOUR CHILDREN AND GRANDCHILDREN GET INTO YOUR DRUGS?

Just because you can't open that childproof cap on your medication bottle, don't assume that your grandchild can't. It's a fact that more kids get into medicines at their grandparents' home than at their own home. Grandparents are more likely to be taking medication and are less likely to be vigilant about keeping it away from curious youngsters. If you have children in your house, even for just a few hours, be sure all your medications are out of reach or inaccessible. This also applies when you're visiting someone who has children—you have to *assume* they will wander into your room and open your bags, and act accordingly. Many pills come in attractive colors and are small enough to be easily swallowed. Some new pills look like small jelly beans and smell like candy.

GUIDELINES FOR SAFE USE OF MEDICATIONS

Patients are rarely given enough information about how to safely and effectively use their medication to avoid addiction. Here are some guidelines.

1. If you have abused any type of drug in the past, including alcohol, or even if you haven't abused drugs but you know you have an addictive personality, tell your physician and your pharmacist and ask directly if the prescribed drug is likely to cause you a problem.
2. Ask your M.D. and your pharmacist if the drug you are being prescribed is addictive, habit-forming or if it could create a dependence.

If the answer is yes, ask for detailed information such as:

- Does this drug create a physical dependence?
- How long does it take to create a physical dependence on this drug?
- Will I have to go through physical withdrawal when I stop taking this drug? (If the answer is yes, ask your M.D. how he plans to help you do that.)
- Is there a drug I could take that is not addictive?

3. Ask your M.D. or pharmacist to explain precisely how you should

take your medicine. Be sure the following information is on the container:

- How often to take it.
- With or without food.
- What it is for, for example, pain or indigestion.

Examples:

- Take one capsule 3 times daily with food for stomach upset.
- Take one capsule a 1/2 hour before bedtime with juice for sleep.
- Take one capsule every four hours between meals for infection until gone.

4. Have your physician put on the label the number of refills you have.

5. When you receive your prescription, read the label out loud to the pharmacist. Make sure you understand how, when, for how long and why you are supposed to be taking the drug. If you have any questions, ask your pharmacist. The container may also contain an expiration date and tell how it should be stored.

6. Tell your physician and your pharmacist about any other drugs (prescription or over the counter) you are taking. If you drink a lot of alcohol, coffee or soft drinks, or if you smoke, be sure to mention it.

7. If you are allergic to any foods or drugs, tell your physician and your pharmacist. If you are pregnant, lactating or trying to become pregnant, tell your physician and your pharmacist.

8. If you notice any side effects after taking a medication such as dizziness, light-headedness, nausea, vomiting, diarrhea, skin rash or any other out-of-the-ordinary symptom, call your physician or pharmacist immediately. You may experience these side effects right away, or in a few days or weeks. You can literally be taking a drug for years without any side effects and then have them suddenly appear.

9. Throw away any medications you are no longer using. Look through your supply of medications, check the expiration dates and throw out any old ones by flushing them (minus the containers!) down the toilet.

10. Keep *all* of your medicines out of the reach of children and never give your prescription drugs to anyone else, even friends or family.

11. Read the labels on all your over-the-counter medicines. Look for cautions or contraindications.

CHAPTER 3

How Your Body Processes Drugs

MOST DRUG TESTING is done on adult men between the ages of 25 and 50, but drugs may act and interact very differently in children, teenagers, women, pregnant and nursing women, menopausal women and particularly in the elderly, where nutrient absorption and liver function is an issue. Your physician's only way of gauging your tolerance to a drug is to begin with a standard dose for an adult male and see what happens. If you don't complain of side effects or no effect, chances are the dose will never be changed.

IF YOU'RE PREGNANT OR BREAST-FEEDING, DON'T TAKE IT

There are virtually no drugs that have no effect on a developing fetus and the effects are nearly always negative. Unless you are in a life-threatening situation, it's just not worth it.

Drug effects are poorly studied in pregnant animals and for all practical purposes, unstudied in humans. An indication on the drug package insert that no negative effects have been found does *not* mean there aren't any. It may just mean it hasn't been studied. You have to assume that any drug you take will hurt your baby.

The same goes for breast-feeding. There are few drugs that don't end up in breast milk. Those that don't may end up there eventually, or affect it in other ways. Something as seemingly harmless as an aluminum-containing antacid taken when a woman is breast-feeding can cause developmental retardation.

Pregnancy and breast feeding are wonderful opportunities to use nutrition as your medicine and to explore safe, gentle alternative approaches such as acupuncture and acupressure, massage, chiropractic and meditation.

There are dozens and dozens of factors that can influence what effect a drug has on you, from how much sleep you got last night and what you had for breakfast, to the condition of your liver and your blood pressure. For example, alcohol abuse can greatly increase or decrease tolerance to a drug, as can obesity, exercise, stress levels and exposure to pollutants such as car exhaust, pesticides or industrial chemicals.

Drugs and nutrients can affect each other in your digestive system, in your bloodstream, in your liver and kidneys, or at the cell level where the drug or nutrient receptor is.

Just as it takes a variety of vitamins, minerals, amino acids and enzymes to process food so that your cells can use it, drugs also go through changes as the body uses them. They are changed as they are made useful, as they are being used and as they are being excreted from the body. Any interference in this process caused by nutritional deficiencies or interference from other drugs, food or alcohol, can raise or lower drug levels.

FACTORS THAT CAN INCREASE OR DECREASE DRUG LEVELS

Sex
Age
Race
Overweight or underweight
Pregnancy and nursing
Illness
Alcohol abuse
Food
Other drugs
Digestion
Kidney or liver damage
Nutritional deficiencies
Supplements
Exposure to toxins such as paint fumes, solvents, pesticides
Over- or under-exercise
Stress
Time of day

DRUGS THAT ARE METABOLIZED DIFFERENTLY IN WOMEN

There are probably many more drugs than these that are metabolized differently in women, but these are the ones we currently know about. If you're given a drug and experience negative side effects, ask your physician to try changing the dosage.

Amitriptyline
Benzodiazepines
Beta-blockers
Chlordiazepoxide
Diflunisal
Imipramine

Methylprednisolone
Oxazepam
Piroxicam
Prednisolone
Trazodone

YOUR BODY'S DRUG DISPOSAL SYSTEMS

The four major routes for excreting a drug from the body are the kidneys, liver, skin and lungs. Most drugs are processed out through the liver and then the kidneys.

If you have kidney or liver disease, how your body handles drugs is profoundly affected. Food, drink or lifestyle habits that stress and damage your kidneys or liver, such as alcohol abuse or chronic exposure to toxins such as solvents and paint fumes, can also affect how you process drugs. Even taking as seemingly harmless a drug as Tylenol (acetaminophen), which is hard on the liver, can affect drug levels. Kidney or liver stress or damage usually raises drug levels higher than normal by slowing down the excretion process.

The aminoglycoside antibiotics such as streptomycin, kanamycin, gentamicin and garamicin cause kidney damage in as much as 15 percent of patients treated with them, but thousands of other drugs cause less obvious stress on your kidneys. When your drug information insert indicates "renal" (kidney) problems, you should be aware that the drug is probably going to be hard on your kidneys.

POTENTIALLY DANGEROUS DRUGS TO AVOID

The following drugs are included on the FDA "watch list" because of concerns about serious side effects.

Drug Name	Use
Parlodel	Mainly to suppress lactation
Protropin	Growth failure
Serevent	Asthma attack prevention
Ticlid	Stroke prevention
Ampicillin	Antibiotic
Augmentin, Timentin	Antibiotic
Biaxin	Antibiotic
Cefotaxime	Antibiotic
Cipro (ciprofloxacin)	Antibiotic
Vantin	Antibiotic
Chlorzoxazone	Muscle pain
Etodolac	Osteoarthritis, pain
Nabumetone	Osteoarthritis, rheumatoid arthritis
Oxaprozin	Arthritis
Piroxicam	Osteoarthritis, rheumatoid arthritis
Clozapine	Schizophrenia
Tacrine	Alzheimer's disease
Ticlopidine hydrochloride	Stroke preventive
Albuterol	Asthma
Aprotinin	Reduce blood loss in bypass surgery
Digoxin	Heart failure, rhythm disturbances
Diltiazem	Hypertension, angina
Lisinopril	Hypertension, heart failure
Questran	High blood cholesterol
Terazosin	Benign prostate enlargement and hypertension

SOURCE: *U.S. News and World Report*, 1995

DRUGS THAT CAN STRESS OR DAMAGE THE KIDNEYS

ACE inhibitors
Acyclovir
Allopurinol
Aminoglycosides
Amphotericin
Beta-blockers
Captopril
Cephalothin
Chemotherapy drugs
Chlorothiazide
Chlorpropamide
Clofibrate
Cyclosporine
Diuretics
Furosemide
Isoproterenol
Lithium

Macanylamine
Methotrexate
Methysergide
Morphine
NSAIDs (acetaminophen, aspirin, ibuprofen)
Penicillins
Phenylbutazone
Phenytoin
Piperidine
Probenecid
Procaine
Quinidine
Salicylate
Sulfonamides
Tolazoline

Keeping Your P-450 Pathways Clear

Many types of drugs are prepared for clearance out of the body through the liver using the cytochrome P-450 enzymes, also known as the cytochrome P-450 pathways.

In a drug-free body, or in the presence of only one drug, the P-450

COMMON DRUGS THAT CAN CAUSE BREAST ENLARGEMENT IN MEN

ACE inhibitors
Amitryptyline (Elavil)
Cimetidine (Tagamet)
Digoxin (Lanoxin)
Famotidine (Pepcid)
Ibuprofen and related NSAIDs
Indomethacin

Ketoconazole
Ketoprofen
Methyldopa
Naproxen
Spironolactone
Terfenadine (Seldane)

DRUGS THAT CAN CAUSE DIARRHEA

Antibiotics
Antidepressant/Anti-anxiety drugs (benzodiazepines, lithium, valproic acid)
Antihypertensives (reserpine, guanethidine, methyldopa)
Cholesterol-lowering drugs (clofibrate, gemfibrozil, the statins)
Cholinergic drugs (metoclopramide)
Gastrointestinal drugs (laxatives, antacids)
Heart drugs (digitalis drugs, quinidine, hydralazine, beta-blockers, ACE inhibitors, diuretics)

---

pathways can handle the load. When you have more than one drug cleared through the same pathway, the system quickly gets overloaded, stalling the removal of the drugs from the system. The result is an overdose that can be life-threatening.

Some examples of drugs that either use the P-450 pathways or block their action are cimetidine (Tagamet), cisapride (Propulsid), the cholesterol-lowering drugs in the statin family, the macrolide antibiotics such as erythromycin and clarithromycin, most antifungal drugs such as ketoconazole and miconazole, antiarrhythmic drugs such as disopyramide (Norpace), the seizure drug phenytoin (Dilantin), the anti-Parkinson's drug bromocriptine (Parlodel), the benzodiazepine anti-anxiety drugs such as diazepam (Valium) and nefazodone (Serzone), the calcium channel blockers such as nifedipine (Procardia), the theophyllines used to treat asthma, the tricyclic antidepressants such as Elavil, the blood thinner warfarin (Coumadin), tacrine (Cognex) used to treat Alzheimer's, the antihistamines terfenadine (Seldane) and astemizole (Hismanal) and caffeine. And these are just the most commonly used drugs. Grapefruit juice also uses this pathway, which is why drinking it is contraindicated with some drugs.

Are you getting the picture? This is a very popular pathway through the liver for clearing certain types of waste matter from the body. I'd like to see the FDA require a warning on the outside of every medication that is cleared through the P-450 pathways or that blocks P-450 pathways, so that every consumer is protected against unintentionally mixing these types of drugs.

How many people do you suppose have been killed in a scenario similar to this one: Joe is taking a calcium channel blocker long term,

---

COMMON DRUGS THAT CAN DECREASE THE EFFECT OF ORAL CONTRACEPTIVES

If you're taking oral contraceptives and are prescribed one of these drugs, be sure to use an alternative form of birth control during the time you're taking these drugs and for at least two weeks afterwards.

Antibiotics	Griseofulvin
Anticonvulsants	Rifampin
Azole antifungals	Ritonavir

---

is temporarily put on a macrolide antibiotic to treat chronic bronchitis, then has a glass of grapefruit juice and a cup of coffee with breakfast, raising his levels of the calcium channel blocker so high that his blood pressure drops precipitously, causing heart failure. It's not an unlikely scenario. Or let's say it's in the evening and he takes some Tagamet (which is available over the counter) for heartburn and a Valium to help him sleep. Our guess is that this type of mis-matching kills hundreds of people every day.

Since it's unlikely that the package insert on the drug you're taking is going to tell you it's cleared through the P-450 pathways, your best bet is to check with your pharmacist before mixing any drugs, even over-the-counter drugs. Labels that warn of such things as hepatic (liver) toxicity, injury, dysfunction or function impairment, which is medical-ese for liver poison, should flash a red light in your head. This doesn't necessarily mean it's a P-450 drug, since most prescription drugs are hard on the liver in some way, but it should make you very wary if you're taking other drugs.

Drugs That Use the Liver's P-450 Pathways or Block Their Action

Mixing these drugs could result in high drug levels and/or liver damage:

Antiarrhythmic drugs (disopyramide)
Antihistamines (terfenadine, astemizole)

Benzodiazepines (diazepam, nefazodone)
Bromocriptine (Parlodel)
Caffeine
Calcium channel blockers (nifedipine)
Cholesterol-lowering drugs in the statin family
Cimetidine (Tagamet)
Cisapride (Propulsid)
Macrolide antibiotics (erythromycin, clarithromycin)
Most antifungal drugs (ketoconazole and miconazole)
Phenytoin (Dilantin)
Tacrine (Cognex)
Theophyllines
Tricyclic antidepressants
Warfarin (Coumadin)

TAKING CARE OF YOUR LIVER WHEN YOU TAKE DRUGS

Your liver is one of the busiest organs of the body, working constantly to process food for transport through the bloodstream and to metabolize waste matter for excretion through urine or feces. The list of prescription drugs that stress or damage the liver is probably longer than those that don't. If you drink alcohol in excess and take liver-stressing drugs, you could be doing substantial damage to your liver.

Some symptoms of liver toxicity are swelling and redness in the palms of the hands, yellowish skin and whites of eyes, itching, small benign fatty tumors and reddish spots on the skin or lumps under the skin of damaged blood vessels.

DRUGS THAT CAN CAUSE WEIGHT GAIN

Anafranil	Lithium
Antidepressants (Wellbutrin)	NSAIDs (ibuprofen, naproxen)
Antihistamines	Oral contraceptives
Corticosteroids (prednisone)	SSRIs (Prozac, Zoloft, etc.)

Use Caution with Acetaminophen

One of the most commonly used drugs that damages the liver is acetaminophen (Tylenol), which is loudly touted in advertising for pain relief because it doesn't upset the stomach the way aspirin or ibuprofen do. What those ads neglect to tell you is that acetaminophen is very hard on the liver.

Recent research has shown that acetaminophen may inflict most of its damage on the liver by blocking the production of the important antioxidant glutathione. Without glutathione, the liver's ability to break down toxins for elimination is impaired. According to a study published in the journal *Free Radical Biology & Medicine*, one hour after an injection of acetaminophen, glutathione levels decrease as much as 83 percent! That is a vulnerable liver. If some type of stress is placed on the liver (i.e., alcohol, pesticides) at the same time the acetaminophen hits it, the damage could be considerable.

If you're in pain you may be in the position of having to pick your poisons, so here's a health-protecting strategy: If you're going to take acetaminophen, take the liver-protective herb milk thistle beforehand (follow directions on the bottle) and add 500 mg of the amino acid cysteine to your daily vitamins. Cysteine is the precursor to glutathione. Also be sure to avoid alcohol when you're taking acetaminophen.

Because drugs have potent and specific actions, they can easily be-

DRUGS THAT ARE HARD ON THE LIVER

Nearly all prescription drugs are hard on your liver, but these are at the top of the list:

Acetaminophen	Chemotherapy drugs
Analgesic painkillers	Cholesterol-lowering drugs
Anesthetics (given during surgery)	Diabetes drugs (oral)
Antibiotics	Heart disease drugs
Anticoagulants	Oral contraceptives
Antihistamines	Parkinson's drugs
Anti-inflammatory drugs	Tuberculosis drugs
Blood pressure-lowering drugs	

come toxic in excess. One of the biggest reasons that natural remedies are preferable to use over prescription drugs whenever possible is that the natural remedies tend to be much gentler and safer if you take too much.

DRUGS THAT CAN SINK YOUR SEX LIFE

If you're a guy, maybe you think that your sex drive has dropped just because you've passed the age of 50. Not necessarily so! Although a man of 50 doesn't have the energy of an 18-year-old, most male impotence after the age of 50 has to do either with clogged arteries or with the drugs physicians love to hand out to men at that age.

If you're suffering from impotence and are taking a prescription drug, call your pharmacist or your physician and ask if one of the side effects of the drug is impotence. If you're taking more than one drug, including over-the-counter drugs, it could be causing your impotence even if that is not listed as a side effect.

Drugs that can sink your sex life include:

Antibiotics
Anticholinergics (used for ulcers and other gastrointestinal disorders, to suppress nausea, for tremors caused by Parkinson's and psychiatric drugs, sometimes for asthma)
Anticonvulsants
Antidepressants
Antihistamines (for allergies and sinus congestion)
Antihypertensives (drugs that lower blood pressure)

DOES THE DRUG YOU'RE TAKING CAUSE DROWSINESS? IF THE ANSWER IS YES, DON'T DRIVE!

According to an organization called CANDID (Citizens Against Drug-Impaired Drivers), prescription and over-the-counter medications that cause drowsiness contribute to more than 100,000 car crashes a year. If your drug insert warns against driving while under the influence of the drug, please take that warning seriously!

Antipsychotics
Appetite suppressants
H2 blockers such as Tagamet, Pepcid and Zantac
Many drugs used to treat heart disease, including beta-blockers, calcium channel blockers, ACE inhibitors and anti-angina drugs
Painkillers such as indomethacin, naproxen and naltrexone
Prostate drugs such as Proscar
Sedatives, tranquilizers, sleeping pills

CHAPTER 4

How Drugs Interact with Food, Drink and Supplements

EVERYTHING YOU PUT IN your mouth has some effect on your body, so it makes sense that drugs would have an effect on what you eat, and what you eat would have an effect on how your body processes drugs. Although the possible interactions and effects of drugs, food, drink and supplements on your unique biochemistry are nearly infinite, there are some generalizations we can make and some dangerous combinations to watch for.

A nutrient can increase the effect of a drug, decrease it, or delay its action, and a drug can interfere with the absorption of nutrients. Deficiencies in a vitamin, mineral or other nutrient such as protein can increase or decrease a drug's action.

TAKING MEDICATION WITH OR WITHOUT FOOD

When you fill a prescription it should always say either, "Take with food," or "Take between meals" (without food). Some drugs will be virtually ineffective if you take them with food and others will give you an upset stomach unless you take them with food. Most drug absorption takes place in your small intestine and how your digestion is working will have a major impact on how the drug is absorbed. If you take a medication with a very fatty meal it will take your stomach longer to empty and that will delay the action of the drug. If you eat a small, acidic meal with very little fat, your stomach may empty very quickly and the drug will take effect more quickly than usual. Some drugs will bind to your food, others will compete with nutrients for receptor sites and others will stimulate digestion.

The tables on the following pages give you lists of drugs that react with food. Some drugs are absorbed more quickly when you take them with food, mainly because they increase the production of bile which speeds up digestion, or because they change the pH of the stomach, again speeding or slowing digestion. If you have been taking a drug between meals and then suddenly take it with food, or vice versa, you could get an overdose or not enough.

DRUGS AND NUTRIENTS

Although not many nutrients such as vitamins, minerals and amino acids, taken in normal doses such as a daily multivitamin, will adversely affect drugs, many drugs can cause nutritional deficiencies. Antacids deplete calcium; aspirin depletes vitamin C and folic acid; diuretics deplete minerals (especially calcium, magnesium, potassium and zinc); cholesterol-lowering drugs interfere with the absorption of fat-soluble vitamins such as A, D and E; corticosteroids such as prednisone deplete vitamin D, potassium and some of the B vitamins; and synthetic hormone replacement therapy depletes the B vitamins and folic acid. (It is ironic that physicians often justify prescribing hormone replacement therapy for women to reduce the risk of heart disease, and yet depletion of these vitamins raises homocysteine levels, which significantly raises the risk of heart disease.)

Drugs that block folic acid production include the arthritis and chemotherapy drug methotrexate, anticonvulsants such as phenytoin and carbamazepine, and the bile acid sequestrants for lowering cholesterol levels, cholestipol and cholestyramine.

Both excess potassium (such as is caused by ACE inhibitors) and cimetidine (Tagamet) and proton pump inhibitors such as omeprazole can interfere with the absorption of vitamin B12. A deficiency of B12 can cause symptoms of senility. How many older people have been put into nursing homes because they were taking cimetidine long term, which blocked B12 absorption? We see ads on TV for these drugs over and over and over again, and eventually, even though we know better, we think the drugs are harmless because that's how they're portrayed in the advertising.

The tuberculosis drug isoniazid depletes vitamin B6, as do the yellow dyes called tartrazines found in 60 percent of all prescription drugs, as well as in most processed foods. Among the many symptoms of a B6 deficiency are hormonal imbalances and carpal tunnel syndrome.

Grapefruit juice can increase the strength of many drugs, by blocking the liver enzymes that are used to clear the drug out of the body.

Many, many drugs will increase the strength of alcohol and vice versa. Always use caution when combining any drug with alcohol.

DRUGS THAT INTERACT DANGEROUSLY WITH ALCOHOL

If the drug you're taking isn't on this list, don't assume it doesn't interact with alcohol.

Drugs That Interact with Alcohol

Drug	Effect
acetaminophen	can cause liver damage
aspirin	stomach bleeding
barbiturates	can cause extreme sedation
benzodiazepines	can cause extreme sedation
codeine	low blood pressure, slowed breathing
diabetes drugs	upset stomach, hypoglycemia, headache
ibuprofen	internal bleeding
phenytoin	can cause extreme sedation
reserpine	increases effects of drug and alcohol
tetracycline	reduces the effect of the tetracycline
tricyclic antidepressants	can cause extreme sedation

Fiber can block absorption of a drug and may even carry most of it right through the digestive tract. If you're taking any type of fiber

NEVER MIX DRUGS AND ALCOHOL

As much as we might like to think alcohol is simply a social lubricant or pleasant accompaniment to dinner, it is a drug and has profound effects on the body. When you mix alcohol with *any* drug, prescription or over the counter, you are entering into the no man's land of drug-drug interactions. If you use alcohol, even just a glass of wine with dinner, *always* ask your physician or pharmacist how a drug interacts with alcohol. If they don't know, ask them to look it up for you.

The drugs listed here are known to either increase the effects of the alcohol, are increased themselves by the alcohol, or have the potential to cause liver damage when combined with alcohol.

Acetaminophen may cause liver damage
Antidepressants
Antifungal drugs such as ketoconazole (Nizoral) may cause liver damage
Antihistamines
Aspirin
Barbiturates
Benzodiazepines and other anti-anxiety drugs
Bromocriptine (Parlodel)
Calcium channel blockers such as verapamil (Verelan, Calan, Isoptin)
Cephalosporin antibiotics—don't drink alcohol for at least three days after taking these drugs
Diabetes drugs (oral)
H2 blockers such as cimetidine (Tagamet) and ranitidine (Zantac)
Indomethacin and other anti-inflammatory drugs (Indocin)
Methotrexate may cause liver damage
Narcotics (Darvon, Empirin, Talwin)
Nitroglycerin
Tranquilizers and sleeping pills

such as psyllium or Metamucil to treat constipation and irregularity, take medications at least an hour before or two hours after you take the fiber.

DRUGS THAT INTERACT WITH MINERALS

Drugs can have a profound effect on how the body handles nutrients. Some reduce mineral absorption, others cause minerals to be excreted in the urine in higher than normal quantities, and others interfere with how the body processes minerals.

- Antibiotics: The antibiotic Neomycin interferes with the absorption of iron. Tetracycline blocks the absorption of dietary minerals; conversely, taking minerals with an antibiotic will also block the action of the antibiotic. The quinolones (i.e., Noroxin, Penetrex, Cipro) block the absorption of iron and zinc.
- Anticonvulsants such as carbamazepine, phenobarbital, phenytoin (Dilantin) or primidone lower levels of copper and zinc.
- Arthritis medications such as D-penicillamine (Cuprimine) can reduce absorption of zinc, iron and probably other minerals as well.
- Aspirin and indomethacin (Indocin) can cause enough blood loss through the stomach over time to cause an iron deficiency.
- Cholesterol-lowering drugs such as cholestyramine (Questran) and colestipol (Colestid) can lower the body's stores of iron.
- Corticosteroids such as cortisone and prednisone may deplete zinc.
- Diuretics, frequently used in the treatment of high blood pressure and heart failure, can cause minerals to be lost in urine.
- Laxatives reduce absorption of minerals.
- Oral contraceptives tend to increase levels of copper, which in excess can cause a decrease in blood levels of iron and zinc.
- Alcohol depletes iron, selenium, zinc and magnesium, in addition to many other important nutrients. Alcoholic drinks like wine and whiskey are also relatively high in the toxic element cadmium which is taken up in greater quantities when zinc levels are low.

DRUGS THAT ARE ABSORBED MORE QUICKLY WHEN TAKEN WITH FOOD

Carbamazepine
Diazepam
Dicumarol
Erythromycin
Griseofulvin
Hydralazine
Hydrochlorothiazide
Labetalol

Lithium citrate
Metoprolol
Nitrofurantoin
Phenytoin
Propoxyphene
Propranolol
Spironolactone

DRUGS THAT ARE ABSORBED MORE SLOWLY WHEN TAKEN WITH FOOD

Acetaminophen (take with food anyway to avoid stomach upset)
Amoxicillin
Ampicillin
Aspirin (but take with food anyway to avoid stomach upset)
Atenolol (can upset the stomach when taken without food)
Cephalosporins
Cimetidine (Tagamet)
Digoxin
Furosemide
Glipizide
Metronidazole
Piroxicam (Feldene)
Quinidine (take with food anyway if it causes an upset stomach)
Sulfonamides
Valproic acid

DRUGS THAT ARE NOT ABSORBED AS WELL WHEN TAKEN WITH FOOD

Ampicillin
Atenolol
Captopril
Chlorpromazine
Erythromycin
Isoniazid
Levodopa (don't take with high-protein foods because it competes
    with amino acids for absorption)
Lincomycin
Methyldopa (don't take with high-protein foods because it competes
    with amino acids for absorption)
Nafcillin
Penicillamine (don't take with dairy products, iron-rich foods or
    vitamins because it binds with some minerals, including calcium)

Penicillin G
Penicillin VK
Propantheline
Rifampin
Tetracyclines (don't take with dairy products, iron-rich foods or
  vitamins because it binds with some minerals, including calcium)

CHAPTER 5

How Drugs Interact with Other Drugs

ONCE YOU REACH THE age of 50, you are almost guaranteed to walk out of a physician's appointment with a prescription for a drug. At the very least, women will get a prescription for hormone replacement therapy and both men and women will be told to take an aspirin every day.

When you start taking any type of drug, you are heading down a long road full of potentially dangerous drug interactions and side effects. Some 36 percent of all hospitalizations are due to drug reactions and of those, at least 25 percent are caused by adverse drug interactions. There are approximately 13,000 prescription drugs available in the U.S. and yet the FDA does not require drug interaction studies as part of its drug approval process. New drugs have been studied by themselves, but not in combination with other drugs.

When you take a new drug in combination with another drug, you're a guinea pig for the drug companies and the FDA. Thousands of people die each year in these hidden human experiments. Our educated guess is that tens of thousands of deaths in older people attributed to "natural causes" or heart failure are actually caused by drug reactions or interactions. Even when a physician becomes aware that a hospitalization or death is the result of a drug reaction, he or she will probably not report it, to avoid lawsuits.

If you have any new health complaints, be suspicious of the drugs you're taking. Ask your pharmacist to inform you of any known interactions when you are taking a new drug or experiencing new symptoms; and carefully read the patient insert that should come with *every* new medication (you may have to use a magnifying glass to do this).

Be extremely conservative and cautious about taking prescription drugs. It is not just a matter of life and death, it's a matter of quality of life. One of the most common side effects of a drug-drug interaction is mental fogginess or confusion. Tragically, many older people are put on as many as eight or a dozen drugs and when they become lethargic and confused they are diagnosed as senile and stuck in a nursing home, when a simple change of medication could have remedied the problem and kept them independent.

The other very common scenario is the drug treadmill, where you are given two or more drugs and when you have side effects from them, you are given more drugs to treat the side effects, which creates more side effects and so on.

NOT ONLY PRESCRIPTION DRUGS

It's not just prescription drugs that can dangerously interact with each other. Over-the-counter drugs can react with prescription drugs, causing them to be stronger, weaker or producing a new symptom. For example, if you're taking the corticosteroid prednisone and you start taking ibuprofen or aspirin every day to treat chronic headaches, the combination could cause gastric (stomach) bleeding. Combining ACE inhibitors with ibuprofen can increase potassium to dangerous levels, causing side effects such as muscular weakness, numbness and an irregular heartbeat.

If you suddenly find yourself suffering from urinary retention or incontinence, it may be because you're combining an antihistamine such as Benadryl that you bought in the drugstore for your allergies, with an anticholinergic drug to treat Parkinson's disease.

If the drug you have been taking is no longer working, it may have to do with using an H2 blocker such as cimetidine (Tagamet), sold over-the-counter for heartburn. Cimetidine interacts with dozens of drugs, either increasing or decreasing their action.

If you're taking an asthma drug such as theophylline, caffeine can cause an overdose of theophylline, with symptoms of a rapid or irregular heartbeat, nausea, dizziness, headache and shakiness. Caffeine is present in coffee, most soft drinks, many over-the-counter headache remedies and in Midol. Theophylline levels in the body can also be increased by capsaicin, found in Tabasco sauce, chili peppers and sometimes used in natural arthritis formulas, and it can be decreased by eating charbroiled meats. Many, many common drugs increase or decrease levels of theophylline.

THE MOST COMMON DRUG OFFENDERS

Because of the thousands of drugs on the market, it is literally impossible for any physician to know all of the possible drug-drug interactions that could threaten your health and even your life. And that doesn't count the interactions with food, over-the-counter drugs and supplements. That means it's up to you to minimize your drug intake and keep close track of what you are taking.

In Part II of this book you'll find lists of drug interactions, but remember these are *known* interactions. Any drug combination can cause a new interaction because your body and your biochemistry are unique.

When prescribing a drug, your physician should take into account not only interactions between drugs, but also how various drugs are going to interact with your unique health profile. If you have an irregular heartbeat and high blood pressure, if your physician prescribes a diuretic that depletes magnesium it will only make the irregular heartbeat worse. If you have asthma and high blood pressure and your physician prescribes an inhaler for the asthma, it could raise your blood pressure even more.

Here are the classes of drugs most often associated with serious interactions with other drugs, foods and supplements:

- Benzodiazepines used as antidepressants such as Ativan, Valium
- Ephedrine and pseudoephedrine, found in most over-the-counter allergy, cough, cold and decongestant medicines
- Heart drugs, including digoxin, calcium channel blockers, beta-blockers and diuretics (especially the "loop" diuretics such as furosemide and the thiazide diuretics)

- H2 blockers such as cimetidine (Tagamet)
- MAO inhibitors such as Marplan and Nardil used as antidepressants
- NSAIDs (nonsteroidal anti-inflammatory drugs, e.g., ibuprofen)
- Steroids (such as prednisone)
- Theophylline, an asthma drug
- Warfarin (Coumadin), a blood thinner

If you are on any of these types of drugs, it is extremely important to be watchful at all times for drug interactions. For example, if you're taking an MAO inhibitor and eat foods that are high in the amino acid tyrosine (i.e., avocados, aged cheese, not-quite-fresh liver or paté, nuts, pickled foods, processed meats such as salami and bologna, wine, yogurt, soy sauce and bananas), the interaction could cause life-threatening high blood pressure, severe headaches, dizziness, mental confusion, visual disturbances and fever. MAO inhibitors are outdated drugs that also react with dozens of over-the-counter drugs. These drugs should be taken only as a very last resort.

CHAPTER 6

Surgery, Drugs and Nutrition: Minimizing the Damage and Maximizing Your Recovery

AMERICAN PHYSICIANS ARE generally way too eager to use the surgeon's knife to carve up and chop out whatever they think is ailing you, at great expense to you and great profit to them and the hospitals they work for. Sometimes when you have a chronic illness, it may seem like having surgery will be a quick and easy end to the pain. But if you don't address the problems that caused the pain in the first place, you'll wind up sick again within a few months, with nothing to show for your surgery but a huge medical bill, a missing organ and a scar.

Of the 750,000 hysterectomies done every year, it is estimated that 650,000 of them are unnecessary. U.S. physicians perform some 300,000 Caesareans a year, most of them unnecessary. Carving up men's prostate glands started to be big business, but men caught on that it wasn't necessary and squawked loudly, and the practice has rapidly declined. (Women need to learn to protest louder when mainstream medicine mistreats them.) Other surgeons' favorites that are often unnecessary are surgery for gallstones and heart disease (especially bypass operations).

Having surgery of any kind is not something to take lightly. There is always a risk of dying in surgery, and the risk of a life-threatening infection is also very real. Hospitals are one of the best places to pick up an infection that is resistant to antibiotics. That alone is reason enough to avoid them unless absolutely necessary.

Keep in mind when you see a physician who is recommending surgery that surgeons like to do surgery. That is their business, that is what they are good at, and that is how they make the big bucks to pay for their Mercedes and Porsches. Always get a second opinion from someone not connected to your physician or the same hospital or HMO and go to a naturopathic doctor or an M.D. who practices alternative medicine, and find out if they think the problem can be solved without surgery. Even if the visit is not covered by insurance, it may be one of the best investments you ever make.

Having given you all the warnings, there are times when surgery is definitely necessary. Dental surgery, appendicitis and some cancers come to mind. Only you can make the final decision about whether surgery is truly necessary, and when you do choose to have it, go into it fully prepared and in optimal health.

In addition to the list of supplements you can take to support your body, it's also important to support yourself emotionally and get plenty of rest before and after surgery. Be sure you have plenty of help at home, and stock the kitchen with nutritious fruit and vegetable drinks and soups. If you are experiencing a lot of anxiety in the week or so prior to surgery, you can use the anti-anxiety herb St. John's wort to help you through. Follow the directions on the container and don't overdo it, please.

PREPARING FOR SURGERY

The two biggest challenges of surgery for your body, besides that of healing the actual wound, are the threat of infection and the stress on your liver. There's no way around it: When you have surgery you will be given lots of drugs, and most of them are very hard on your liver. This especially applies to anesthesia drugs. Take extra good care of your liver before, during and after surgery. Your liver is responsible for taking nutrients and farming them out to the rest of the body, and it is also responsible for breaking down or neutralizing toxic waste products such as excess hormones and pesticides. If your liver is busy fighting damage from drugs, it won't be able to heal your body as quickly or effectively.

One of the most irresponsible practices in mainstream medicine is giving people large doses of acetaminophen (i.e., Tylenol) after surgery. This pain killer is notoriously hard on the liver and is the last thing your body needs after surgery. Avoid this drug both before, during and after surgery. Make it clear to your physician and your anesthesiologist that you are not interested in being given acetaminophen after surgery.

To spare your liver, you should also avoid alcohol for the week before surgery, as well as foods high in fat (especially hydrogenated oils and fried foods). Other factors that can stress the liver include exposure to pesticides, solvents, paints and gasoline.

Many prescription drugs can harm the liver. These include steroids (prednisone), antifungal drugs such as ketoconazole (Nizoral), and tuberculosis drugs (Laniazid). If you are taking any kind of prescription or over-the-counter drug, get out a magnifying glass and read the package insert for warnings about "hepatic function impairment" or "hepatoxicity." This is medical-ese for liver damage.

I want you to support your liver by taking some special supplements before and after surgery.

- **Milk thistle** *(Silybum marianum)* is an herb that is very supportive of the liver. Take it as a tincture, one dropperful three times daily, or as tablets or capsules (follow directions on the container), in a standardized product (meaning the amount of the active ingredient, silymarin, is guaranteed). Take it between meals for a week before surgery and for two weeks after.
- **Alpha lipoic acid** (also called thioctic acid), a substance made by the body which directly supports the detoxifying abilities of the liver. Diabetics should use alpha lipoic acid with caution as it can cause hypoglycemia. You can take two 100-mg capsules three times a day, with meals, for a week before surgery and for two weeks after.
- **N-acetyl-cysteine** is an amino acid precursor to the important liver antioxidant glutathione. It is commonly used in hospital emergency rooms to treat patients with acetaminophen-induced liver poisoning. It will also help stimulate your immune system. You can take one 500-mg capsule three times daily between meals for the week before surgery and for two weeks after.
- **Fiber** is important to good bowel function, which is important to a healthy liver. If your colon is not effectively eliminating toxins, they will be sent back to the liver. Eating plenty of fiber will

assure that your bowels are moving well. This means eating plenty of whole grains, fresh fruits and vegetables.

AVOID INFECTION, SPEED HEALING AND BOOST THE IMMUNE SYSTEM

Infection is a major risk of surgery. The sooner you get yourself out of the hospital the lower your risk of getting an infection. You can help avoid infection and speed up the healing process by keeping your immune system strong. In addition to the vitamins you're taking as part of the Six Core Principles for Optimal Health (see Chapter 8), you will support your body if you take the following supplements.

- **Your biggest ally in fighting infection and speeding healing is vitamin A.** Take 15,000 IU of vitamin A (not beta-carotene) daily for a week before surgery, and 50,000 IU the two days before and after surgery, then continue with 15,000 IU daily for about 10 days. (If you're pregnant, don't take more than 15,000 IU daily.) If you're having dental surgery you can rub it on your gums before and after surgery to greatly speed up the healing process.
- **Take extra antioxidants, zinc and a B50 complex** for two weeks before and after surgery. They will support your immune system and the healing process. Take an extra 400 IU of vitamin E, an extra 1,000 to 2,000 mg of vitamin C (don't take so much you get diarrhea), 200 mcg extra of selenium, and 15 mg extra of zinc. Also take a bioflavonoid antioxidant such as grapeseed extract and green tea extract, to help speed wound healing.
- **Glutamine** is a nonessential amino acid that becomes essential when we're under certain types of stress, such as surgery. The immune system can't function without glutamine. It speeds up the healing process, aids in detoxification in the liver and kidneys, and supports the health of the small intestine. Take 500 mg twice daily between meals for a week before and two weeks after surgery.

HOMEOPATHIC REMEDIES FOR SURGERY

Homeopathic remedies are particularly effective for helping cope with surgery, and you can safely take them just before surgery and just after since they are tiny sugar pellets or tablets that dissolve under the tongue.

Homeopath Dana Ullman, author of *The Consumer's Guide to Homeopathy* (Tarcher/Putnam, 1996), recommends arnica in a 30C dose before and after surgery. Take four pellets under the tongue the night before, the morning of the surgery and just before the surgery.

Homeopathics also work well to treat the nausea that almost always occurs after surgery. Ullman recommends Nux vomica in a 6C or 30C dose. You can refer to Ullman's book for homeopathic remedies for specific types of nauseas and treatment for different types of surgery.

CHAPTER 7

How to Read Drug Labels and Information Inserts

EVERY PRESCRIPTION DRUG has what is called a "drug information insert" or "package insert" that comes with it. You will rarely see this when you fill a prescription at a pharmacy, but you should never take a drug without reading it first. Ask your pharmacist for a copy. The drug companies don't really want you or the physician to read these inserts, because no drug looks good after you've read all its possible side effects and adverse reactions, so it is printed in extremely tiny, hard-to-read type. At the same pharmacy where you fill your prescriptions you can buy a magnifying glass for a few dollars, so that you can read your drug insert. It will be one of the best investments you've ever made in your health.

You absolutely cannot count on the FDA, the drug company, your physician or your pharmacist to keep you safe from dangerous drugs and their interactions. Your pharmacist is your greatest ally when it comes to protecting you from drugs, but ultimately it's up to you to stay informed and to make decisions about your health. Your physician doesn't want to tell you about possible drug side effects because he or she has been programmed in medical school to believe that if you're told about side effects you'll become a hypochondriac and get them. That is a condescending attitude that is unlikely to change any time soon. You are the best judge of whether you are having a bad reaction to a drug. Please trust your body's feedback and pay attention to it.

Every year tens of thousands of people take home a prescription drug for a minor ailment and end up very ill, sometimes permanently, or even dead, because they weren't aware of the risks associated with the drug. A dangerous side effect or adverse reaction may happen in less than one percent of the people who took the drug in testing, but if you happen to be in that one percent it could save your life to be informed.

For new drugs, the information listed on the package insert comes primarily from FDA-required studies on the drug. But don't think that just because the drug company has spent tens of millions of dollars jumping through FDA-required hoops that the drug is well-studied. In fact, many studies use patients in mental institutions, nursing homes, homeless shelters, universities and other places with untypical test subjects. Anyone in a mental institution is already going to be thoroughly drugged, making any study results virtually useless because of drug interactions. Those in homeless shelters are often abusing street drugs or alcohol, again creating unpredictable reactions, not to mention a population impossible to follow up on. University students may or may not be taking drugs and using alcohol, but in any case they are generally young and healthy, unlike the majority of people who take prescription drugs.

Another factor making drug studies less than meaningful is that few drugs are studied for more than three months, making long-term side effects unpredictable.

The Public Citizen Health Research Group, which publishes the book and newsletter, *Worst Pills, Best Pills*, suggests avoiding any drug that hasn't been on the market for at least five years. Before that time, you are, in effect, a guinea pig for the FDA and the drug company. And even then, as our tragic experience with fen-phen has shown us, five years may not be enough.

A GUIDE TO YOUR DRUG INSERT

The *Physician's Desk Reference* is a large volume that you've probably seen on the shelf in your physician's office. It is updated every year, and in it is printed the drug information insert for nearly every prescription drug on the market. Here are the categories of information provided and a translation of some of the medical terms that make it difficult to understand without a medical dictionary.

Brand Name

Generic Name

Form (Capsules, Tablets, Liquid, etc.)

Description This describes the drug in chemical terms, often with an accompanying molecular diagram. It also lists fillers, binders, dyes and other nondrug ingredients in the medication. This is important if you are allergic to food dyes, preservatives or even ingredients such as corn which may be used as a filler. If you find you are sniffling, sneezing, wheezing, coughing or experiencing fatigue or puffiness after taking a medication, it could be due to an allergic reaction to a preservative or food dye, especially the yellow and red dyes, which are used in the majority of prescription medications.

Clinical Pharmacology This is a description of what the drug does in the human body. Most of these descriptions conclude with a paragraph stating that the action or mechanism of the drug is not fully understood. Always keep that in mind—even the drug company often doesn't really know how the drug works.

Indications and Usage This tells you what the drug is prescribed for. If your specific ailment isn't listed here that's called an "unlabeled use," meaning the drug hasn't been studied or approved by the FDA for that use. Once a drug is approved by the FDA for any use, physicians are free to prescribe it for any reason they choose.

DRUGS THAT CAN CAUSE INCONTINENCE

Antibiotics	Lithium
Atropine	Misoprostol
Benzodiazepines	Nicardipine
Beta-blockers	Nifedipine
Bupropion	Prazosin
Diuretics	Sleeping pills
Doxazosin	Spironolactone
Fluoxetine	Terazosin
Isradipine	Tranquilizers
Levobunolol	

Physicians frequently prescribe drugs for unlabeled uses, and drug companies frequently cleverly market drugs for unprescribed uses even though they legally aren't supposed to. For example, the antidepressant Prozac is approved by the FDA for treating depression, but for years it has also been marketed for obsessive-compulsive disorder and premenstrual syndrome. The drug companies spread the word about these unlabeled uses through drug company reps. Another common ploy is to fund a so-called "study" showing that the drug works for an unlabeled use and then releasing the results of the study to the media (TV news programs such as "20/20" are favorites for this type of marketing). Another tactic they use is to find a few people who experienced a "cure" for the disease by taking the medication and then they take those stories to the media. This type of media coverage, as well as articles that are "planted" in magazines by public relations companies or departments, create what is known as patient demand. You see a story on a news program about the unlabeled use of the drug and next time you go to your physician you mention it. It's a very effective form of marketing.

Don't be overly concerned if your ailment isn't listed here—chances are the labeled use hasn't been very well-studied either!

Contraindications This is where the drug maker is supposed to say, "If you have ——————— (disease), don't take this drug." Most of the time what's listed here is something useless like, "a known allergy or sensitivity to ——————— (drug name).

Warnings This is where you want to pay close attention. This section lists a variety of conditions that might make taking the drug dangerous. For example, the warnings section for the drug Procardia (nifedipine) warns that it can cause "excessive hypotension (low blood pressure)" which can be life-threatening. It also warns of the possibility of increased angina, myocardial infarction (heart attack), a withdrawal syndrome and congestive heart failure. Our guess is that only a handful of the hundreds of thousands of people taking this drug are ever aware of these dangers.

This is also the place to look for warnings about using the drug with patients who have renal or hepatic impairment, dysfunction or disease. Renal refers to the kidneys and hepatic refers to the liver.

Nearly all prescription drugs are hard on your liver, but this type of warning should alert you to added risk.

Precautions This is another section of the drug insert where your physician may be warned about prescribing the drug to people with renal or hepatic dysfunction, or it may advise them to frequently monitor kidney and liver function. Again, a red flag should go up—this drug is particularly hard on those organs.

This section also lists drug interactions. If you are taking any other type of drug, read carefully and if you find you are already taking a drug on the list, do *not* take the new drug until you have spoken with your physician or your pharmacist about the interaction.

If the drug you're taking has caused cancer, genetic mutations or impaired fertility in laboratory animals, this is the place to find it. Physicians like to pooh-pooh this type of research, but I'd like you to take it very seriously. If the cancer, mutation or impaired fertility wasn't significant, it wouldn't have made it onto the drug information insert. While rodents aren't an ideal model of what happens in a human, it's an accurate enough indicator to cause concern.

This is also where warnings about taking the drug if you're pregnant show up. However, it's safest to consider *all* drugs unsafe during

---

DRUGS THAT CAN CAUSE PHOTOSENSITIVITY

Amantadine	Diuretics
Antibiotics	Etretinate
Antidepressants	Isotretinoin
Antifungals	NSAIDs
Antihistamines	Oils and chemicals used in perfumes
Antihypertensives	and cosmetics
Antipsychotics	Oral contraceptives
Benzocaine	Oral diabetes drugs
Benzodiazepines	Promethazine
Carbamazepine	Quinidine
Chemotherapy drugs	Tretinoin
Clofibrate	Trimeprazine
Disopyramide	

pregnancy. Drugs should be completely avoided during pregnancy unless the mother or child's life is at risk.

Adverse Reactions When a drug company is testing a drug on humans, it is required to record all the adverse reactions or side effects a patient has to it. The adverse reactions may have nothing to do with the drug, but there is no way of separating an authentic adverse reaction from a coincidental reaction. On the other hand, adverse reactions are notoriously underreported, so for example if a drug is reported to cause dizziness in 13 percent of the people taking it, it's likely to be much higher than that.

The bottom line is that if you experience any of the side effects/ adverse reactions listed on the drug insert you should tell your physician. If the side effect is even remotely life-threatening, get medical attention right away.

M.D.s have a way of making patients feel as if they are responsible for drug side effects and minimizing the discomfort they can cause. If this happens to you, please either stand up for yourself, have someone such as a spouse do it for you or find another doctor. You should not ever have to suffer from drug side effects, nor should you ever allow your physician to get you onto the drug treadmill by prescribing new drugs to treat the side effects of the first or second one.

Overdosage This section gives the symptoms of an overdose of the drug and if available, an antidote to an overdose. Many heart drugs, such as ACE inhibitors, beta-blockers, digitalis drugs and the blood-thinning drugs can be fatal if levels are even a little bit too high. There are many factors that can raise levels of these drugs, including drug-drug interactions, drug-food interactions, alcohol consumption and stress. Knowing the symptoms of an overdose can be life-saving if you catch it early.

Dosage and Administration This section lists the amounts the drugs come in, and in what form they are delivered, for example, capsule, tablet, oral, liquid.

OTHER WORDS YOU SHOULD KNOW

It's preferable not to take any prescription drug long term, but if you do it's wise to purchase a medical dictionary and use it to look up words in the drug information insert that you don't understand. You can find a paperback medical dictionary in almost any bookstore.

Medical Terms Frequently Found in Drug Information Inserts

Adenomas: Benign tumors.

Agranulocytosis: A sudden drop in white blood cells called granulocytes, indicating a serious dysfunction of the immune system.

Alopecia: Hair loss.

Amenorrhea: Absence of menstruation.

Anaphylaxis: A severe allergic reaction that can be fatal.

Anemia: Deficiency of red blood cells in the blood.

Angina: Chest pain.

Anorexia: Loss of appetite.

Arrhythmias: Irregular heartbeats.

Arthralgia: Joint pain.

Bradycardia: Slow heartbeat.

Cerebral: Having to do with the brain.

Clinical trials: Drug studies on humans, versus rodents or in a test tube.

CNS: Central nervous system; refers to the nerves of the brain and spinal cord, which is to say those nerves which regulate almost everything in the body.

Dermatitis: Skin rash.

Dys as a prefix: Dysfunction, difficult, painful.

Dyspepsia: Indigestion, heartburn, bloating.

Dyspnea: Difficult breathing.

Dysuria: Painful urination.

Edema: Water retention, bloating, swelling due to water retention.

Electrolyte: In the human body this usually refers to the minerals calcium, potassium and sodium.

Fibromyositis: Joint or muscle pain and swelling.

Gastrointestinal: Having to do with the digestive system.

Glossitis: Inflammation of the tongue.

Hemorrhage: Uncontrolled bleeding or loss of a large amount of blood.

Hepatic: Having to do with the liver.

Hirsutism: Excessive hair growth.

Hyper as a prefix: Too much.

Hypo as a prefix: Too little.

Hyper- or hypocalcemia: Too much or too little calcium in the blood.

Hyper- or hypoglycemia: Too much or too little sugar in the blood.

Hyper- or hypokalemia: Too much or too little potassium in the blood.

Hyper- or hypomagnesia: Too much or too little magnesium in the blood.

Hyper- or hyponatremia: Too much or too little sodium in the blood.

Hyper- or hypotension: High or low blood pressure.

Hyperkinesia: Restlessness or jerky, rapid movements.

In vitro: In a test tube.

In vivo: In a body.

IV: Intravenous, usually referring to a drug given through a needle into a vein.

Jaundice: Yellowing of the skin and sometimes the whites of the eyes usually caused by liver or gallbladder dysfunction.

Leukopenia: An abnormal drop in white blood cells, indicating a compromised immune system, often caused by an adverse drug reaction.

Malaise: Weakness, discomfort as in feeling a flu or fever coming on.

Myocardial infarction: Heart attack caused by blockage of an artery.

Orthostatic hypotension: Dizziness when standing from a sitting or lying position.

Neuritis: Swelling of a nerve.

Neuropathy: Nerve pain, swelling, degeneration.

Neutropenia: An abnormal drop in white blood cells called neutrophils.

Pallor: Pale skin.

Palpitations: Pounding or racing heart.

Parenteral: Substances going into the body other than via the mouth and digestive system. It usually refers to drugs or nutrients given intravenously, through a vein.

Paresthesia: Numbness, tingling.

Photosensitivity: Sensitivity to sunlight which can cause a rash, hives or swelling.

Porphyria: Abnormal pigmentation of the skin.

Pruritus: Itching.

Pulmonary: Having to do with the lungs.

Renal: Having to do with the kidneys.

Stomatitis: Inflammation in the mouth.

Syncope: Fainting.

Tachycardia: Rapid heartbeat.

Thrombophlebitis: Swelling of a vein, often associated with the formation of a blood clot.

Thrombosis: Blood clot.

Tremor: Shakiness or quivering, often seen in the hands of older people.

Urticaria: A skin rash usually caused by an allergic reaction.

Vertigo: Dizziness.

KNOW YOUR GENERIC NAMES

Throughout Part II of this book you will find hundreds of drug names. Although in some cases both the generic name and the brand name will be listed, most often only the generic name will be listed. If you are taking a generic version of your drug it will often just be called by its generic name. But if not, you can usually find the generic name on your pill bottle or the container it came in. If the generic name is not on the bottle, ask your pharmacist to write it on. The generic name will also be found on the drug insert information.

Remember, always ask for a generic drug when you get a drug prescription. They are nearly always much less expensive, and in spite of drug company marketing to the contrary, they are the same.

GENERIC AND BRAND NAMES OF COMMONLY USED DRUGS
(Not all brands names are listed.)

Acetaminophen (Tylenol)
Albuterol (Ventolin, Proventil)
Amlodipine (Norvase)
Amoxicillin (Amoxil, Trimox, Augmentin)
Ampicillin (Polycillin, Amicillin)
Aspirin (Bayer, Bufferin)
Atenolol (Tenormin)
Captopril (Capoten)
Carbamazepine (Tegretol, Atretol)
Cephalosporins (Cefaclor, Cephalexin, Duricef)
Chlorpromazine (Thorazine)
Cimetidine (Tagamet)
Clarithromycin (Biaxin)
Diazepam (Valium)
Digoxin (Lanoxin)
Diltiazem (Cardizem)
Erythromycin (Ery-Tab, E-Mycin)
Fluoxetine (Prozac)
Furosemide (Lasix)
Glipizide (Glucotrol)
Griseofulvin (Fulvicin, Grifulvin)

Hydralazine (Apresoline)
Hydrochlorothiazide (Reserpine)
Labetalol (Normodyne, Trandate)
Levodopa (Larodopa, Dopar)
Lisinopril (Prinivil, Zestril)
Medroxyprogesterone (Provera)
Methyldopa (Aldomet, Amodopa)
Metoprolol (Lopressor, Toprol)
Nifedipine (Procardia)
Omeprazole (Prilosec)
Paroxetine (Paxil)
Phenytoin (Dilantin)
Piroxicam (Feldene)
Propoxyphene (Darvon)
Propranolol (Inderal)
Sertraline (Zoloft)
Simvastatin (Zocor)
Spironolactone (Aldactone)
Terazosin (Hytrin)
Triamterene (Dyrenium)
Valproic acid (Depakote)
Warfarin (Coumadin)

II

PRESCRIPTION DRUGS AND THEIR NATURAL ALTERNATIVES

CHAPTER 8

The Six Core Principles for Optimal Health

THE NUMBER OF WAYS to stay healthy is at least as great as the number of ways to get sick. Because everyone is unique in their genetic, physical, emotional and mental makeup, there's no one program that will completely cover everyone. You will discover for yourself, through trial and error, what works for you and what doesn't, and hopefully with the help of a competent health-care professional, you can create a lifestyle that rewards you with vibrant good health and energy.

However, there are some guidelines that everyone can use to lay a solid foundation for good health and they are summarized in the Six Core Principles for Optimal Health. These six core principles are basic and simple and anybody can follow them.

While this book is not a substitute for the individual medical care your health-care professional provides, it can help empower you to become a more active and knowledgeable participant in your own health care.

The Six Core Principles for Optimal Health are simple and effective whether you do one step or all six. The more steps you take, the better you'll feel. Optimal health is like driving a finely tuned automobile instead of an old clunker. Either one might be able to get you from place to place, but what a difference in the drive!

STEP 1: DRINK SIX TO TEN GLASSES OF CLEAN WATER DAILY

Two-thirds of the human body is water, yet water is our most neglected nutrient. Of course water is a nutrient. It's more necessary for sustaining life than food. You can survive more than a month without food. But without water, the human body can function for only about a week. You cannot expect to enjoy optimal health if you deprive your body of the water it needs. (By the way, juices, milk, tea, coffee and soft drinks don't count.)

If you drink six to 10 glasses of clean water daily (more or less depending on your size, lifestyle and individual biochemistry), your body will thank you in so many ways. For one thing, your skin will be glowing with good health in just a month or so. And constipation will be a thing of the past, especially if you also exercise and eat fiber-containing foods. You will find controlling your weight easier. Many times when you think you're hungry, a glass of water will suffice.

Because water is a solvent, it helps rid your bloodstream of excess fat, which can help to reduce your blood serum cholesterol level. It's possible that 99 percent of all kidney stones result from not drinking enough water.

Make It Sparkling Clean

Notice that the recommendation is to drink *clean* water. In most places in the world these days, including North America, drinking clean water means avoiding tap water. To ensure that your water supply is clean, use a filtration system. You can purchase an inexpensive water filter or a complete household unit, depending on your needs and your budget.

The least expensive route is a pitcher with a filter attached. All you do is pour the water through. Ideally I'd like to see you with a more sophisticated filtration system in your home that eliminates heavy metals, chlorine, benzene and other carcinogens. Prices start around $200 for the original unit, then about $70 a year to replace the filter. You can easily install sink top units yourself.

Water filtration companies can install water filtration units in your home. Many companies have units large enough to serve a whole house, apartment or condominium, and others small enough to fit under or above the kitchen sink. Shop around for the best price. Ask for an analysis of what remains in your water after it has been filtered.

If the salesperson doesn't give you a detailed answer or starts to hem and haw, find another company fast.

There are currently three types of reasonably priced water filtration systems that eliminate most pollutants from your water. One combines reverse osmosis with carbon filters. Another uses a zinc/copper and charcoal filter and the third is a ceramic filter. Check your local telephone book under "Water Filtration" to find companies that sell these systems.

These systems enable you to filter your tap water for pennies a gallon. It tastes great, which makes it easy for you to drink the six to 10 glasses recommended.

STEP 2: GET BACK TO BASICS AND REDISCOVER DELICIOUS WHOLE FOODS

You are what you eat, but if you eat a lot of refined foods you won't be a more refined person, you will be a drastically less healthy person. Our national health began a dramatic decline when refined and processed foods were introduced. The rise in chronic degenerative diseases such as heart disease and diabetes correlates with the rise in consumption of foods that have all the nutrients stripped out of them and harmful preservatives and additives put in. If you're eating lots of canned, packaged, preserved and frozen foods, gradually switch to whole foods. Whole foods are essentially as nature made them. Foods packaged by nature come complete with all the nutrients you need. You get enzymes, vitamins, minerals, amino acids and hundreds of other nutritional substances you need for a healthy, energetic body capable of handling stress and fighting off disease.

Go for the Whole Grains and Legumes

Grains such as wheat, corn, millet, barley, oats, quinoa, amaranth and rice are not only delicious, they contain a wonderful potpourri of nutrients, as well as fiber. Get reacquainted with whole grains. Try oatmeal or a whole-grain cereal or bread for breakfast. For lunch, have a salad on a bed of brown rice or millet. Add barley to soups and stews and try corn tortillas with your vegetables. If any new grain upsets your digestion, introduce it more gradually or skip it.

Fresh Vegetables and Fruits: Your Ticket to Longevity

People who eat plenty of fresh vegetables and fruits have a lower cancer risk, as well as less heart disease and a lower risk of diabetes. Instead of the canned and frozen varieties, head for the fresh produce section. Treat yourself and your family to daily salads, lightly steamed vegetables seasoned with olive oil and lemon and a delicious dessert of fresh fruit. Not only will you live longer, you'll feel better along the way.

Healthy Oils

One of the primary causes of heart disease in this country is bad fats. This doesn't just apply to saturated fats (which really aren't bad for you unless you eat too much of them). It applies much more to the trans fatty acids found in hydrogenated oils and margarine-type products, which are bad for you in any amount. These partially saturated, manmade fats were designed not to go rancid, but they have been found to actually cause heart disease. Please avoid them. Since hydrogenated oils are found in most chips, cakes, cookies and other processed foods, this is another great reason to go for the whole foods.

Most of the unsaturated fats found in vegetable oil are rancid, which is also a major health risk. For cooking it's best to stick to the monounsaturated fats, olive and canola oil. Olive oil is the best—it's delicious and extra virgin olive oil is largely unprocessed, so you get all the good nutrients in it. Although canola oil is also processed, it's the best oil to use in baking and other uses where you want a very light oil.

Become a Label Reader

The best way to avoid processed foods and hydrogenated oils is to read labels. Don't be fooled by products that say "all natural" or "no cholesterol" or "no sugar added" on the front of the package. These terms are misleading. Checking out the nutrition content label is the only way to really know what you're getting.

Processed foods are high in fat, high in sodium and high in sugar. So, you say, you'll fix that by purchasing low-fat or low-sodium foods. Okay, but watch out for the old shell game. When manufacturers cut down on one of these three, they usually add more of one of the others. For example, nonfat yogurt is usually loaded with sugar.

If you're eating processed foods, you're not tasting real food. There's no taste left. That's why they add all the fat, salt and sugar. Again, the only way you'll know what you're getting is not by reading the front of the package, but by reading the label. The nutritional labels used today are more helpful than labels were in the past. Although these labels aren't perfect (the big food companies don't want you to see what you're really buying), they are a step in the right direction.

Label reading is really like detective work. For example, sugar goes under lots of names. "Ose" at the end of a word stands for sugar. There's sucrose (common table sugar), dextrose and fructose (fruit sugar). Watch out for highly refined fructose, which is used in cola drinks and many of the so-called natural soft drinks. Basically, it's so refined that it is no different from regular white sugar. By the way, brown sugar is just good old white sugar with molasses coloring. Of course, it's best to cut down on the sugar in your diet. It's just empty calories; there's no nutrition, plus it zaps your energy.

Simple sugars enter your bloodstream quickly, giving you that much-touted lift. But the catch is that your pancreas is caught off guard by the sugar rush and it releases too much insulin. The result is an in-body processing error that lets you down the hard way: a drop in blood sugar, usually within the hour, that leaves you feeling less energetic, less alert and more irritable than you were before.

STEP 3: ADD MOVEMENT TO YOUR LIFE

Movement is essential for optimal health. For some of you, exercise is a four-letter word. But once you start moving, you will get more out of life. You'll notice that your mood is brighter and that life's little annoyances don't get to you the way they once did. You'll have more energy and sleep better than you have in years. Since exercise

MOVEMENT HELPS PREVENT

Arthritis	Osteoporosis
Back pain and injuries	Stroke
Heart diseases	Type II diabetes

IT DECREASES

Blood pressure	Cholesterol
Body fat	Rate of cancer

IT INCREASES/IMPROVES

Balance	Muscular strength and flexibility
Circulation	Reflexes
Energy	Self-esteem
Immune system	Sex life

improves circulation and endurance, you may even find your sex life has renewed vigor—in fact you may start finding you're getting as much exercise from your midnight aerobics as from your daily walk.

Brisk walking at least three days a week for 30 minutes (about two miles) is all you need to do. If you can take a brisk walk every day, so much the better. If you have any medical condition that might make brisk walking hazardous to your health, consult your doctor first. If you haven't been exercising at all, start slowly until you have increased the distance to at least two miles.

You can walk any time of the day. If you're a morning person, your energy will be high at that time of day and if you're a city dweller, pollution levels are lowest before rush hour begins. Taking a walk in the evening can help you relax and you'll sleep like a baby.

While you are walking, move your arms in time with your walking pace. Most of you should be perspiring a bit after your walk. Your pace should reach 3 to 4 miles per hour. That means you'll cover a mile every 15 to 20 minutes. Stretching before exercise and cooling down afterward are very important for safe, effective exercise.

STEP 4: MAINTAIN A HEALTHY WEIGHT

You can lose weight and never go hungry when you cut the fat, focus on vegetables and move your body. The goal is to gradually create a new, healthier lifestyle. As you change your eating habits and exercise more, the weight will naturally come off. There is way too much pressure on women in our culture to have the body of a teenager for life. Women and men naturally put on weight as they age, which is fine. What you want to avoid is obesity, and we all know what that is.

Lose the Fat

You don't need to cut fat completely out of your diet; that's not good for you either. But you do need to keep it lower than our national average, which is 40 percent of our daily calories.

Think of it, if you're 15 pounds overweight, you're carrying around a bowling ball with you. Do you have one, two or three bowling balls? That weight puts extra stress on your heart, plus you're using up precious energy that could be used doing something you really enjoy. If you reduce the fat in your diet to 25 to 30 percent of your total calories, you will probably lose weight. For most Americans, this means cutting fat consumption nearly in half.

Saturated fat has gotten a bad name. It is not bad for you except in excess. In fact it's necessary for good health. The problem is that most Americans eat way too much of it. Saturated fat is usually solid at room temperature. It includes butter, marbled meat, and tropical oils such as coconut, palm kernel or palm oil. To cut back on saturated fat, use olive oil instead of butter. Use canola oil in your cooking rather than unstable unsaturated vegetable oils. When you stir fry vegetables, use water at the beginning, at high heat, then throw in a small amount of oil at the last minute. When you cut the fat, you dramatically decrease your chances of obesity, heart disease, diabetes, high blood pressure and stroke.

Make Your Carbs Complex

Complex carbohydrates such as whole grains, brown rice and legumes (beans) are metabolized much more slowly in your body than refined carbohydrates.

When you eat refined grains such as white flour and white rice, your body treats them as if they're sugar and if you don't burn them off right away, they go directly to fat. When you eat complex carbohydrates, your body tends to use them for energy more slowly, so you have a better chance of burning them off. Complex carbohydrates are also much higher in vitamins and minerals. The refining process strips the fiber and nutrients out of grains.

And watch out, whole wheat does not necessarily mean whole grain. Read labels. Many whole-wheat breads are not much better for you than the infamous Wonder Bread. It's easy to find whole-grain cereals in the supermarket these days—just beware of high levels of salt and sugar.

Potatoes and the new types of whole-wheat pasta and Jerusalem artichoke pasta count as complex carbohydrates, but they tend to be broken down into sugars faster than the others mentioned, so eat them in moderation.

Sugar Is Fat Too

As far as calories are concerned, sugar that isn't burned off right away might as well be fat. All sugars are turned into fat when they can't be utilized by your body fairly quickly. That's why you want to turn to fresh, raw vegetables when you want to munch on something. Vegetables are nature's perfect source of vitamins, minerals and fiber. Next time you get a snack attack, try some carrot or celery sticks. Also try jicama (hick-ah-ma) sticks, a starchy Mexican vegetable that looks like a big potato and has a mild, sweet taste. When you cook vegetables, lightly steam or stir fry them. If you've been used to boiled vegetables, you'll be amazed at how tasty and flavorful lightly cooked vegetables are.

If you have a sweet tooth, switch to fruit. Grapes are especially sweet. Apples and pears make good afternoon snacks. Although the sugars in fruit are still sugar, they aren't absorbed as quickly as re-fined white sugar and unlike white sugar, a piece of fruit has vitamins, minerals and fiber. (If you have a craving for chocolate, you may be deficient in magnesium—try munching on some figs or almonds.) When you get an afternoon or evening craving for fat, try a handful of unsalted nuts such as almonds or cashews. But don't overdo it—nuts are packed with calories.

Keep Proteins Low-Fat and Learn to Love Soy

Proteins are essential for good health, but most Americans get too much protein and with it, too much saturated fat. Too much protein also increases your risk of osteoporosis. The average adult only needs about 1.5 to 2 oz. of protein a day. One 1/4-pound hamburger con-tains about 1.5 oz of protein. Most of us are eating three or four times that. Dairy products also tend to be high in fats and most adults cannot digest milk products properly, so I'd like you to minimize those.

Fish is a good source of low-fat protein, as are chicken and turkey. Soy products such as tofu, tempeh and miso are high in protein and calcium. Soy also contains substances that can protect you against breast and prostate cancer. It's easy to learn to love soy products. Read *Earl Mindell's Soy Miracle* (Simon & Schuster, 1995) to find out how to make soy a daily part of your diet.

Double the Fiber and Absorb Fewer Fats

You've probably heard a lot about how good fiber is for you. It's true! The American Cancer Institute recommends 25 to 30 grams of fiber a day, yet most people only get half of that. I'd like you to get 30 to 35 grams, or approximately 1 oz. of fiber every day, and here's why. Fiber speeds up the movement of food through the intestinal tract. The faster the food moves through, the less time there is for your body to absorb fats. Fiber also acts like a whisk broom to sweep the small intestine clean, keeping it free of infection. In the large colon it absorbs the toxins being removed from the body.

The good news is that increasing your fiber is a piece of cake (so to speak). If you're eating whole foods and plenty of fresh vegetables, it's easy to get your fiber every day. If you're over the age of 50 and need a little help, you can add anywhere from 1 teaspoon to 1 table-spoon of psyllium seed or psyllium husk (pronounced silly-um) to your diet daily. You know this fiber as Metamucil, but unfortunately Metamucil has a lot of sugar or artificial sweeteners and food color-ings. Pure psyllium is better for you and it's cheaper. You can buy psyllium in health food stores.

Psyllium is easy to use. Just stir it into juice or water and drink immediately. Then drink a glass of water immediately afterward. (You can count these toward your six to 10 glasses of water per day.) Be sure to drink plenty of water. Start with a teaspoon of psyllium and if necessary, work your way up gradually to a tablespoon.

If you have a bowel disorder, check with a doctor first before using psyllium or increasing the fiber in your diet. It's important to add fiber to your diet gradually if you're not used to it, or you could experience gas and bloating.

STEP 5: GET ACQUAINTED WITH NATURAL HEALING REMEDIES

Over the past few decades it's become clear that synthetic drugs are not the magic bullets we thought they would be. It's true that these drugs have saved many lives, but it's also increasingly true that they are taking a great many lives and ruining even more with debilitating side effects. One quarter of the elderly population, or 6.6 million peo-ple, are taking a drug they should never take. There's a good chance that the side effects of prescription drugs cause most symptoms of aging such as fatigue, forgetfulness and impotence. Take as few pre-scription drugs as possible and learn to treat common problems such as indigestion and allergies with common sense and practical, natu-ral alternatives.

You can avoid the vast majority of prescription drugs simply by following the Six Core Principles for Optimal Health. When you do need to treat a cold, allergy, illness or symptom of aging, you can nearly always use simple, effective natural remedies and herbs. High blood pressure, high cholesterol, diabetes, prostate troubles, menopause symptoms, allergies, arthritis, indigestion and many of our other common illnesses can all be avoided with a healthy lifestyle, or treated very safely and effectively with natural remedies.

Make a list of all the over-the-counter and prescription medications you're taking. Next to each one, write down the reason you're taking it. Next time you visit your physician, bring the list with you and ask your physician to circle the medications that are really necessary and cross off the ones you could do without. You might be surprised at how many you can do without. Any medications crossed off, throw away when you get home.

Next, find the drugs you're taking in this book and read that chapter, especially the section on the natural alternatives. If you decide to go off of a prescription drug and try the natural remedies, please work with a health-care professional, especially if you want to stop a drug that could be dangerous to go off of suddenly, such as drugs for heart disease.

If you're not taking any prescription drugs, congratulate yourself. And if your physician wants to put you on one, go on the defensive. Ask important questions such as: Exactly what will this drug do? How long will I need to take it? Are there any safe, effective ways to treat this problem without drugs? Is this the lowest dose I can take? What are the side effects?

STEP 6: GET ON THE PRESCRIPTION ALTERNATIVES VITAMIN AND MINERAL PLAN

The first six Core Principles lay the foundation for your optimal health. But optimal health is more than just not being sick. When you are radiantly healthy your body becomes a finely tuned instrument beautifully designed to fight off just about anything that comes its way. Nutritional supplements such as vitamins and minerals are health insurance. You are making sure your body has everything it needs to stay balanced and tuned.

A lot of people ask, "Why do I need to take vitamins if I eat well?" First, the soil our food is grown in is badly depleted of many essential minerals. Second, by the time food gets on your table, sometimes weeks after it has been picked, it has lost many of its important vitamins, such as vitamin C. Third, our bodies are so assaulted these days by environmental pollutants that we need extra vitamins and minerals to boost our immune systems. And, realistically, very few of us eat a truly balanced diet.

You would need to eat huge quantities of fresh, organic produce to get the vitamins and minerals present in a few vitamin supplements. For example, you'd have to drink eight glasses of fresh-squeezed orange juice every day in order to get just 1,000 mg of vitamin C.

The Basic Plan

Here's the basic program: A high-potency multiple vitamin with minerals (minerals also enable your body to use the vitamins). Be sure to read the label. With many multivitamins you need to take up to 12 a day to get the amounts listed below. Here's what your daily multivitamin intake should contain:

Vitamin A, 1,000 to 5,000 IU
Beta-carotene or carotenoids, 10,000 to 15,000 IU
The B vitamins, including:
  B1 (thiamin), 25 to 100 mg
  B2 (riboflavin), 25 to 100 mg
  B3 (niacin), 25 to 100 mg
  B5 (pantothenic acid), 25 to 100 mg
  B6 (pyridoxine), 50 to 100 mg
  B12, 100 to 1,000 mcg
  Biotin, 100 to 300 mcg
  Choline, 25 to 100 mg
  Folic acid, 400 mcg
  Inositol, 100 to 300 mg
Vitamin C, 100 to 300 mg
Vitamin D, 100 to 400 IU
Vitamin E, at least 100 IU
Minerals
  Boron, 1 to 5 mg
  Calcium (citrate, lactate or gluconate), 100 to 500 mg (women should take a total of 600 to 1,200 mg daily)

Chromium, 200 to 400 mcg

Copper, 1 to 5 mg

Magnesium (citrate or gluconate), 100 to 500 mg (women should take a total of 300 to 600 mg daily)

Manganese (citrate or chelate), 10 mg

Selenium, 200 mcg

Vanadium (sulfate), 25 to 200 mcg

Zinc, 10 to 15 mg

If your multivitamin doesn't contain the following, add them separately to your daily vitamin intake:

1,000 mg vitamin C, twice daily

400 IU vitamin E

A formula of 600 mg calcium and 300 mg magnesium

Antioxidant Vitamins and Bioflavonoids for Youthful Good Looks and Pollution Protection

The antioxidant vitamins such as beta-carotene, C and E, combined with antioxidant bioflavonoids such as grapeseed extract and green tea extract, will help you feel better and look better. Antioxidants and bioflavonoids counteract the effects of vitamin robbers such as pollution, pesticides, rancid fats and alcohol. Antioxidants and bioflavonoids also protect you from indoor pollution. The majority of pollution you're exposed to is indoors. It comes from paints, waxes, solvents and synthetic fibers in your home and office.

Antioxidants protect you from premature aging by neutralizing molecules that damage your healthy cells. These molecules, called free radicals, are made in your body and are normally easily disposed of. Exposure to pollution increases the number of free radicals. How does this age you? Free radicals cause your cells to die off faster than they would otherwise. And as you get older, your body produces fewer new cells to replace the ones that die, resulting in aging. The vitamins recommended reduce the number of free radicals, which slows the process of aging.

VITAMIN C: MORE THAN A VIRUS FIGHTER

Vitamin C is one of the few known antiviral substances. It helps form the collagen (glue) between cells, which helps prevent viruses from piercing cell walls. Viruses can multiply only after they have entered a cell. In addition, vitamin C is a boon to allergy sufferers. At a dosage of 2,000 mg per day, vitamin C decreases histamine levels in the bloodstream by 40 percent. Histamine is the substance that causes watery eyes, sneezing and congestion—the nasty symptoms of colds and allergies.

Vitamin C and vitamin E prevent the oxidation of so-called bad (LDL) cholesterol, which is very detrimental to the arteries.

What to take: Take an esterfied form of vitamin C which is specially buffered. To really take advantage of vitamin C, take it with bioflavonoids (peel of lemon, lime and grapefruit), rutin (from buckwheat), hesperidin and rose hips. This is called the C complex. Vitamin C complex is similar to what is found in nature.

Good foods for vitamin C: most fresh fruits and vegetables, such as apricots, asparagus, cantaloupe, cauliflower, citrus fruits, guava, mango, strawberries, broccoli, mustard greens and tomato juice.

VITAMIN E: THE HEART AND BLOOD VESSEL HELPER

The Shute brothers, both M.D.s, recommended vitamin E in the 1940s as a prevention against heart disease and were nearly thrown into jail for their trouble. Today, wonder of wonders, we are scientifically proving that vitamin E prevents heart disease. Recent research has shown that you must consistently take a vitamin supplement to receive the long-term benefits for the heart, so be sure to get your vitamin E daily.

Because it improves blood flow to the extremities, vitamin E is also wonderful for leg pains, such as charley horse leg cramps and for warming feet and hands. Studies have shown that vitamin E helps lower blood pressure, speeds wound healing and can slow the progression of Parkinson's disease and cataracts.

What to take: 400 IU of natural vitamin E daily in the dry form (succinate) for better absorption. Natural vitamin E is also called d-alpha tocopherol. Start with low doses, 100 IU daily and work up to 400 IU daily after a month or so.

Good foods for vitamin E: almonds, asparagus, bran, brown rice, cucumbers, dark green vegetables, herring, kale, peanuts, seeds, soybeans, unrefined vegetable oils, wheat germ and wheat germ oil and whole grains.

THE ANTIOXIDANT BIOFLAVONOIDS: GRAPESEED EXTRACT & GREEN TEA

Bioflavonoids are organic compounds found in plants that are key to the power of antioxidants. These powerful substances reduce inflammation and pain, strengthen blood vessels, improve circulation, fight bacteria and viruses, improve liver function, lower cholesterol levels and improve vision.

Bioflavonoids are found in a wide variety of plants. Some of the best food sources are the white material underneath citrus fruit peels, peppers, and berries. Although bioflavonoids are not considered essential to life, and therefore are not classified as vitamins, it is becoming clear that they *are* essential to good health. Two of the most potent antioxidant bioflavonoid supplements are grapeseed extract and green tea.

For maxiumum antioxidant bioflavonoid protection, include 50 mg of the active ingredient in grapeseed extract, proanthocyanidins (PCOs) in your daily supplement regimen as an anti-aging and preventive measure. To use therapeutically for a specific ailment such as heart disease or eye disease, take 150 to 300 mg daily.

You need to drink a lot of green tea—10 to 20 cups a day—to take complete advantage of green tea's protective properties. Since that's way too much for most people (and too much caffeine), you're better off using the extract. You can take one to two tablets or capsules of 30 percent polyphenol green tea extract daily, with meals.

THE RELAXATION FORMULA: CALCIUM/MAGNESIUM

For natural relaxation and a healthier heart, take a mix of calcium, magnesium and other essential minerals. Calcium is nature's sleep aid. Take it just before bedtime. It is absorbed well at that time and will relax you. In addition, calcium regulates your heartbeat and is essential for proper muscle function, bone health and blood clotting.

Magnesium works in synergy with calcium and has dozens of important jobs of its own to perform in the body, including regulating fluid balance in your cells and acting as a cofactor for many enzyme reactions. One of magnesium's major roles is to strengthen and regulate the heart muscle. Diets deficient in magnesium can lead to heart spasms. In fact, some physicians are giving their patients magnesium before heart operations. Magnesium also helps relieve most types of muscle spasm.

What to take: A multiple mineral mix of 400 to 600 mg calcium, 300 to 400 mg magnesium, twice daily.

Good foods for calcium and magnesium: Sardines, salmon, collard greens, kale, broccoli and dairy products are rich in calcium. Foods rich in magnesium include unmilled grains, figs, almonds, seeds, dark green vegetables and bananas.

Assimilate Your Food with Digestive Enzymes

Eating good foods won't help much if your body can't assimilate them. This is where good digestion comes in. If you have gas, bloating or cramps after eating, or if your food sits in your stomach for more than 45 minutes, you may be a candidate for a digestive enzyme supplement. (Long-term use of antacids can also block your digestive enzymes.)

There are three major types of enzymes that break down a specific food type for absorption into the body: amylase for digesting carbohydrates, protease or proteolytic enzymes for digesting protein and lipase for digesting fat. If you want help digesting lactose you can get an enzyme supplement that contains lactase.

It's also important to include betaine hydrochloride (HCl) with your digestive enzymes. This will supplement your stomach's acid, an important part of good digestion. You should be able to find a good formula that combines digestive enzymes and HCl. (See Chapter 10 on digestion for details.)

CHAPTER 9

Drugs for Heart Disease and Their Natural Alternatives

Pick almost anyone in North America over the age of 50 off the street and chances are they can tell you the major causes of heart disease: obesity, a high-fat diet, not enough exercise, stress, high cholesterol, high blood pressure. Right? Well, partially.

As you'll discover later in this chapter, high cholesterol and high blood pressure don't directly *cause* heart disease, they are more like indicators that heart disease exists. An analogy would be that a fever doesn't cause the flu, but it's a good indicator that it's there. Another way of putting it is that high blood pressure and high LDL cholesterol are *symptoms* of heart disease rather than primary causes. Knowing you have these so-called risk factors for heart disease is useful only if you track down their underlying causes and treat them.

Drugs that lower cholesterol and blood pressure *may* reduce your risk of heart disease, but they tend to simultaneously raise your risk of other diseases because they don't treat the underlying problem. If you try to force a symptom away with a powerful drug, the underlying problem is just going to pop up somewhere else until you treat the cause. We now know that other factors such as your homocysteine levels and your antioxidant levels are just as important, if not more so, than cholesterol and blood pressure. You'll find out more about them later in the chapter.

The American Heart Association estimated that the cost of cardiovascular disease in 1994 was $128 billion. This includes the cost of physicians and nursing services, hospital and nursing home services, the cost of medications and loss of productivity. The personal cost of heart disease is the biggest loss of all. Yet heart disease is one of the easiest diseases of all to *prevent*. Even if your parents and grandparents had heart disease, you can still prevent it in yourself.

If heart disease kills more people every year than anything else, why aren't these simple cures being shouted from the rooftops? Why isn't it the biggest topic of discussion on all the talk shows? First of all, it's too simple, too inexpensive and not nearly dramatic enough for a talk show. Heart disease treatment in the U.S., consisting mainly of surgery and drugs, is a *multi-billion* dollar industry. Why would those with a vested financial interest in heart disease treatment give it up for simple, natural, inexpensive remedies? That means that preventing and treating your heart disease is in your hands. It's your responsibility.

Simple cures seem to be the hardest thing to do for many people, because they involve a change in lifestyle and daily habits. The only way to *cure* heart disease is to work on its *causes*. If you take the initiative to make positive changes in your diet, get some exercise, lose some weight and take some supplements, you will begin to see improvement in your health very rapidly.

The single biggest factor contributing to heart disease in America is our poor diet. We eat too much fat, too many processed foods, and not enough fresh vegetables. In the 1950s, the Japanese diet was 16 percent fat and they had almost no incidence of heart disease. Today their diet is 26 percent fat and heart disease is the second leading cause of death in Japan. In the U.S. the average diet contains 36 to 40 percent fat.

There is no question that people who eat less meat and more fish, fruits and vegetables, and drink more wine, have significantly lower rates of death from heart disease. Furthermore, there is a strong correlation between diets high in polyunsaturated fatty acids (vegetable oils prone to oxidation/rancidity) and a high rate of death from heart disease, and correspondingly less death in those cultures that eat more monounsaturated fats such as olive oil. Those countries with the highest intake of antioxidants and bioflavonoids have the lowest death rates from heart disease.

SHOULD YOU BE TAKING AN ASPIRIN A DAY?

If you read the headlines and listen to conventional physicians you'll be convinced that aspirin is the miracle drug of the century. Not only does it banish pain and reduce inflammation and fever, it prevents heart disease. And now we're hearing that it prevents colon cancer. Yes, aspirin is a wonder drug. For short-term use there's nothing like a couple of aspirin to knock out a headache, reduce the pain of a sprain, and even to quickly reduce heart disease risk while working on safer and more effective long-term solutions.

Used long term, aspirin does more harm than good. It causes gastric bleeding, ulcers, suppresses the immune system and promotes macular degeneration, an irreversible eye disease. And while it decreases the risk of some types of strokes, it increases the risk of other types.

Aspirin essentially works by blocking the production of hormone-like substances called prostaglandins, which constantly regulate every cell in the body in many of their complex interactions. Some prostaglandins, when made in the body in excess, play a role in promoting heart disease, inflammation and pain. The fact that aspirin very effectively blocks these prostaglandins would be good news, except that it blocks the formation of both "good" and "bad" prostaglandins, and in the process of suppressing the good prostaglandins, also suppresses the immune system. (A little aside—some of aspirin's benefit may also come from the use of magnesium in buffered aspirin, the form most often used in heart disease studies. A little magnesium every day could provide major benefits to the heart.)

While the bad prostaglandins can make your blood more likely to aggregate or clump together and cause a stroke or heart attack, good prostaglandins lower blood pressure, inhibit blood aggregation and the production of cholesterol, and reduce inflammation reactions. Hmmmm. Sounds like "good" prostaglandins provide the same heart benefits that aspirin does. And they do. Much of heart disease has to do with the fact that bad prostaglandins are outweighing good prostaglandins.

If we encourage the good prostaglandins and discourage the bad, we can prevent heart disease without aspirin's side effects. Most of the good and all of the bad prostaglandins are made from GLA oils, or gamma linoleic acid, a type of essential fatty acid found in fruits, vegetables and grains. You need GLA to make the majority of the good prostaglandins, but then you need to make sure it goes down the good prostaglandin pathway. What drives GLA down the wrong pathway to the bad prostaglandins? The biggest culprits are dietary: hydrogenated oils such as margarines, and a diet high in refined carbohydrates and sugar will drive GLA oils down the bad pathways. Viral illnesses and excessive adrenal hormones secreted in response to stress can also create more bad prostaglandins and a deficiency of good ones.

There are small amounts of GLA oils in oatmeal and trace amounts in many fruits and vegetables. You only need minuscule amounts of these oils to drive your prostaglandin pathways. The most significant source of GLA oils is found in borage oil, which is sold in capsules at your health food store. However, your GLA oils should be balanced with EPA oils, so before you go out and buy borage oil capsules, read on.

A specific type of omega-3 oil, eicosapentaenoic acid (EPA), found in fish oil, will inhibit the production of bad prostaglandins without bothering the good ones. This is why it's important to eat cold water, deep sea fish such as salmon, cod, bass, halibut, sardines, albacore tuna and flounder at least twice a week. You can also take fish oil capsules, but the highest benefit definitely comes from eating fish.

In a nutshell, get your GLA oil by avoiding things that deplete it and by eating oatmeal, and get your EPA oils by eating fish regularly. If you want to take GLA (borage oil) and EPA (fish oil) supplements for a few months to get your prostaglandin pathways in good working order, you should be taking 50 to 100 more EPA than GLA. You only need 1 to 2 mg of GLA and 50 to 100 mg of EPA.

There is an amazing amount of misinformation out there about fats and oils and what they do in the body. If you'd like a clearly written, well-researched book on prostaglandins and essential fatty acids, try *Enter the Zone* by Barry Sears (Regan Books, 1995).

NATURAL ALTERNATIVES FOR TREATING HEART DISEASE

In this section you'll find general suggestions for preventing and treating heart disease, angina and irregular heartbeats, and later in the chapter, in the sections on high cholesterol and high blood pressure, you'll find specific suggestions for treating the underlying causes of those conditions.

Your number-one, most important step in preventing and treating heart disease is to follow the Six Core Principles for Optimal Health. That is your foundation for all-around optimal health. Every single step in the plan is vitally important to a healthy heart.

Here are some further steps you can take to take care of your heart.

Use Alcohol in Moderation

Caution and moderation are the watchwords for drinking alcohol. Studies show that a low alcohol intake, particularly of red wine, protects against heart disease when included as part of a healthy diet. However, even just a bit too much alcohol can bump up blood pressure and help create nutritional deficiencies which increase your risk of heart disease.

Make Garlic a Staple of Your Diet

Garlic is the herb of legend and myth. It is mentioned in the Bible, in Homer's Odyssey, in ancient Chinese texts, and has been found in the tombs of ancient Egyptians. Now we have *dozens* of scientific studies to back up the folklore claims for garlic's prowess in keeping us healthy.

While garlic may or may not work to ward off vampires, it does a great job at neutralizing three risk factors for heart disease: high blood fats, high blood pressure and blood clotting. After raw garlic, the most effective form of garlic appears to be aged extract of organic garlic with a high allicin content, but they all have some beneficial effects.

Keep Your Fibrinogen Low

You may not have heard a lot about fibrinogen as a risk for heart disease, but it is a key factor. Fibrinogen is a protein substance found in blood that plays an important role in blood clotting. In effect, it makes the blood sticky or gummy, but too much makes the blood too sticky. Fibrinogen is an important substance in the body, being the precursor of fibrin, a nondissolving protein that plays a major role in the ability of blood to clot. As with so many substances in our body, having enough fibrinogen is essential to good health, but too much is not healthy.

In nearly every study done on heart disease, high levels of fibrinogen in the blood were found to be directly related to coronary artery disease, probably by interfering with blood flow. Excess fibrinogen is also related to atrial fibrillation, strokes, intermittent claudication (pain in the legs when walking) and high blood pressure. Reducing fibrinogen levels may be your single best protection against having a stroke. The good news is that most of the factors that raise or lower fibrinogen are the same ones that raise or lower other risk factors for heart disease.

WHAT MAKES FIBRINOGEN LEVELS RISE?

- Psychological and mental stress can increase fibrinogen levels.
- High blood sugar raises fibrinogen levels.
- Very high LDL cholesterol levels will raise fibrinogen levels.
- Estrogen, which is found in birth control pills and in hormone replacement therapy, raises fibrinogen levels, which make it ironic that the pharmaceutical industry is making claims that estrogen prevents heart disease. It may slightly lower your risk of dying from a heart attack, but it raises your risk of dying from a stroke and from cancer. (More about that in the chapter on hormone replacement therapy.)
- Smoking has a direct effect on raising fibrinogen levels.
- Obesity significantly raises fibrinogen levels.

WHAT LOWERS FIBRINOGEN LEVELS?

- Exercise is the single biggest factor in lowering fibrinogen levels.
- A glass of wine with dinner may slightly lower fibrinogen levels.
- Fish oil supplementation may lower fibrinogen levels.

- Eating plenty of garlic lowers fibrinogen.
- Olive oil lowers fibrinogen.
- Vitamin E lowers fibrinogen.
- A vegetarian diet lowers fibrinogen.

Keep Your Homocysteine Low

In the past few years it has been very well scientifically documented that high levels of homocysteine, a byproduct of metabolism of the amino acid methionine, is an important risk factor in heart disease and strokes associated with narrowed blood vessels. In fact, high homocysteine levels will turn out to be a much more accurate marker of heart disease risk than cholesterol or blood pressure.

Researchers currently believe that excess homocysteine damages blood vessels, so it may turn out to be a primary cause of heart disease and not just an indicator. Homocysteine is an amino acid meant to exist only temporarily in the body as a byproduct of methionine (another amino acid) metabolism. In a healthy body it's quickly transformed into harmless substances. If you have a deficiency of certain B vitamins or a genetic predisposition that interferes with the metabolism of homocysteine, the levels of it in your blood will rise, and so will your risk of heart disease and stroke.

According to a study done at Tufts University School of Medicine in Boston, if your homocysteine levels are just 20 percent above normal, your risk of cardiovascular disease is significantly increased. If your physician wants to measure your homocysteine levels, a normal homocysteine level is about 12 umol/L, and cardiovascular risk increases at about 14 to 16 umol/L.

Scientists know that homocysteine damages arteries, but haven't been able to determine how. The best evidence suggests that it causes certain kinds of arterial cells (endothelial cells) to literally fall apart. This is the type of damage that attracts cholesterol to the artery walls in an attempt to patch things up. But the "bad" cholesterol accumulates and eventually clogs up the arteries. Antioxidants will help significantly in reducing the amount of bad cholesterol in the blood, but if homocysteine levels remain high, the damage to arterial walls will continue.

Some drugs can cause high homocysteine levels, particularly those that interfere with folic acid. Those that interfere with folic acid include methotrexate, an immunosuppressive drug given to cancer, rheumatoid arthritis and psoriasis patients; the anticonvulsant drugs phenytoin (Dilantin) and carbamazepine (Tegretol, Epitol); and the bile acid sequestrants for lowering cholesterol levels, cholestipol (Colestid) and cholestyramine (Questran). It's ironic that these cholesterol-lowering drugs, given to reduce heart disease, may actually cause it by raising homocysteine levels!

Other research has shown that homocysteine levels rise when daily folic acid intake is 200 mcg per day or less. This is a typical example of how inadequate the RDA (Recommended Daily Allowance) amounts are, because the current recommended daily allowance for folate is 200 mcg.

Fortunately for nearly everyone, homocysteine can be easily and inexpensively lowered by taking some B vitamins. If you're taking a daily multivitamin that includes 400 mcg of folic acid, 50 mg of vitamin B6 and 1,000 mcg of vitamin B12, you should be covered. If your homocysteine levels are high, you should be getting an additional 200 mg daily of vitamin B6 (pyridoxine), and 1 to 4 mg of folic acid daily until your homocysteine levels are back to normal.

Since a deficiency of vitamin B12 can also indirectly raise homocysteine levels, and since a high intake of folic acid can mask a vitamin B12 deficiency, make sure your intake of vitamin B12 is at least 1,000 mcg per day. Vitamin B12 is best taken sublingually (under the tongue), in a nasal gel or spray, or as an injection.

Get Plenty of Magnesium

Arnold is a fairly healthy guy in his mid-sixties, who wound up in a hospital emergency room in the middle of the night, frightened and in pain, wondering if he was having a heart attack. It turned out he was suffering from a type of angina that causes spasms of the heart muscle. After giving him some drugs and monitoring him for a few hours, they sent him home that night, telling him to make an appointment with his physician.

A few weeks later Arnold's angina pain was returning, and his physician wanted to put him on a beta-blocker. Now Arnold takes pretty good care of himself (he does have a weakness for good ice cream), he hates going to the physician, and really dislikes taking drugs. Finally he got the name of a physician using alternative health-care approaches who gave him some intravenous magnesium and prescribed a daily magnesium supplement. Not only did Arnold's angina pain totally disappear after the intravenous magnesium, his energy level was higher than it had been in years. This was a happy guy!

The essential mineral that's the biggest key to prevention and treatment of heart disease is magnesium. Several recent studies have shown that when people come into an emergency room with a heart attack, if they are given intravenous magnesium right away, their chances of survival go way up, and if they continue to receive it their survival rate continues to improve. It has been shown to help with angina and to improve the symptoms of congestive heart failure.

Magnesium works on several levels to keep the heart in good working order:

- **Prevents muscle spasms:** According to several Japanese studies published in the *American Journal of Cardiology*, the oxygen deficiency and spasms caused by magnesium deficiency narrows the coronary arteries, leading to angina. A great deal of angina pain could be relieved simply by bringing magnesium levels up to normal.
- **Keeps blood flowing smoothly:** Magnesium helps keep the blood from getting "sticky," a condition which can contribute to having a stroke.
- **Keeps cholesterol under control:** Another Japanese study found that patients with low HDL ("good") cholesterol had low magnesium levels, and that when they took magnesium supplements their HDL levels increased. In addition, animal studies have shown that when magnesium is deficient, the amount of oxidized LDL cholesterol increases, with a corresponding increase in arterial damage.
- **Maintains normal blood pressure:** There have been at least 28 independent studies showing that patients with hypertension (high blood pressure) have a magnesium deficiency. People who

have long term high blood pressure have magnesium levels that average 15 percent below normal.

- **Keeps the heartbeat regular:** A magnesium deficiency can lead to irregular heartbeat (arrhythmia). If you're on the medicine digitalis to treat heart disease, the medication can be toxic if you are deficient in potassium or magnesium.

It looks like magnesium is involved in just about every aspect of keeping a healthy heart, yet most Americans are deficient in this essential mineral. A large survey done by the U.S. Department of Agriculture found that only 25 percent of 37,785 individuals had magnesium intakes at or greater than the Recommended Daily Allowance, which is too low to begin with. Some 20 to 65 percent of critically ill hospitalized patients have a magnesium deficiency. A normal blood serum magnesium test will not give you an accurate indication of your magnesium levels. It's more accurate (and unfortunately more expensive) to measure intracellular magnesium levels.

Early symptoms of a magnesium deficiency can include muscle and nerve pain and an irregular heartbeat. A magnesium deficiency can also create potassium and calcium deficiency. Magnesium can be depleted by stress, excessive alcohol, sugar, diabetes, kidney disease, chronic diarrhea, not enough protein in the diet, too much protein in the diet and thyroid disorders. Alcoholics are at a much greater risk for heart disease. Many researchers believe the increased risk is caused by the depletion effect excess alcohol has on magnesium.

Good food sources of magnesium include whole grains (especially oats, brown rice, millet, buckwheat and wheat), legumes (lentils, split peas and beans), bran, almonds and peanuts, and broccoli. Chocolate contains large amounts of magnesium, and a craving for chocolate may be an indicator of a magnesium deficiency.

Drugs That Deplete Magnesium

Aminoglycosides	Diuretics
Cisplatin	Foscarnet
Corticosteroids	Gentamicin
Cyclosporine	Pentamidine

Magnesium by itself can cause diarrhea, so unless you are constipated, be sure to take it in a multivitamin, in combination with calcium, or in the form of magnesium glycinate, gluconate or citrate. You can take 300 to 400 mg of magnesium daily as a supplement.

Antioxidants, Antioxidants, Antioxidants

When a squirt of lemon juice helps food stay fresh it is working as an antioxidant, protecting against the harmful effects of oxygen. Oxygen harmful? When an oxygen molecule loses an electron, it becomes an unstable molecule called a free radical, which tries to stabilize itself by grabbing another oxygen from any body substance or tissue nearby, causing that molecule in turn to become unstable. Antioxidants are molecules that are able to donate an oxygen molecule to the free radical without becoming destabilized themselves.

This process of free radical creation is called oxidation, a normal and important part of your body's metabolism. It's when oxidation reactions overwhelm your body's ability to stabilize them that they do damage. Oxidation does damage when we're under a lot of stress, exposed to a heavy load of toxins, or don't have enough antioxidants in our diet.

Out-of-control oxidation is a causative factor in illness, including heart disease and strokes. Today's polluted world means our bodies have to cope with far higher levels of free radicals than ever before. Free radical culprits include smog, cigarette smoke, pesticides and food additives. The average American doesn't eat nearly enough antioxidant-rich fresh fruits and vegetables to counteract these environmental toxins. Our bodies are in double oxidant jeopardy, which makes taking antioxidant supplements an important part of preventing heart disease.

Antioxidants come in many forms, from teas and herbal tinctures to foods and vitamins. Their marvelous power gives a shielding, protective effect against heart disease. Some work better than others to protect against heart disease.

Ginkgo biloba extract is made from the tree of the same name. It is particularly rich in antioxidant substances which act synergistically. One of its properties leads to improvement in circulation to the heart. As might be expected, it also reduces oxidized LDL cholesterol levels and lowers LDL cholesterol generally. In addition, it raises "good" HDL cholesterol, and lowers blood fat levels.

Ginkgo biloba takes time to produce its effects and should be taken in repeated doses for a fairly long period of time. Ginkgo biloba extract (GBE) with at least 24 percent ginkgoflavoglycosides, is the best form to take. Standardized, semi-purified and concentrated, GBE provides consistent levels of its most active compounds. Take the recommended dosage on the package.

Glutathione, also known as GSH, is a tripeptide made from the amino acids cysteine, glycine and glutamic acid. This humble little protein is found in the cells of nearly all living organisms on Earth, and its primary job is waste disposal. GSH has three main detox jobs in the body:

1. When there are free radicals lurking about, threatening to start an oxidation reaction, GSH catches them, neutralizes them, passes them on (often to another antioxidant such as vitamin E), and begins the cycle anew;
2. In the liver, GSH latches on to toxic substances and binds to them, so the liver can excrete them without being damaged; and
3. GSH prevents red blood cells from being damaged by neutralizing unstable forms of oxygen. We literally cannot survive without this miraculous antioxidant.

Glutathione's antioxidant work is the front line defense for preventing oxidation of LDL cholesterol which damages the arteries. It's also crucial in protecting the lymphatic system and the digestive system from an overload of unstable lipids (fats and oils). If glutathione levels drop anywhere in the body, the burden of toxic stress goes up.

GSH is one of the most abundant substances in the body, and as long as we have a good supply of its building block cysteine (glycine and glutamic acid are rarely in short supply) and its cofactor selenium, it will be hard at work doing its detoxifying chores. GSH levels drop as we age, and can be depleted by an overload of rancid oils (such as polyunsaturated and partially hydrogenated vegetable oils), overexposure to poisons such as pesticides, and pharmaceutical drugs that stress the liver such as acetaminophen and aspirin. Since glutathione often passes off its neutralized waste products to antioxidants such as vitamin C and vitamin E, a deficiency of these vitamins can impair its function.

Measuring glutathione levels is expensive at this time, but if you have heart disease, are at a high risk for it, or have high LDL cholesterol levels, try raising your glutathione levels. The best way to raise glutathione levels is by taking a cysteine supplement, preferably in the more stable form of N-acetyl cysteine. Follow directions on the container for dosages. Foods with high levels of cysteine include onions, garlic, yogurt, wheat germ and red meat.

Green tea is a polyphenol, an aromatic, organic compound that acts as a potent antioxidant in the body. Like others in this family it prevents the oxidation of LDL cholesterol, lowers cholesterol, raises "good" HDL levels and lowers triglyceride levels. It also reduces blood coagulation and prevents the clumping of red blood cells, both good steps for the prevention of heart disease. Green tea extract is available in tablet form, without caffeine.

PCOs are procyanidolic oligomers, which are bioflavonoids found in grapeseed, lemon tree bark, peanuts, cranberries and citrus peels. Known to improve circulation, PCOs strengthen blood vessel walls and prevent the clumping of blood clotting substances, protecting against stroke. These properties come on top of PCOs' very strong antioxidant powers that pre-empt LDL oxidation.

To address high cholesterol with PCOs, 150 to 300 mg per day is recommended. Otherwise, 50 mg of PCOs daily makes a good supplement if you're over 50. Many studies have shown that PCO extract from grapeseed is one of the most powerful antioxidants known. It also increases the performance of other antioxidants.

Vitamin E is your greatest ally and protector when it comes to vitamins and heart health, and yet most people are deficient in vitamin E. In one study, the vitamin E intake of elderly, affluent Americans was less than three-quarters of the RDA.

Impressive results were shown in two major Harvard University studies of health professionals. A survey of over 39,000 male professionals showed that they enjoyed a 37 percent lower risk of coronary artery disease when they took 100 IU or more of vitamin E daily. The Nurse's Health Study of 87,000 women showed a 40 percent lower risk of heart disease for women on the same dose of vitamin E.

A European population study looked at 100 apparently healthy men aged 40 to 49 years old. Blood levels of vitamin E were found to be the most important risk factor for heart disease, even beyond smoking. There is evidence, too, that vitamin E can dissolve clots, helps the heart pump more efficiently, naturally makes arteries widen and increases the oxygen available in the blood.

Vitamin E is a fat-soluble oil found in many foods, including unrefined vegetable oils, whole grains, butter, organ meats, eggs, a variety of nuts, sunflower seeds, fruit, soybeans and dark green leafy vegetables.

I recommend you take vitamin E either as mixed tocopherols or d-alpha tocopherol. Do not use the synthetic form of vitamin E, called dl-alpha tocopherol.

Although vitamin E is very safe even at high doses, 400 IU (dry form) daily should be an adequate dose for adults. The dry or succinate form is recommended for anyone sensitive to oils or with problems absorbing nutrients (if you're over the age of 65 you probably fall into the latter category). Vitamin E works well taken with its partners in the body, the nutrients vitamin C, beta-carotene and other flavonoids, and selenium.

NATURAL REMEDIES FOR A STRONGER HEART

Natural remedies for strengthening the heart tend to help significantly with symptoms such as arrhythmia and angina, and can also make a big difference in people with congestive heart failure. Three of the most effective are coenzyme Q10, hawthorn and carnitine.

COENZYME Q10 (CoQ10)

CoQ10 has the ability to protect and strengthen the heart and lower blood pressure. CoQ10 is a vital enzyme, a catalyst to the production of energy in our cells. Without it, our cells simply won't work. It's chemical name is *ubiquinone*—it is ubiquitous, or everywhere, where there is life. Its levels in the human body are highest in the heart and liver. When we are ill or stressed, and as we age, our bodies are less able to produce CoQ10.

According to a study done by CoQ10 expert Karl Folkers, published in the *International Journal of Vitamin and Nutrition Research*, patients with a variety of cardiac disorders consistently demonstrate a blood deficiency of CoQ10. A double-blind Japanese study with 100 patients who had cardiac failure showed that only 30 mg per day of CoQ10 for two to four weeks produced a measurable improvement in symptoms. Many older people whose heart function has degenerated and who try CoQ10 report an almost immediate boost in their energy levels.

People who suffer from angina report that the pain disappears and they can exercise. In a double-blind placebo study using CoQ10 and other drugs traditionally used to treat angina, it was found that CoQ10 was far more effective in reducing or eliminating angina pain than any of the other medications. Other studies have shown that people on heart medications can greatly reduce their dosage of medicine if it is combined with CoQ10.

The best way to take CoQ10 is in a gel capsule, which is much stronger than the powder form. You can take one 30 to 60 mg capsule up to three times a day with meals. If you have serious heart disease you can double that amount for a few months.

If you want to know more about CoQ10, get a paperback book called *The Miracle Nutrient: Coenzyme Q10*, by Emile G. Bliznakov, M.D. and Gerald L. Hunt (Bantam Books, 1987).

HAWTHORN BERRIES (*Crataegus oxyacantha*)

Hawthorn berries have been used as a heart tonic for centuries and are widely used in Europe for angina and for lowering blood pressure. They are rich in bioflavonoids which help strengthen the blood vessels. They are also a vasodilator, which increases the flow of blood and oxygen to the heart, lowers blood pressure and strengthens the heart muscle.

Hawthorn berries work gradually, and you may not notice a difference for a month or so. You can find hawthorn berry extract in capsule or tincture forms. Because the amounts vary widely, follow directions for use on the bottle. Some of the tinctures can be very powerful, so it is very important that if you're already on heart medicine you work with your doctor. However, in and of themselves, hawthorn berries are nontoxic and very safe.

CARNITINE

This amino acid is another heart-strengthening nutrient that appears to be especially useful for treating angina and congestive heart failure. You can take 500 mg twice a day, preferably between meals.

BAN PESTICIDES FROM YOUR LIFE

Chronic exposure to pesticides is a known heart disease risk, but one that most people never think of when they have their lawn doused with chemicals or spray their garden, go after bugs in the house with a can of spray, or have their house fumigated. If you're pouring poisons down gopher or mole holes, dousing your aphids with pesticides and your dog with flea dip, you're exposing yourself, and your heart, not to mention your dog, to unacceptable levels of poisons.

These poisons may not kill you on the spot, but they will create free radical damage in your tissues and accumulate in the body. A study done in the Ukraine of agricultural workers showed that those frequently exposed to pesticides had a higher rate of heart disease as well as a higher rate of abortions and birth defects. There is also evidence that fetal exposure to pesticides can cause congenital heart disease.

Pesticides aren't the only toxins that can cause heart disease. Others found in the workplace and also in the garage include: solvents, glues and other binding materials, dyes, lacquers, paints, PCBs, metals and vinylchloride. In many cases, workers only need to be exposed to *fumes* or *dust* from these materials to increase their risk of heart disease.

Don't take it for granted that, just because you buy a pesticide, herbicide, fungicide, cleaning solvent, paint or other chemical from the hardware store, it's safe. The industries that use these substances are largely unregulated. There are literally thousands of these products on the shelves that have never been tested for safety. In fact, you should assume they are harmful unless you find out otherwise, and avoid contact with skin and avoid breathing the fumes. Even such simple household chemicals as ammonia and chlorine can be harmful.

Reduce Your Exposure to Toxins

Here are some tips for reducing your exposure to pesticides and other environmental toxins:

- Control fleas on your pets and in your home with substances such as boric acid compounds (now found in most pet stores or call Flea Busters) and aromatic oils such as pennyroyal, rather than flea powders.
- If you're a gardener, do it the organic way. There are plenty of books and magazines on the subject, and local classes are easy to find. You can create a beautiful lawn and garden without chemicals and in the long run you'll have far fewer pest problems.
- Don't drink tap water.
- If you are exposed to pesticides, take a cool shower and drink plenty of clean water to help flush out the poisons.
- Wash, peel or even scrub fruits and vegetables well and eat organic produce whenever possible.
- If you think something at work is making you sick, pursue it. It could be mold or fungus in the heating or cooling system, fumes from wall paneling or carpets, or a coworker's cigarette smoke.
- Stop using fungicides, herbicides and pesticides. Get out of the habit of blasting indoor and outdoor pests with a can of spray. Learn how to control pests naturally.
- Don't move in next door to an agricultural field or orchard unless you know it's organic and likely to stay that way.

TRY NOT TO USE COMBINATION DRUGS

There are some drugs that combine the different types of heart drugs listed below. It is not advisable to take the combination heart drugs. It's difficult enough to combine and track the effects and side effects of these drugs without putting them all in one pill. If they come in separate pills you can take more or less of one (with your physician's supervision) if you're experiencing side effects, to track down a cause. Remember, side effects are never your fault, and you should never feel you just have to suffer them.

DRUGS FOR ARRHYTHMIA, ANGINA AND CONGESTIVE HEART FAILURE

Arrhythmia and angina (pain in the chest area) are symptoms of heart disease. They are together here because the drugs used to treat them are often the same. Digoxin is the fourth most-prescribed drug in America.

Cardiac Glycosides (Digitalis Drugs)

DIGITOXIN (Crystodigin)
DIGOXIN (Lanoxicaps, Lanoxin)

WHAT DO THEY DO IN YOUR BODY?

The digitalis drugs are derived from the plants *Digitalis purpurea* and *Digitalis lanata*, otherwise known as foxglove. Although an exact description of their action on the heart is complicated and technical, in essence what they do is make the heartbeat strong and increase its ability to pump blood.

WHAT ARE THEY PRESCRIBED FOR?

Congestive heart failure and irregular heartbeat (arrhythmia).

WHAT ARE THE POSSIBLE SIDE EFFECTS?

Although the digitalis drugs are used to treat irregular heartbeat, they can also cause it. Other adverse effects can include nausea, vomiting, loss of appetite, diarrhea and stomach pain.

The primary danger of these drugs is too high a dose. Since there are many ways in which the dosage can be inadvertently increased, overdosage is a very real concern. A long list of drugs can slow clearance of the drugs from the body or increase the effect of the drugs. People taking this medication need to be very alert to what they are eating and drinking. The early symptoms of an overdosage are nausea, vomiting, diarrhea, stomach pain and loss of appetite. Other symptoms include headache, weakness, fatigue, sleepiness, confusion, restlessness, visual disturbances such as blurred vision, depression, skin rash, hives and irregular heartbeat. Your physician should be notified if you have any of these symptoms.

WHAT ARE THE INTERACTIONS WITH OTHER DRUGS?

Note: All of these interactions should be considered dangerous.

Digitalis drugs may raise levels or prolong the effects of these drugs:

↑ Thiazide and loop diuretics

These drugs many increase the effects or prolong the action of digitalis drugs:

↑ Alprazolam
Aminoglycosides
Amiodarone
Anticholinergics
Benzodiazepines
Bepridil
Captopril
Cyclosporine
Diltiazem
Diphenoxylate
Erythromycin
Esmolol
Felodipine

Flecainide
Hydroxychloroquine
Ibuprofen
Indomethacin
Itraconazole
Nefazodone
Nifedipine
Omeprazole
Propafenone
Quinidine
Tetracycline
Tolbutamide
Verapamil

These drugs may reduce the effects of digitalis drugs:

↓ Aminoglutethimide
Aminoglycosides
Aminosalicyclic acid
Antacids (aluminum or magne-
    sium salts)
Antihistamines
Antineoplastics
Barbiturates

Cholestyramine
Colestipol
Hydantoins
Hypoglycemic agents (oral diabetes
    drugs)
Kaolin/pectin
Metoclopramide
Neomycin

Penicillamine   Sucralfate
Phenytoin   Sulfasalazine
Rifampin

WHAT ARE THE INTERACTIONS WITH FOOD?

Food in general slows the absorption rate of the drug, but doesn't necessarily decrease levels. A high fiber meal can slow absorption of the digitalis drugs *and* reduce levels, by absorbing the drugs and carrying them through the intestines unabsorbed. High carbohydrate meals may slow absorption more than a balanced meal. High fat meals may cause the body to reabsorb the drug, slightly increasing levels.

WHAT NUTRIENTS DO THEY THROW OUT OF BALANCE OR INTERACT WITH?

The digitalis drugs increase the excretion of magnesium and potassium.

WHAT ELSE TO TAKE IF YOU TAKE THESE DRUGS

Be sure to take a good mineral supplement if you're taking digitalis drugs. Low potassium combined with high digitalis can be a deadly combination, causing irregular heartbeats, so it's especially important to keep your potassium levels high by eating potassium-rich foods such as bananas, nuts, avocados, figs, prunes, tomatoes and meat.

Along with diuretics, laxatives and licorice root can also deplete potassium.

Nitrates (Nitroglycerin)

AMYL NITRATE

ISOSORBIDE DINITRATE (Isordil, Sorbitrate, Isosorbide, Dilatrate)

ISOSORBIDE MONONITRATE (Monoket, ISMO, Imdur)

NITROGLYCERIN (Nitrostat, Nitrolingual, Nitrogard, Nitrong, Nitro-Bid, Nitrocine, Nitroglyn, Minitran, Nitrodisc, Deponit, Nitro-Dur, Nitrol)

There are no specific natural alternatives to this drug. In other words, if you have such severe angina that not taking this drug could put your life in jeopardy, it's important to keep taking it while you work to reduce your angina symptoms naturally. Since this drug is most often taken only when an angina attack occurs, you'll naturally wean yourself off it as your angina is reduced. These drugs are somewhat outdated as heart attack and angina preventives; if you're taking daily doses whether or not you have an angina attack, ask your physician about switching to a safer drug.

What Do They Do in Your Body?

Reduce or relieve spasms in the heart muscle, thereby dilating blood vessels and lowering blood pressure.

What Are They Prescribed For?

Angina attacks.

What Are the Possible Side Effects?

Postural hypotension (feeling dizzy or faint when you stand from a sitting or lying position) can be a dangerous and possibly fatal side effect. It can also damage organs. Other side effects include aggravation of some types of angina (chest pain) and some types of glaucoma, and it may cause severe headaches, blurred vision and dry mouth.

Adverse reactions can include nausea, vomiting, diarrhea, heartburn, involuntary passing of urine and feces, impotence, urinary frequency, anxiety, restlessness, agitation, weakness, dizziness, fainting, rebound angina and hypertension, irregular heartbeat, insomnia, pounding heart, rash, flushing, twitching muscles, joint aches, bronchitis, sinus infection, sweating, water retention.

Caution: Think Twice About Taking These Types of Drugs If . . .

- You have existing hypotension.
- You have kidney or liver disease.
- You have glaucoma.

WHAT ARE THE INTERACTIONS WITH OTHER DRUGS?

Nitrates may reduce the effects of this drug:

↓ Heparin

These drugs may increase the effects or prolong the action of nitrates:

↑ Alcohol*
Aspirin
Calcium channel blockers

DRUGS FOR PREVENTING STROKE AND BLOOD CLOTS

Blood Thinners

COUMARINS: Warfarin (Coumadin), Anisindione (Miradon)

HEPARINS: Enoxaparin (Lovenox), Dalteparin (Fragmin)

WHAT DO THEY DO IN YOUR BODY?

They are known as anticoagulants or blood thinners, and although their actions are complicated, in essence they thin the blood, reduce its stickiness and its tendency to clot.

WHAT ARE THEY PRESCRIBED FOR?

To reduce the risk of stroke or blood clots, for treatment after a stroke or heart attack; they are sometimes prescribed during or after surgery.

WHAT ARE THE POSSIBLE SIDE EFFECTS?

The major risk in taking the anticoagulants is that they will work too well and not allow the blood to clot when it needs to, causing a

---

* Potentially dangerous interaction.

hemorrhage or uncontrolled bleeding. This can happen internally or externally. The anticoagulants are also affected by a wide range of other drugs, making dangerous drug interactions common. Easy bruising, nosebleeds, dark urine and tarry or red stools may be the first signs of too high a dose or uncontrolled bleeding. People with bleeding ulcers can die if given anticoagulants.

CAUTION: THINK TWICE ABOUT TAKING THESE TYPES OF DRUGS IF . . .

- You have a bleeding ulcer.
- You have adrenal insufficiency.
- You have heavy bleeding during menstruation.
- You have liver or kidney problems.
- You have diarrhea.

Women and the elderly are more sensitive to these drugs.

WHAT ARE THE INTERACTIONS WITH OTHER DRUGS?

If you are taking anticoagulants, do not take *any* new drug, even over-the-counter drugs, without checking first with your physician or pharmacist.

These drugs may increase the effects or prolong the action of anticoagulants:

↑ Acetaminophen
Alcohol
Amiodarone
Aminoglycosides
Androgens (testosterone, DHEA)
Beta-blockers
Cephalosporins
Chloral hydrate
Chloramphenicol
Cimetidine
Clofibrate
Corticosteroids (prednisone)

Cyclophosphamide
Dextrothyroxine
Diflunisal
Disulfiram
Erythromycin
Fluconazole
Flu vaccines
Gemfibrozil
Glucagon
Hydantoins
Ifosfamide
Isoniazid

Ketoconazole
Loop diuretics
Lovastatin
Metronidazole
Miconazole
Mineral oil
Moricizine
Nalidixic acid
NSAIDs
Omeprazole
Penicillins
Phenylbutazones
Propafenone

Propoxyphene
Quinidine
Quinine
Quinolones
Salicylates (aspirin)
Sulfinpyrazone
Sulfonamides
Tamoxifen
Tetracycline
Thioamines
Thyroid hormones
Vitamin E

These drugs may reduce the effects of anticoagulants:

↓ Aminoglutethimide
Ascorbic acid (vitamin C)
Barbiturates
Carbamazepine
Cholestyramine
Dicloxacillin
Ethchlorvynol
Etretinate
Glutethimide
Griseofulvin

Nafcillin
Oral contraceptives
Rifampin
Spironolactones
Sucralfate
Thiazide diuretics
Thiopurines
Trazodone
Vitamin K

WHAT ARE THE INTERACTIONS WITH FOOD?

Alcohol can increase the time it takes to clear anticoagulants from the body, increasing the risk of bleeding. Over time the opposite can happen; the drug may be cleared out faster than usual.

Cooking oils that contain silicone additives, such as sprays, may bind with these drugs and decrease their absorption. Eating a lot of foods very high in vitamin K could theoretically block the actions of these drugs. Foods high in vitamin K include dark, leafy green vegetables, lettuces, potatoes, fish and fish oils, fruits, especially citrus fruits, egg yolks, dairy products, the cruciferous family of vegetables including broccoli, cauliflower, cabbage and Brussels sprouts. Onions and soy foods may increase the action of anticoagulants. If you eat lots of vegetables, don't stop because you're taking this drug! Have your physician adjust the drug levels accordingly.

Don't drink tonic water if you're taking an anticoagulant. It contains an ingredient called quinine that can enhance the action of anticoagulants.

What Nutrients Do They Throw Out of Balance or Interact With?

Anticoagulants may attach to the metals in mineral supplements and not be absorbed. Take separately from mineral supplements. Vitamin C interferes with the action of these drugs, reducing their effects. Vitamin E, which by itself "thins" the blood, may increase the effects of anticoagulants, although to date no studies have shown that it's harmful to combine vitamin E and anticoagulants.

Natural Alternatives to Drugs for Treating Strokes and Blood Clots

Your foundation for preventing strokes and blood clots is to follow the Six Core Principles for Optimal Health, and to follow the guidelines earlier in the chapter for a healthy heart. Getting plenty of exercise, drinking plenty of water, avoiding "bad" fats and oils, and keeping blood pressure moderate are especially important.

A stroke can either be caused by a blood vessel breaking, or a blood clot blocking a blood vessel. Estrogens, including those used in birth control pills and for hormone replacement therapy, greatly increase the risk of some types of strokes. See the chapter on hormones for safe approaches to hormone replacement therapy.

Garlic, onions, berries and fish are foods that keep the blood and blood vessels healthy. The most important supplements for strong blood vessels are the bioflavonoids, including grapeseed extract, rutin, hesperidin, ginkgo biloba, green tea and bilberry. Supplements important for healthy, "slippery" blood (follow dosage recommendations for daily vitamins in this book) include magnesium, vitamin B6, folic acid, vitamin B12, vitamin E, selenium, N-acetyl cysteine, lysine and garlic.

If you have high levels of vitamin C, your risk of dying from a stroke may be half that of those with lower levels. This is according to a major study published in the *British Medical Journal* that tracked 730 elderly men and women for 20 years. Low levels of vitamin C were a strong predictor of death from stroke. You're doing just fine if you're on the Prescription Alternatives Vitamin Program and taking your 2,000 mg of vitamin C daily.

Some Drugs Delay Stroke Recovery

A stroke causes damage to the brain that can often be reversed with time and physical therapy. But it can be a long, slow, difficult road to healing, and those who are on that journey should be given every advantage. That's why you should know that some drugs can actually slow recovery after a stroke. The brain is particularly vulnerable after a stroke, and a recovering stroke patient shouldn't be given any drugs that aren't absolutely necessary.

According to a study done at North Carolina's Duke University that analyzed 96 stroke patients, 37 of them who were taking drugs such as benzodiazepines (Valium, Oxazepam, Serax, Ativan, Xanax, Diazepam, etc.) took significantly longer to recover. In fact, even one dose of a drug such as the dopamine antagonist haloperidol (Haldol) can delay recovery by as much as two weeks. These human studies were a follow-up to animal studies which demonstrated the same result. Other drugs that appeared to delay recovery included prochlorperazine (another dopamine antagonist), antihypertension drugs such as clonidine and prazosin, and anticonvulsant drugs such as phenytoin and phenobarbital.

Having a stroke can be a very frightening and disorienting experience, but sedatives shouldn't be used unless it's absolutely necessary. Before you resort to prescription drug sedatives, try some of the natural anti-anxiety remedies such as kava and St. John's wort.

Your first attempts at reassuring and calming a stroke victim should be the best sedatives of all: loving, supportive family and friends, gentle massage, humor, beautiful music, a good view out the window, good nutrition and competent medical care and physical therapy.

DRUGS TO LOWER HIGH BLOOD PRESSURE

The dangers of high blood pressure (hypertension) have been extremely well-publicized over the past decade. It's the dreaded silent killer, with no symptoms until you've got congestive heart failure (CHF), dropped dead of a heart attack or suffered a stroke.

One could hardly call high blood pressure "silent" these days, because drug companies have spent millions and millions of dollars over the past few decades to make sure everyone knows about it and to make it so scary that you'll take their hypertension drugs at the first sign of a higher-than-normal blood pressure reading. Any time you walk into a physician's office, clinic or hospital of any kind, the first thing they do is take your blood pressure.

While it's very true that extremely high blood pressure can be dangerous and should be treated aggressively, millions of North Americans with moderately high blood pressure are unnecessarily bullied by physicians into taking hypertension drugs without first making the diet and lifestyle changes that will lower almost all high blood pressure. This is a perfect example of how much quicker and easier it is to write a prescription for a drug that will make the numbers look better, without getting involved with the complexities of helping a person make lifestyle changes.

Hypertension drugs usually lower high blood pressure, but they have significant side effects and they treat the symptom, not the underlying cause. When you take them, the symptom of high blood pressure is suppressed and your numbers look good for your HMO (health maintenance organization) and insurance company, but your disease continues to progress. It's important for you to be aware that unless you're one of the few people who have high blood pressure caused purely by genetics or an illness such as kidney disease, your high blood pressure is caused by diet and lifestyle choices and you can certainly do something about those!

If you're already on blood pressure-lowering drugs, do not go off them suddenly. Work with an experienced health care professional to lower your blood pressure naturally while you wean yourself off the drugs.

The Facts on Blood Pressure

Your blood pressure rises above normal when too much fluid is being pumped through the blood vessels, or the blood vessels constrict, putting greater pressure on your heart and blood vessels. It can also be caused when the arteries lose their elasticity. If you think of the plumbing in a house, when water pressure is high it comes out of the faucets with great force. When water pressure is low it may only trickle out of the faucet.

Blood pressure readings show two numbers: the systolic pressure, which is the greatest amount of pressure exerted when the heart pumps or contracts, and the diastolic pressure, which is the lowest amount of pressure when the heart is in-between beats, or relaxed. A "normal" blood pressure reading for an adult is 130 (systolic) over 85 (diastolic), also shown as 130/85 mm Hg (millimeters of mercury, under pressure). A high diastolic blood pressure is more indicative of heart trouble in an older adult than a high systolic blood pressure.

But don't let these numbers bully you. A sudden rise in blood pressure is something to see your doctor about, but otherwise keep in mind that everyone is different and your blood pressure will rise naturally as you age. This does not necessarily mean you need drugs to lower it! Your body is effectively compensating for changes in your body that happen with aging. If you're over the age of 60, your systolic blood pressure may safely be as high as 180 mm Hg and your diastolic as high as 100 mm Hg.

Should you worry if your blood pressure varies some from these numbers? If you're overweight, stressed out, smoking, eating poorly, drinking too much alcohol or coffee, or not exercising or have heart disease, lung disease or diabetes, yes, because these are the risk factors for high blood pressure and you need to get to work changing them—now. If you are following the Six Core Principles for Optimal Health and don't have any of the above risk factors or a family history of very high blood pressure, be aware that it's high and treat it naturally.

Don't ever start taking a blood pressure drug based on one reading. Your arteries are muscular and flexible, designed to change blood pressure constantly in response to the needs of your body. Blood pressure readings taken in a physician's office are usually higher than normal and those taken in a drug store are inaccurate as much as 60 percent of the time. If your physician feels your hypertension is severe enough to warrant taking drugs, you should be monitoring your blood pressure at home.

Your physician is in a very tough position when it comes to treating your high blood pressure. If your blood pressure numbers don't fit into the charts and your physician doesn't prescribe the drugs, he or she can be penalized by an HMO or insurance company and is vulnerable to malpractice suits. But the practice of prescribing drugs to treat hypertension just doesn't fit the facts.

Numerous studies, including the famous Multiple Risk Factor Intervention Trial in the U.S. and the large Australian Medical Research Council Trial, have shown that people with mild to moderate high blood pressure who *don't* take prescription drugs to lower their blood pressure do *better* than those who do take drugs. At a recent American Heart Association Meeting it was reported that without treatment 1 percent of people with high blood pressure have a heart attack, but

---

Drugs That Can Raise Your Blood Pressure

NSAIDs (nonsteroidal anti-inflammatory drugs such as aspirin, acetaminophen, ibuprofen)

Bronchodilators such as epinephrine and ephedrine

Corticosteroids (prednisone)

Etidronate (used to treat osteoporosis)

Nasal decongestants (phenylpropanolamine)

The migraine drug sumatriptan (Imitrex)

The benzodiazepine anti-anxiety drugs (Valium)

Many of the antidepressants but especially venlafaxine (Effexor) and the MAO inhibitors (Nardil, Parnate)

with treatment with a calcium channel blocker, 1.6 percent had a heart attack! That's a 60 percent increase.

Unless you're under the age of 60 and your blood pressure is "severe" (above 180/110), there is little evidence that blood-pressure lowering drugs (also called antihypertensives) actually reduce the risk of heart attack and stroke, or even the risk of dying. If you're in your seventies or older it's clear that the drugs will do you more harm than good. At that age there is no evidence that blood pressure as high as 220/120 is more harmful than taking hypertension drugs. Don't ignore blood pressure that high, but be aware that taking drugs isn't likely to prolong your life.

Nearly all of the studies showing that antihypertensives do more harm than good were done with a placebo, meaning the group that did better did *nothing* to improve their blood pressure. Now imagine how bad the antihypertensives would look if they were measured against natural methods of lowering blood pressure such as weight loss, exercise, diet and stress reduction!

TYPES OF ANTIHYPERTENSIVES

There are four major types of drugs prescribed to lower blood pressure: diuretics, beta-blockers, ACE inhibitors and calcium channel blockers. Diuretics lower blood pressure by reducing the amount of fluid in the body.

The rest of the drugs listed here lower blood pressure by suppressing body signals that it's time to raise blood pressure. This makes the numbers look good, but when you really need some blood pressure it's not there and that's the underlying cause of the deadly side effects of these drugs. For example, if you need to run or climb stairs, or you get a bad scare, your body will be putting out signals to raise blood pressure and the drug will be blocking those signals. The theory is that this will keep your blood pressure from going so high that it gives you a heart attack, but on the other side of the coin there are good physiological reasons for your blood pressure to go up sometimes and if your body can't meet those demands it could kill you.

All of these drugs are used to control and suppress a wide variety of heart disease symptoms, but none have any healing properties.

Diuretics are often prescribed to treat the water retention caused by liver and kidney disease, but since they can also aggravate kidney and liver disease they can be counterproductive.

Diuretics

Diuretics, which are essentially designed to reduce fluid levels by making you urinate more, are one of the most common blood pressure medicines prescribed. One of the biggest problem with diuretics is the depletion of minerals that you pee away. In addition to losing sodium, you lose most of the other minerals too, including potassium, magnesium and calcium which are essential to proper heart function. There's no sense in lowering your blood pressure to prevent heart disease if your method of lowering it is going to cause it anyway! Numerous studies have shown that people with high blood pressure tend to be deficient in magnesium, so the last thing they need is to lose more.

Diuretics also tend to deplete the B vitamins. If you're on a diuretic be sure you're taking plenty of B vitamins.

One of the most devastating side effects of diuretics for women is their tendency to promote the excretion of calcium in the urine, resulting in bone loss and osteoporosis.

Another side effect of diuretics is a higher susceptibility to heat stroke or heat stress, caused by the body's inability to cool off by sweating. This is particularly important for older people who live in a warm or hot climate. When it's hot and you're taking a diuretic, it's important to drink plenty of fluids.

Thiazide Diuretics

BENDROFLUMETHIAZIDE (Naturetin)

BENZTHIAZIDE (Exna)

CHLORTHALIDONE (Thalitone, Hygroton)

CHLOROTHIAZIDE (Diuril, Diurigen)

HYDROCHLOROTHIAZIDE (Esidrix, HydroDIURIL, Hydro-Par, Oretic, Ezide)

HYDROFLUMETHIAZIDE (Diucardin, Saluron)

INDAPAMIDE (Lozol)

METHYCHLOTHIAZIDE (Aquatensen, Enduron)

METOLAZONE (Zaroxolyn, Mykrox)

POLYTHIAZIDE (Renese)

QUINETHAZONE (Hydromox)

TRICHLORMETHIAZIDE (Metahydrin, Naqua, Diurese)

WHAT DO THEY DO IN YOUR BODY?

Increase urination, reduce fluid and water retention.

WHAT ARE THEY PRESCRIBED FOR?

High blood pressure, edema (swelling, water retention, puffiness), congestive heart failure.

WHAT ARE THE POSSIBLE SIDE EFFECTS?

The most common and dangerous side effect of diuretics is excessive loss of minerals and/or an imbalance of minerals, called an electrolyte imbalance. Signs of a mineral imbalance can include dizziness, dry mouth, weakness, muscle pains or cramps, low blood pressure, rapid heartbeat, sleepiness and confusion.

High uric acid levels can lead to gout, a painful inflammation usually in the big toe. Other possible side effects: kidney damage, hyperglycemia (may increase fasting blood glucose) and/or precipitation of underlying diabetes, raised LDL "bad" cholesterol and triglyceride levels, anemia and sun sensitivity.

These drugs can also cause a wide variety of digestive problems, loss of appetite, vision problems, headaches, skin problems, restlessness and impotence.

CAUTION: THINK TWICE ABOUT TAKING THESE TYPES OF DRUGS IF . . .

- You have lupus.
- You have kidney or liver problems.
- You have diabetes.
- You have urinary tract problems such as enlarged prostate that interferes with urination. Diuretics can make you even more uncomfortable by increasing the number of times you have to urinate.

WHAT ARE THE INTERACTIONS WITH OTHER DRUGS?

Thiazide diuretics may raise levels or prolong the effects of these drugs:

↑ Allopurinol (often used to treat gout, which can be aggravated by some diuretics)
   Anesthetics
   Calcium salts found in calicum supplements
   Chemotherapy drugs
   Diazoxide* (an emergency room drug)
   Digitalis* drugs such as digoxin, digitoxin (Lanoxin)
   Lithium*
   Loop diuretics

The following drugs may be reduced in potency or decreased in the amount of time they are effective:

↓ Anticoagulants
   Antigout
   Insulin
   Some muscle relaxants
   Sulfonylureas (drugs for diabetes)

These drugs may increase the effects or prolong the action of thiazide diuretics:

---

*Potentially dangerous interaction.

↑ Amphotericin B
Anticholinergics
Corticosteriods
Laxatives (can increase loss of potassium)

These drugs may reduce the effects of thiazide diuretics:

↓ Cholestyramine
Colestipol
Methenamines
NSAIDs* (especially indomethacin, naproxen, ibuprofen)

WHAT ARE THE INTERACTIONS WITH FOOD?

If you take too many electrolytes, such as in sports drinks, you may reduce the effectiveness of the drug.

It's good to eat plenty of high-potassium foods when taking diuretics that don't "spare" potassium. Some common high-potassium foods include bananas, citrus fruits, melons, almonds, green leafy vegetables, potatoes, carrots, avocado, soybeans.

Licorice (not the candy made with anise, the herb or root) can be an anti-diuretic and reduce the actions of these drugs. It can also cause you to excrete higher than normal levels of potassium, the last thing you want on a diuretic that doesn't spare potassium.

Eating a lot of meat can increase uric acid even more, increasing the possibility of gout. If you are sensitive to monosodium glutamate (MSG), its negative effects can be exaggerated when you're taking diuretics.

Since the secondary purpose of taking diuretics is to reduce your levels of sodium, it's obviously wise to follow a low-sodium diet, to reduce your need for the diuretics. One of the best ways to do this is to eliminate processed and packaged foods from your diet and concentrate on whole foods such as whole grains and fresh fruits and vegetables. When you do buy processed foods, read labels carefully. Many low-fat or sugar-free foods add lots of salt or MSG to improve taste.

---

* Potentially dangerous interaction.

WHAT NUTRIENTS DO THEY DEPLETE OR THROW OUT OF BALANCE?

Minerals, especially sodium, chloride, potassium, calcium and magnesium. Zinc is one of the important minerals that can be lost along with the other minerals. Zinc is crucial to proper immune system functioning, wound healing and thyroid function.

Diuretics can cause a depletion of vitamin A, which many Americans are already deficient in.

WHAT ELSE TO TAKE IF YOU TAKE THESE DRUGS

A good mineral formula that includes: zinc, copper, boron, iodine, cobalt, manganese, molybdenum, vanadium, chromium, selenium, plenty of calcium and magnesium, and, if you're a premenopausal woman, iron.

Be sure you're getting both beta-carotene and vitamin A in your multivitamin formula. Eat plenty of fresh fruits and vegetables.

OTHER TIPS ON THESE DRUGS

They can skew the results of many blood and urine tests.

Loop Diuretics

BUMETANIDE (Bumex)
ETHACRYNIC ACID (Edecrin)
FUROSEMIDE (Lasix)
TORSEMIDE (Demadex)

WHAT DO THEY DO IN YOUR BODY?

Increase urination, reduce fluid and water retention, largely by reducing sodium chloride (salt) uptake in your cells.

CAUTION!

Signs of a mineral imbalance:

Dizziness	Nausea and vomiting
Dry mouth	Rapid heartbeat
Low blood pressure	Sleepiness and confusion
Muscle pains or cramps	Weakness

WHAT ARE THEY PRESCRIBED FOR?

High blood pressure, edema (swelling, water retention, puffiness).

WHAT ARE THE POSSIBLE SIDE EFFECTS?

One of the most common and dangerous side effects of loop diuretics is dehydration caused by too much fluid loss. This can be deadly. These diuretics are also more likely to cause hypotension, or blood pressure that is too low, which can also be dangerous, and such excessive potassium loss that it becomes life-threatening.

An excessive loss of minerals and/or an imbalance of minerals, called an electrolyte imbalance, may result.

If your blood pressure is reduced too much, you may get dizzy when you stand up.

High uric acid levels can lead to gout, a painful inflammation usually in the big toe.

Other possible side effects: kidney damage, reversible and irreversible hearing problems, diarrhea, hypoglycemia (they increase fasting blood glucose) and/or precipitation of underlying diabetes, raised LDL "bad" cholesterol and triglyceride levels and photosensitivity, a reaction to the sun. These drugs can also cause muscle pain and cramps, restlessness, a wide variety of digestive problems, vision problems and skin problems.

CAUTION: THINK TWICE ABOUT TAKING THESE TYPES OF DRUGS IF . . .

- You have lupus.
- You have kidney or liver problems.

- You have diabetes.
- You have urinary tract problems such as enlarged prostate that interferes with urination. Diuretics can make you even more uncomfortable by increasing the number of times you have to urinate.

WHAT ARE THE INTERACTIONS WITH OTHER DRUGS?

The following drugs may be increased in potency or increased in the amount of time they are effective when combined with loop diuretics.

↑ ACE inhibitors* (use extreme caution)
  Aminoglycosides
  Anticoagulants
  Beta-blockers (propranolol) can be increased by furosemide
  Chloral hydrate
  Cisplatin (increases the risk of hearing problems)
  Digitalis (digoxin)
  Lithium*

  Some muscle relaxants may be increased or decreased
  Theophyllines* can be either increased or decreased

The following drugs may be reduced in potency or decreased in the amount of time they are effective when combined with loop diuretics:

↓ Antigout
  Insulin
  Some muscle relaxants
  Sulfonylureas (drugs for diabetes)

  Theophyllines can be either increased or decreased

These drugs may increase the effects or prolong the action of loop diuretics:

---

* Potentially dangerous interaction.

↑ Cisplatin
Clofibrate (Atromid-S)
Laxatives can increase loss of potassium
Thiazide diuretics

These drugs may reduce the effects of loop diuretics:

↓ Hydantoins such as phenytoin (Dilantin)
NSAIDs, especially indomethacin, naproxen, ibuprofen
Probenecid
Salicylates (aspirin)

WHAT ARE THE INTERACTIONS OF LOOP DIURETICS WITH FOOD?

The absorption of the drug may be reduced if you take it with food.

If you take too many electrolytes, such as in sports drinks, you may reduce the effectiveness of the drug.

It's good to eat plenty of high-potassium foods when taking diuretics that don't "spare" potassium. Some common high-potassium foods include bananas, citrus fruits, melons, almonds, green leafy vegetables, potatoes, carrots, avocado, soybeans.

Licorice (not the candy made with anise, the herb or root) can be an antidiuretic and reduce the actions of these drugs.

Eating a lot of meat can increase uric acid even more, increasing the possibility of gout.

If you are sensitive to MSG, its negative effects can be exaggerated when you're taking diuretics.

WHAT NUTRIENTS DO LOOP DIURETICS DEPLETE OR THROW OUT OF BALANCE?

Minerals, especially sodium, chloride, potassium, calcium and magnesium.

Taken long term, loop diuretics cause a depletion of the vitamin thiamin (B1), which plays a key role in the functioning of the nervous system. A deficiency of thiamine can aggravate congestive heart failure or other heart problems.

Chronic thiamin deficiency can also block enzymes involved in glucose metabolism, which may be why these drugs can cause hypoglycemia.

Zinc is one of the important minerals that can be lost along with the other minerals. Zinc is crucial to proper immune system functioning, wound healing and thyroid function.

Diuretics can cause a depletion of vitamin A, which many Americans are already deficient in.

WHAT ELSE TO TAKE IF YOU TAKE THESE DRUGS

A good mineral formula that includes: zinc, copper, boron, iodine, cobalt, manganese, molybdenum, vanadium, chromium, selenium, and, if you're a premenopausal woman, iron. Eat plenty of fresh fruits and vegetables.

An extra B-complex vitamin supplement that includes at least 50 mg of thiamin. (It's best to take the B vitamins together.)

Be sure you're getting both beta-carotene and vitamin A in your multivitamin formula.

OTHER TIPS ON THESE DRUGS

They can skew the results of many blood and urine tests.
Take them with food or they may upset your stomach.

Potassium-Sparing Diuretics

AMILORIDE (Midamor)

SPIRONOLACTONE (Aldactone)

TRIAMTERENE (Dyrenium)

COMBINATIONS (Dyazide, Moduretic, Aldactazide, Maxzide)

The potassium-sparing diuretics are usually combined with one of the other diuretics to reduce excessive potassium depletion. However, the potassium-sparing diuretics in turn may cause excess potassium, called hyperkalemia, which can also be dangerous. Symptoms of too much potassium include: muscular weakness, fatigue, numbness and tingling, and irregular heartbeat.

WHAT DO THEY DO IN YOUR BODY?

Reduce fluid and water retention in such a way that the body retains potassium.

WHAT ARE THEY PRESCRIBED FOR?

In conjunction with loop and thiazide diuretics prescribed for high blood pressure and congestive heart failure, to reduce the loss of potassium, to treat aldosteronism (an excess of the adrenal hormone aldosterone which causes the body to hold onto salt and excrete potassium) and to treat a variety of conditions involving potassium loss.

Spironolactone reduces the level of aldosterone, an androgen, or male hormone, so it has been used to treat excess hair growth, acne and other symptoms of excess androgens. Considering that this drug promotes tumor growth in rats and can cause unexplained uterine bleeding in women at high doses, it seems frivolous to use it other than short term in life-threatening situations.

Triamterene is mainly used to treat edema or water retention, especially when it is caused by aldosteronism.

WHAT ARE THE POSSIBLE SIDE EFFECTS?

Excess potassium (hyperkalemia). Liver and kidney problems may get worse. The peripheral neuropathy (numbness in the extremities) caused by diabetes may get worse. Dizziness, nausea, vomiting, appetite loss.

Spironolactone: this drug affects sex hormones by reducing aldosterone levels. Aldosterone is an androgen or male hormone. Taking it can cause a reduction in male hormones and as a consequence, breast enlargement and other feminizing effects in men. It also promotes the growth of a variety of malignant tumors in rats.

Spironolactone can cause lethargy, mental confusion, headaches, stomach ache, irregular menstruation and thirst.

Triamterene may promote the formation of kidney stones and can raise blood sugar levels. It can also induce kidney failure.

CAUTION: THINK TWICE ABOUT TAKING THESE TYPES OF DRUGS IF . . .

- You have kidney or liver problems.
- You have diabetes.
- You have urinary tract problems such as enlarged prostate that interferes with urination. Diuretics can make you even more uncomfortable by increasing the number of times you have to urinate.

WHAT ARE THE INTERACTIONS WITH OTHER DRUGS?

AMILORIDE

The effects of these drugs may be increased or prolonged with the use of amiloride:

↑ Any type of potassium preparation* (the symbol for potassium is K, often used for product names on labels)
  Digitalis (digoxin) may be increased or decreased
  Lithium*

The effect of this drug may be decreased or shortened with the use of amiloride:

  Digoxin may be increased or decreased

These drugs may increase the effects or prolong the action of amiloride:

↑ ACE inhibitors*

These drugs may reduce the effects of amiloride:

↓ NSAIDs

---

*Potentially dangerous interaction.

SPIRONOLACTONE

The effects of these drugs may be increased or prolonged with the use of spironolactone:

↑ Any type of potassium preparation (the symbol for potassium is K, often used for product names on labels)
Digitalis (digoxin) may be increased or decreased
Lithium*

The effects of these drugs may be reduced or shortened when combined with spironolactone:

↓ Anticoagulants
Mitotane

Digitalis glycosides may be increased or decreased

These drugs may increase the effects or prolong the action of spironolactone:

↑ ACE inhibitors*

These drugs may reduce the effects of spironolactone:

↓ NSAIDs, especially salicylates*

TRIAMTERENE

The effects of these drugs may be increased or prolonged with the use of triamterene:

↑ Any type of potassium preparation* (the symbol for potassium is K, often used for product names on labels)

*Potentially dangerous interaction.

Amantadine
Lithium*

Digitalis may be increased or decreased

These drugs may increase the effects or prolong the action of triamterene:

↓ ACE inhibitors*
Cimetidine
NSAIDs, especially indomethacin, naproxen, ibuprofen*

What Are the Interactions with Food?

If you take too many electrolytes, such as in sports drinks, you may get too much potassium.

Eating a lot of high-potassium foods in combination with taking the drugs can also raise potassium levels too high. Some common high-potassium foods include bananas, citrus fruits, melons, almonds, green leafy vegetables, potatoes, carrots, avocado, soybeans.

Licorice (the root or herb used medicinally, or the candy with real licorice flavoring) can be an antidiuretic and may decrease potassium levels, reducing the effect of these drugs. Licorice also contains a component called glycyrrhizin which is similar to aldosterone, the very hormone spironolactone is prescribed to reduce, so taking a lot of licorice could negate those effects.

Eating a lot of meat can increase uric acid even more, increasing the possibility of gout.

Spironolactone levels may be increased by eating a lot of protein or fat at one sitting. Levels may be decreased by a high-fiber diet. If you're eating fiber-rich cereals or taking a fiber supplement such as psyllium, take it a few hours apart from taking this drug.

If you are sensitive to MSG, its negative effects may be exaggerated when you're taking diuretics.

WHAT NUTRIENTS DO THEY DEPLETE OR THROW OUT OF BALANCE?

Minerals, especially sodium, chloride, potassium, calcium, magnesium and zinc. Zinc is crucial to proper immune system functioning, wound healing and thyroid function.

Diuretics can cause a depletion of vitamin A, which many Americans are already deficient in.

WHAT ELSE TO TAKE IF YOU TAKE THESE DRUGS

A good mineral formula that includes: zinc, copper, boron, iodine, cobalt, manganese, molybdenum, vanadium, chromium, selenium, and, if you're a premenopausal woman, iron.

Be sure you're getting both beta-carotene and vitamin A in your multivitamin formula. Eat plenty of fresh fruits and vegetables.

Beta-Blockers (Beta-Adrenergic Blocking Agents)

ACEBUTOLOL (Sectral)

ATENOLOL (Tenormin)

BETAXOLOL (Kerlone)

BISOPROLOL FUMARATE (Zebeta)

CARTEOLOL (Cartrol)

ESMOLOL (Brevibloc) used for abnormal heartbeat

METOPROLOL (Lopressor, Toprol XL)

NADOLOL (Corgard)

PENBUTOLOL SULFATE (Levatol)

PINDOLOL (Visken)

PROPRANOLOL (Inderal, Betachron E-R)

SOTALOL HCl (Betapace) used for irregular heartbeat

TIMOLOL MALEATE (Blocadren)

Beta-blockers or beta-adrenergic-blocking drugs are somewhat out-dated, but some physicians still use them to treat high blood pressure. The down side of these drugs is that they can actually *cause* congestive heart failure, heart attacks, strokes and asthma. Beta-blockers can cause serious arrhythmias (irregular heartbeats) and may worsen blood vessel problems that reduce circulation to the extremities, such as in diabetes. Asthmatics should *never* take a beta-blocker as it may trigger life-threatening airway spasms.

Alpha/Beta-Adrenergic Blockers

CARVEDILOL (Coreg)

LABETALOL (Normodyne, Trandate)

WHAT DO THEY DO IN YOUR BODY?

Beta-blockers reduce blood pressure by slowing the heart rate, reducing the force of contractions of the heart muscle and relaxing the arteries.

WHAT ARE THEY PRESCRIBED FOR?

High blood pressure, especially in combination with a thiazide diuretic, and many other heart disease symptoms such as angina, irregular heartbeat and recovery from some types of heart attack, migraines, tremors and anxiety.

WHAT ARE THE POSSIBLE SIDE EFFECTS?

There have been literally dozens of "adverse effects" reported by people taking beta-blockers, which are listed on the drug information insert. If you have any type of new symptoms while on this drug, even if you have been on it for a long time, check with your physician and read the drug information insert. If you don't have the insert, either ask your pharmacist for one or look it up in the PDR (*Physicians' Desk Reference*).

Dizziness and fatigue are two of the most common complaints of people on these drugs. That may mean you're taking too much. These side effects are considered "mild" by drug companies and physicians, but they can cause depression and reduce the activities you can participate in. Yet another good reason to lower your blood pressure naturally!

A large, double-blind, multi-center randomized trial (the National Heart, Lung and Blood Institute's Cardiac Arrhythmia Suppression Trial) found that in certain types of heart attack patients, some beta-blockers caused a significantly higher death rate and risk of a second heart attack compared to patients who did nothing.

Beta-blockers can cause serious arrhythmias and may worsen blood vessel problems that reduce circulation to the extremities, such as in diabetes. They can also lead to cardiac failure by over-depressing the ability of the heart to contract.

Like all drugs that are prescribed to lower blood pressure, beta-blockers can easily send blood pressure too far in the other direction, causing hypotension or low blood pressure. Symptoms of hypotension include dizziness when standing, sweating, fatigue.

Other side effects can include muscle weakness, dizziness, hypo- and hyperglycemia, impotence, eye problems, worsening of lung problems, depression, joint pain and rarely, anaphylaxis, a severe allergic reaction.

Kidney and liver damage may be made worse by beta-blockers and can cause unpredictable increases in drug levels.

Some beta-blockers can send your cholesterol levels in the opposite direction that you want them to go: increased LDL, VDL and triglycerides and decreased HDL.

Sudden withdrawal from beta-blockers can be dangerous.

CAUTION: THINK TWICE ABOUT TAKING THESE TYPES OF DRUGS IF . . .

- You have congestive heart failure or irregular heartbeat.
- You have asthma or other lung diseases such as chronic bronchitis and emphysema.

Most beta-blockers can suppress symptoms of diabetes and an overactive thyroid (hyperthyroidism). Since beta-blockers can cause or prolong hypoglycemia, use caution if you are diabetic.

WHAT ARE THE INTERACTIONS WITH OTHER DRUGS?

Not all of these interactions may happen with all of the beta-blockers. However, just because the interaction isn't listed in sources that list drug interactions doesn't mean it doesn't happen, it may just mean the company hasn't done the research or it hasn't been reported. Use caution with all the possible interactions listed below and have a talk with your physician or pharmacist if a combination is recommended.

The following drugs may be increased in potency or increased in the amount of time they are effective when combined with beta-blockers:

↑ Acetaminophen (Tylenol)
  Anticoagulants such as warfarin (Coumadin)
  Benzodiazepines (diazepam, flurazepam, triazolam)
  Calcium channel blockers with carvedilol
  Clonidine* is dangerous when combined and then withdrawn
  Diabetes drugs, oral, especially with carvedilol
  Digoxin with carvedilol
  Epinephrine* may be followed by increase in beta-blocker effect
  Ergot alkaloids for migraine, e.g., Cafergot, Sansert
  Flecainide
  Haloperidol
  Hydralazine
  Lidocaine*
  Phenothiazines
  Prazosin
  Theophylline may be increased or decreased
  Thioridazine (Mellaril), chlorpromazine (Thorazine)

The following drugs may be reduced in potency or decreased in the amount of time they are effective when combined with beta-blockers:

↓ Clonidine* is dangerous when combined and then withdrawn
  Disopyramide may also increase effect of beta-blocker
  Sulfonylureas
  Theophylline may be increased or decreased

*Potentially dangerous interaction.

These drugs may increase the effects or prolong the action of beta-blockers:

↑ Calcium channel blockers* (diltiazem, felodipine, necardipine)
Disopyramide may also decrease effect of this drug
Diuretics* (excess potassium loss can cause irregular heartbeat, rapid heartbeat)
Epinephrine, including many over-the-counter cough and cold medicines (may be preceded by a rise in blood pressure)
Flecainide
Haloperidol
H2 blockers (Tagamet, Zantac)
Hydralazine
Loop diuretics
MAO inhibitors
Oral contraceptives
Phenothiazines (thioridazine, chlorpromazine)
Propafenone
Quinidine
Quinolones (ciprofloxacin)
Thioamines

These drugs may reduce the effects of beta-blockers:

↓ Aluminum salts
Ampicillin* (also increases allergic reaction to ampicillin)
Barbiturates*
Calcium salts, e.g., calcium supplements, Tums
Cholestyramine (take this drug at least an hour apart from taking a beta-blocker)
Colestipol (take this drug at least an hour apart from taking a beta-blocker)
NSAIDs (ibuprofen, indomethacin, piroxicam)*
Rifampin
Salicylates (aspirin, Alka-Seltzer)
Sulfinpyrazone

---

* Potentially dangerous interaction.

Theophylline (beta-blockers may increase or decrease drug levels)

Thyroid hormones

WHAT ARE THE INTERACTIONS OF BETA-BLOCKERS WITH FOOD?

Taking atenolol (Tenormin) and sotalol (Betapace) with food may reduce or slow their action. Taking labetalol (Normodyne, Trandate), metoprolol (Lopressor, Toprol) and propanolol (Inderal) with food may increase drug levels.

Taking propanolol with a high-protein meal or with alcohol may increase drug levels even more.

OTHER TIPS ON THESE DRUGS

They may interfere with glucose tolerance tests, insulin tests, glaucoma tests and a variety of other blood and urine tests.

Ace Inhibitors

BENAZEPRIL (Lotensin)

CAPTOPRIL (Capoten)

ENALAPRIL (Vasotec)

FOSINOPRIL (Monopril)

LISINOPRIL (Prinivil, Zestril)

MOEIXPRIL (Univasc)

QUINAPRIL (Accupril)

RAMIPRIL (Altace)

TRANDOLAPRIL (Mavik)

Angiotensin Antagonists

LOSARTAN POTASSIUM (Cozaar)

WHAT DO THEY DO IN YOUR BODY?

ACE inhibitors lower blood pressure by blocking the production of a series of chemicals, especially one called angiotensin, that the body releases to raise blood pressure. When blood pressure drops, the kidneys release a hormone called renin, which in turn stimulates the production of angiotensin, which has its own potent actions, including constricting the arteries to raise blood pressure. Angiotensin also stimulates the release of the adrenal hormone aldosterone, which gives cells signals to hold onto sodium and release potassium, thus allowing fluid buildup, another way of raising blood pressure.

Thus taking an ACE inhibitor has a very powerful effect on an important blood pressure control mechanism, which is good news when your blood pressure needs lowering in the moment. But this can be bad news when it needs to rise, because the mechanism that allows it to do so is suppressed.

ACE inhibitors are a classic example of suppressing a symptom to treat a disease. The danger, of course, is that the disease progresses underneath and a whole new set of symptoms and risks are created by the drug.

WHAT ARE THEY PRESCRIBED FOR?

High blood pressure, especially in combination with thiazide diuretics. Some of the ACE inhibitors are prescribed for congestive heart failure and for heart attack patients after a myocardial infarction and sometimes for diabetic nephropathy (kidney disease).

WHAT ARE THE POSSIBLE SIDE EFFECTS?

The most common side effect of ACE inhibitors is an annoying, persistent, nagging cough. While this isn't directly life-threatening, it's a big energy drain and it's enough to create a loss of sleep. ACE inhibitors have probably gotten more people stuck on the drug treadmill than any other single drug. Why? They take an ACE inhibitor, they get a cough and complain to their physician. Instead of taking them off the ACE inhibitor the physician prescribes a cough suppressant, which causes insomnia, so the physician prescribes a sleeping pill, which is addictive. And so on.

The ACE inhibitor captopril (Capoten) can cause a large reduction of white blood cells (neutropenia), seriously compromising the immune system. This seems like an unacceptably severe side effect when there are so many alternatives. The risk of neutropenia is especially high for people with some kinds of kidney problems. There is some evidence that other ACE inhibitors could also cause neutropenia, although not as frequently. Captopril may also cause kidney damage.

ACE inhibitors can cause a serious allergy-type reaction (anaphylactic) which causes swelling, especially around the head and neck, that can be fatal when it obstructs airways.

Because ACE inhibitors block the release of the adrenal hormone aldosterone, which is an androgen, or male hormone, they have been known to cause symptoms of feminization in men such as breast enlargement. This same mechanism also blocks signals telling the body to release potassium, which can result in excessively high levels of potassium.

As with all drugs that lower blood pressure, there is always the risk that the blood pressure is lowered too much, or that some other factor such as food, another drug, diarrhea, dehydration, exercise or overheating will combine with the drug to lower blood pressure too far.

The ACE inhibitors ramapril (Altace) and fosinopril (Monopril) can aggravate existing liver disease. There have been a couple of cases where people taking ACE inhibitors suffered from liver damage and liver failure (death), as well as kidney damage and kidney failure.

The ACE inhibitor trandolapril hasn't been on the market long enough for us to have a good grasp of its side effects.

Other side effects of ACE inhibitors are dizziness (common with all drugs that lower blood pressure), headaches, irregular heartbeat, chest pain, diarrhea, nausea, fatigue, shortness of breath, rash, sexual dysfunction, vision disturbances, taste disturbances and weakness.

There have been dozens of "adverse effects" reported by people taking ACE inhibitors so don't rule out a symptom as a side effect of this drug just because it's not on this list.

These types of drugs can cause injury and death to a developing fetus when taken in the second and third trimesters. For this reason, there doesn't seem to be any reason whatsoever for a woman of child-bearing age to take them.

CAUTION!

Please think twice about taking an ACE inhibitor no matter what, especially captopril. They are especially risky for people with some types of kidney or liver disease, and the elderly, who tend to have decreased kidney function as a matter of aging. Don't go near this drug if there is any possibility of pregnancy.

WHAT ARE THE INTERACTIONS WITH OTHER DRUGS?

The following drugs may be increased in potency or increased in the amount of time they are effective when combined with ACE inhibitors:

↑ Allopurinol*
Diabetes drugs (oral, e.g., glyburide, glipizide)
Digoxin (digitalis)
Lithium
Loop diuretics
Potassium products*
Potassium-sparing diuretics*

The following drugs may be reduced in potency or decreased in the amount of time they are effective when combined with ACE inhibitors:

↓ Tetracycline antibiotics (with quinapril)

These drugs may increase the effects or prolong the action of ACE inhibitors:

↑ Cyclosporine
Erythromycin, an antibiotic

---

*Potentially dangerous interaction.

Phenothiazines (e.g., Thorazine)
Probenecid (with captopril)

These drugs may reduce the effects of ACE inhibitors:

↓ Antacids (take at least two hours away from taking an ACE inhibitor)
NSAIDs* (e.g., indomethacin, ibuprofen, naproxen, aspirin)
Rifampin (with enalapril)

WHAT ARE THE INTERACTIONS OF BETA-BLOCKERS WITH FOOD?

Capsaicin or cayenne, used as a spice and as an alternative medicine treatment for a variety of ailments, may make an ACE inhibitor-caused cough worse. Capsaicin is also used topically to treat herpes zoster (shingles). Levels of captopril may be significantly reduced if it is taken with food, so take it an hour away from eating. Other ACE inhibitors may be reduced less significantly. (Enalapril, benazepril and lisinopril *do not* seem to be affected by food.)

Calcium Channel Blockers (Calcium Antagonists)

AMLODIPINE (Norvasc)

BEPRIDIL (Vascor)

DILTIAZEM (Cardizem, Dilacor, Tiazac)

FELODIPINE (Plendil)

ISRADIPINE (DynaCirc)

NICARDIPINE (Cardene)

NIFEDIPINE (Adalat, Procardia)

NIMODIPINE (Nimotop)

*Potentially dangerous interaction.

NISOLDIPINE (Sular)

VERAPAMIL (Calan, Isoptin, Verelan, Covera)

WHAT DO THEY DO IN YOUR BODY?

The movement of calcium in and out of some cells of the heart and arteries plays an important role in their contraction. Calcium channel blockers block the movement of calcium, lowering blood pressure by suppressing the contraction of artery muscles, dilating the arteries and reducing arterial resistance to blood flow.

WHAT ARE THEY PRESCRIBED FOR?

Calcium channel blockers are prescribed for a variety of heart problems, including angina, arrhythmias (irregular heartbeat), rapid heartbeat, high blood pressure and congestive heart failure. They are also prescribed for migraine headaches and Raynaud's syndrome. Those prescribed for high blood pressure include amlodipine, verapamil, SR diltiazem, nicardipine, SR nifedipine, isradipine, felodipine and nisoldipine.

WHAT ARE THE POSSIBLE SIDE EFFECTS?

Calcium channel blockers are among the most widely prescribed drugs in North America and yet they are also among the most dangerous drugs you can take. Although they can be very useful in normalizing an irregular heartbeat and spasms in the heart muscle, their long-term use for lowering blood pressure is very questionable.

They can cause serious new arrhythmias, dangerously low blood pressure, abnormally slow heart rates, congestive heart failure, heart attacks, gastrointestinal bleeding, liver and kidney damage and reduced white blood cell count and they interact dangerously with many drugs.

In test rats they caused cancer and the fast-acting forms of nifedipine have been shown in studies conducted by the National Heart, Lung and Blood Institute to *increase* the risk of a fatal heart attack.

Some of the more common "adverse reactions" include dizziness, swollen hands and feet (edema), chronic headaches, nausea, giddiness, nervousness, numbness and tingling, diarrhea, constipation, digestive problems such as stomach cramps, gas and heartburn, dry mouth, flushing, urinary tract problems, sexual problems, shortness of breath, muscle cramps and pains and a cough.

The different types of calcium channel blockers can vary in their actions and side effects quite a bit, so if you must take one, be sure your physician is experienced in prescribing them and be sure to read the drug insert carefully for yourself.

CAUTION: THINK TWICE ABOUT TAKING THESE TYPES OF DRUGS IF . . .

- You have kidney or liver disease. Calcium channel blockers are contraindicated with some types of heart disease, such as sick sinus syndrome. This differs with the type of calcium channel blocker. Talk to your physician and read your drug insert. Dangerous side effects tend to occur more often in patients who are also on beta-blockers. This is a potentially dangerous combination.

WHAT ARE THE INTERACTIONS WITH OTHER DRUGS?

Note: Not all calcium channel blockers may have all of these interactions. Check with your pharmacist and read the drug information insert.

Calcium channel blockers may raise levels or prolong the effects of these drugs:

↑ Anticoagulants, e.g., warfarin
　Beta-blockers*
　Carbamazepine* (this interaction does not seem to happen with nifedipine)
　Cyclosporine* (this interaction does not seem to happen with nifedipine)
　Digitalis glycosides, e.g., digoxin
　Encainide
　Etomidate

---

*Potentially dangerous interaction.

↑ Fentanyl
Lithium (may also decrease levels)
Magnesium sulfate (intravenous)
Prazosin
Some muscle relaxants
Tricyclic antidepressants, e.g., imipramine

Theophyllines* may be increased or decreased

The following drugs may be reduced in potency or decreased in the amount of time they are effective when combined with calcium channel blockers:

↓ Quinidine*

Lithium may be increased or decreased
Theophyllines* may be increased or decreased

These drugs may increase the effects or prolong the action of calcium channel blockers:

↑ Dantrolene
Erythromycin*
Fluoxetine, e.g., Prozac; this could happen with other drugs of
    this type as well
H2 blockers, e.g., Tagamet, Zantac, Pepcid
Quinidine* (may also be reduced in potency by calcium channel
    blockers)

These drugs may reduce the effects of calcium channel blockers:

↓ Barbiturates
Calcium salts, e.g., calcium supplements, Tums
Carbamazepine*
Hydantoins
Rifampin*
Sulfinpyrazone

---

*Potentially dangerous interaction.

WHAT ARE THE INTERACTIONS WITH FOOD?

Some calcium channel blockers are unaffected by food, some are decreased and some are increased. Ask your pharmacist and read your drug information insert. Some calcium channel blockers, including nifedipine and verapamil, may bind with minerals in food or supplements, reducing the availability of the drug. Taking felodipine and nifedipine with grapefruit juice can double drug levels, a potentially deadly interaction, and it can also affect the levels of other types of calcium channel blockers. It's best in general not to take medicine with grapefruit juice unless your physician asks you to. Some calcium channel blockers may increase the amount of alcohol that gets into the blood when you have a drink or take medicine containing alcohol.

WHAT NUTRIENTS DO THEY THROW OUT OF BALANCE OR INTERACT WITH?

Excess vitamin D may reduce the effectiveness of verapamil. Some calcium channel blockers, including nifedipine and verapamil, may bind with minerals in food or supplements, reducing the availability of the drug.

OTHER TIPS ON THESE DRUGS

Calcium channel blockers can affect the results of blood and urine tests.

If you're taking a calcium channel blocker in the dihydropyridine class (i.e., felodipine-Plendil, nifedipine), watch out for dangerous interactions with erythromycin, an antibiotic, which can double felodipine levels. High felodipine levels can cause heart palpitations and low blood pressure.

OTHER ANTIHYPERTENSIVE (BLOOD PRESSURE-LOWERING) DRUGS

None of these drugs is considered a primary or single treatment for high blood pressure. They are almost always used in combination with other drugs.

Anti-Adrenergic Agents, Centrally Acting

METHYLDOPA, METHYLDOPATE (ALDOMET)

WHAT DO THEY DO IN YOUR BODY?

Methyldopa and methyldopate lower blood pressure, probably by reducing levels of serotonin, dopamine, norepinephrine and epinephrine and possibly by lowering renin, a substance released by the kidneys in response to low blood pressure.

WHAT ARE THEY PRESCRIBED FOR?

High blood pressure.

WHAT ARE THE POSSIBLE SIDE EFFECTS?

Liver disease is a direct contraindication to taking methyldopa. This drug carries a high risk of damaging the liver, a high risk of causing blood disorders including anemia, and can cause a syndrome of symptoms that resembles lupus. Other side effects include sedation (which may impair coordination and the ability to think clearly), fatigue, depression, fever, headache, dizziness, weakness, abnormally slow heartbeat, nausea, rash, breast enlargement in men and women, impotence and decreased libido. As with all antihypertensive drugs, it carries the risk of abnormally low blood pressure.

CAUTION!

Please think twice about taking these drugs, period. There are many other newer drugs that can do the same job without the high risk. They have too many potent and negative effects on too many important bodily systems. If you have any type of liver disease, don't take them.

WHAT ARE THE INTERACTIONS WITH OTHER DRUGS?

Methyldopa may raise levels or prolong the effects of these drugs:

↑ Levodopa
Lithium
Sympathomimetics

The following drug may be reduced in potency or decreased in the amount of time it is effective when combined with methyldopa:

↓ Tolbutamide (Orinase)

This drug may increase the effects or prolong the action of methyldopa:

↑ Haloperidol (Haldol)

These drugs may reduce the effects of methyldopa:

↓ Sympathomimetics
Propranolol

WHAT ARE THE INTERACTIONS WITH FOOD?

Methyldopa levels will be decreased if it is taken with food, especially protein.

Eating too much salt while taking methyldopa could increase fluid retention and cause edema or water retention.

WHAT NUTRIENTS DO THEY THROW OUT OF BALANCE OR INTERACT WITH?

Methyldopa decreases vitamin B12 levels and probably decreases folic acid levels as well.

WHAT ELSE TO TAKE IF YOU MUST TAKE THESE DRUGS

Preferably, intravenous vitamin B12 and folic acid, but these drugs can cause sensitivity reactions so even that may be risky. At the very least, take sublingual vitamin B12 and folic acid supplements. Be aware that the folic acid may hide evidence of anemia, a side effect of the drugs.

OTHER TIPS ON THESE DRUGS

They affect many blood and urine tests.

Clonidine

CLONIDINE (Catapres)

WHAT DOES IT DO IN YOUR BODY?

It has many effects on the body, including lowering blood pressure; reducing renin, aldosterone and catecholamines (all important to normal bodily function); and stimulating growth hormone.

WHAT IS IT PRESCRIBED FOR?

Hypertension and many other miscellaneous conditions such as menopausal flushing (hot flashes) and diabetic diarrhea, reflecting its wide spectrum of effects on the body.

WHAT ARE THE POSSIBLE SIDE EFFECTS?

The most dangerous part of this drug is that if you miss a dose or two you could experience sudden and dangerously high blood pressure. Since everyone misses medication occasionally, this alone makes it not worth taking this drug. It has also caused degeneration of the retina in animals and has a long list of unpleasant side effects including: dry mouth, dizziness, depression, sedation, constipation, fatigue, loss of appetite, nausea, rash, impotence, decreased libido, muscle weakness, dry eyes, and an odd mix of brain dysfunction symptoms such as hallucinations and nightmares.

CAUTION!

Think twice about taking this drug, period. It's way too dangerous and there are other, better alternatives.

WHAT ARE THE INTERACTIONS WITH OTHER DRUGS?

Beta-blockers combined with clonidine may cause high blood pressure. Beta-blockers also make the rebound high blood pressure worse when a dose or two of medication is missed. Tricyclic antidepressants can block the blood pressure-lowering effect of clonidine.

WHAT ARE THE INTERACTIONS WITH FOOD?

If you eat too much salt when you're taking clonidine it can cause fluid retention.

Guanfacine

GUANFACINE (Tenex)

WHAT DOES IT DO IN YOUR BODY?

Lowers blood pressure and affects many other bodily systems, including the stimulation of growth hormone and the reduction of renin activity and catecholamine levels.

WHAT IS IT PRESCRIBED FOR?

High blood pressure, heroin withdrawal and migraine headaches.

WHAT ARE THE POSSIBLE SIDE EFFECTS?

Sedation, drowsiness, depression, fatigue and if you forget to take a dose it can cause nervousness, anxiety and rebound high blood pressure. Other side effects are dry mouth, weakness, dizziness, constipation, impotence, vision and taste disturbances, palpitations and rash.

CAUTION!

This is another drug that simply seems outdated and unnecessary most of the time. Don't use it.

Guanabenz

GUANABENZ (Wytensin)

WHAT DOES IT DO IN YOUR BODY?

Reduces blood pressure by acting on the brain centers that reduce blood pressure.

WHAT IS IT PRESCRIBED FOR?

High blood pressure.

WHAT ARE THE POSSIBLE SIDE EFFECTS?

The most dangerous side effect of guanabenz is its tendency to rebound high blood pressure if you miss a dose or two. This makes it a potentially dangerous drug. It also can cause drowsiness, sedation, depression, fatigue, dry mouth, dizziness, weakness and headache.

CAUTION!

Please think twice about taking this drug at all.

Anti-Adrenergic Agents, Peripherally Acting

RESERPINE (Reserpine)

WHAT DOES IT DO IN YOUR BODY?

Lower blood pressure by lowering levels of catecholamine and 5-hydroxytryptamine in many parts of the body, including the brain and adrenal glands.

WHAT IS IT PRESCRIBED FOR?

High blood pressure, psychosis, schizophrenia.

WHAT ARE THE POSSIBLE SIDE EFFECTS?

Depression is the most common and most damaging side effect of reserpine. It shouldn't be used at all by people with any type of depression. It's also not a good drug for people with ulcers or kidney damage or disease, and it causes cancer in animals. Other side effects include dry mouth, dizziness, headache, irregular heartbeat, abnormally slow heartbeat, shortness of breath, a set of symptoms resembling Parkinson's, impotence, rash.

CAUTION!

Please think twice about taking this drug, period. Major depression is too serious and insidious a side effect to take lightly.

WHAT ARE THE INTERACTIONS WITH OTHER DRUGS?

Reserpine should never be taken within three weeks of taking an MAO inhibitor. This type of combination can produce a severe and even fatal reaction.

Reserpine may raise levels or prolong the effects of these drugs:

↑ Digitalis (digoxin)
   Quinidine
   Sympathomimetics (direct acting)

The following drugs may be reduced in potency or decreased in the amount of time they are effective when combined with reserpine:

↓ Sympathomimetics (indirect-acting)

These drugs may reduce the effects of reserpine:

↓ Tricyclic antidepressants

Guanethidine and Guanadrel

GUANADREL (Hylorel)

GUANETHIDINE (Ismelin)

WHAT DO THEY DO IN YOUR BODY?

Lower blood pressure.

WHAT ARE THEY PRESCRIBED FOR?

To lower blood pressure.

WHAT ARE THE POSSIBLE SIDE EFFECTS?

These are dangerous and potent drugs that frequently cause orthostatic hypotension, which is a failure of the blood pressure to rise when you stand up from a sitting or lying position. This is dangerous and often causes dizziness and weakness that can result in falls.

They have many other effects on the body, including fever, catechol-

---

* Potentially dangerous interaction.

amine depletion, impairment of kidney function and inability to ejaculate.

Adverse reactions include dizziness, weakness, abnormally slow heartbeat, fluid retention, angina, fatigue, muscle tremors, depression, vision disturbances, incontinence, anemia, shortness of breath and nasal congestion.

The rate of side effects with guanadrel is extremely high during the first eight weeks of taking it. These include shortness of breath on exertion, palpitations, chest pain, coughing, shortness of breath at rest, fatigue, headache, faintness, drowsiness, visual disturbances, loss of feeling, numbness, tingling, confusion, psychological problems, depression, sleep disorders, increased bowel movements, gas, indigestion, constipation, loss of appetite, inflammation of the tongue, nausea/vomiting, dry mouth and throat, stomach pain, urinary tract problems, sexual problems, excessive weight gain or loss, aching limbs, leg cramps.

CAUTION!

Please think twice about taking this drug, period. Take a look at all those side effects again and think about whether feeling that bad for eight weeks could possibly be worth it!

WHAT ARE THE INTERACTIONS WITH OTHER DRUGS?

Guanethidine and guanadrel may raise levels or prolong the effects of these drugs:

↑ Sympathomimetics (direct-acting)

This drug may increase the effects or prolong the action of guanethidine:

↑ Minoxidil*

These drugs may increase the effects or prolong the action of guanadrel:

↑ Beta-blockers*
Sympathomimetics (direct-acting)
Vasodilators*

These drugs may reduce the effects of guanethidine:

↓ Anorexiants
Haloperidol
MAO inhibitors
Methylphenidate
Phenothiazines
Sympathomimetics

These drugs may reduce the effects of guanadrel:

↓ Phenothiazines, Tricyclic antidepressants

Alpha-1 Blockers (Alpha-1-Adrenergic Blockers)

DOXAZOSIN (Cardura)

PRAZOSIN (Minipress)

TERAZOSIN (Hytrin)

WHAT DO THEY DO IN YOUR BODY?

Lower blood pressure.

---

*Potentially dangerous interaction.

WHAT ARE THEY PRESCRIBED FOR?

Lowering blood pressure, benign prostatic hyperplasia, some types of congestive heart failure, Raynaud's disease.

WHAT ARE THE POSSIBLE SIDE EFFECTS?

Prazosin tends to cause sodium and water retention, something that is important to avoid when lowering blood pressure.

Like some of the other hypertensive drugs, prazosin, terazosin and doxazosin can cause rebound hypertension if a few doses are missed and can caused dizziness and even fainting upon standing from a sitting or lying down position.

These drugs should not be given to people who have liver damage.

Doxazosin reduced fertility in male rats and testicular atrophy has occurred in dogs and cats given terazosin or prazosin.

Doxazosin can cause an abnormal reduction in white blood cell count.

People taking terazosin tended to gain weight.

These drugs affect cholesterol levels, but how they affect them seems to vary. Other side effects include dizziness, fatigue, weakness, drowsiness, headache, heart palpitations, nausea, shortness of breath, nasal congestion, vision disturbances.

CAUTION: THINK TWICE ABOUT TAKING THESE TYPES OF DRUGS IF . . .

- You have liver disease or damage.
- Your immune system is compromised or suppressed.
- You are obese.
- Your cholesterol is high.

WHAT ARE THE INTERACTIONS WITH OTHER DRUGS?

The following drug may be reduced in potency or decreased in the amount of time it is effective when combined with alpha-1 blockers:

↓ Clonidine

These drugs may increase the effects or prolong the action of alpha-1 blockers:

↑ Beta-blockers* (prazosin)
   Verapamil (prazosin)

This drug may reduce the effects of alpha-1 blockers:

↓ Indomethacin (prazosin)

Vasodilators

HYDRALAZINE (Apresoline)

WHAT DOES IT DO IN YOUR BODY?

Lowers blood pressure by interfering with the ability of calcium to move in and out of cells and effect the contraction of some parts of the heart and artery muscles. At the same time it increases heart rate and output. It also increases renin levels, which stimulates the production of angiotensin, which is exactly what other hypertensive drugs block.

WHAT IS IT PRESCRIBED FOR?

High blood pressure.

WHAT ARE THE POSSIBLE SIDE EFFECTS?

Hydralazine can cause a set of symptoms that resembles lupus, which may not necessarily all go away when the drug is stopped. This happened in 5 to 10 percent of patients, which is a high number.

   It can cause nerve pain in the hands and feet, blood abnormalities

---

*Potentially dangerous interaction.

and angina and has been implicated in myocardial infarctions, a type of heart attack.

Side effects include headache, loss of appetite, digestive problems, angina, vision problems, numbness and tingling, dizziness, tremors, depression, anxiety, rash, nasal congestion, flushing, water retention, muscle cramps, shortness of breath, difficulty urinating and of course abnormally low blood pressure (hypotension).

CAUTION: THINK TWICE ABOUT TAKING THESE TYPES OF DRUGS IF . . .

- You have coronary artery disease, have had a stroke or are at risk for one, have lung disease, have blood abnormalities or have lupus.

WHAT ARE THE INTERACTIONS WITH OTHER DRUGS?

Hydralazine may raise levels or prolong the effects of these drugs:

↑ Beta-blockers
   Metoprolol
   Propranolol

These drugs may increase the effects or prolong the action of hydralazine:

↑ Beta-blockers
   Metoprolol
   Propranolol

This drug may reduce the effects of hydralazine:

↓ Indomethacin

WHAT ARE THE INTERACTIONS WITH FOOD?

Taking with food will increase drug absorption. Eating a lot of salty foods will increase water retention.

WHAT NUTRIENTS DOES IT THROW OUT OF BALANCE OR INTERACT WITH?

Hydralazine depletes vitamin B6. Foods containing a relative of hydralazine called tartrazine, a yellow dye, will also deplete vitamin B6. Symptoms of B6 deficiency are numerous and include depression, memory loss, pain in the fingers and feet, carpal tunnel syndrome, menstrual symptoms, to name a few.

WHAT ELSE TO TAKE IF YOU TAKE THIS DRUG

Take 50 mg of vitamin B6 daily in addition to your daily multivitamin.

MINOXIDIL (Loniten)

WHAT DOES IT DO IN YOUR BODY?

Lowers blood pressure, grows hair.

WHAT IS IT PRESCRIBED FOR?

High blood pressure, male pattern baldness.

WHAT ARE THE POSSIBLE SIDE EFFECTS?

This is such a dangerous drug that it is only recommended as a last ditch effort if no other hypertensive drugs have worked. It can cause a serious condition called pericardial effusion and it can make angina worse. In animals it caused all kinds of gross abnormalities of the heart, including lesions and infertility.

It can cause fluid and mineral imbalances that are the opposite of what would benefit someone with high blood pressure, as well as an abnormally strong heartbeat and kidney impairment.

CAUTION: THINK TWICE ABOUT TAKING THIS DRUG IF . . .

- You have kidney problems.
- You have angina or have had a heart attack.

Please think twice about taking this drug, period. It's way too dangerous and there are many better alternatives.

WHAT ARE THE INTERACTIONS WITH OTHER DRUGS?

This is a bad drug to combine with guanethidine, because it can make the already considerable orthostatic hypotension risks of guanethidine even worse.

NATURAL ALTERNATIVES TO HIGH BLOOD PRESSURE DRUGS

High blood pressure is caused by arteries in distress and is one of the easiest symptoms of poor health to treat with simple, natural remedies.

Since medicines that lower blood pressure do have side effects—some of them risky and unpleasant—it's important to always *begin* by treating high blood pressure with nondrug methods. If you're taking medicine for high blood pressure, your physician should be monitoring you regularly and should have a goal of getting you off the medication.

When you're taking drugs to lower blood pressure, it's important not to take herbs that directly lower blood pressure such as hawthorn, without checking with your doctor and monitoring your blood pressure so you can make the necessary reductions in medication. Since the following blood-pressure lowering program works effectively to lower blood pressure, if you are also taking a hypertension drug you will need to measure your blood pressure daily at home to be sure it doesn't drop too low.

If you suddenly find you have high blood pressure, be sure to check with your doctor to rule out heavy metal poisoning (i.e., lead, mercury, cadmium) and kidney disease.

Weight Loss and Exercise

If you are overweight the first and most important step in lowering blood pressure, even if it is genetic, is to lose weight. People with high blood pressure weigh an average of 29 pounds more than people with normal blood pressure. For every two pounds of weight you drop, your blood pressure will drop at least one point in both the systolic and diastolic readings.

The natural partner of weight loss is exercise, which also improves circulation. If you exercise you are 34 percent less likely to develop hypertension than if you're a couch potato. Just a brisk half hour walk three or four times a week can lower blood pressure from 3 to 15 points in three months. Exercise will also help reduce stress, an important component in hypertension.

The Six Core Principles for Optimal Health are your foundation for treating hypertension naturally. When you're treating hypertension it's especially important to keep your antioxidant levels high, to eat plenty of fiber-filled vegetables and whole grains and drink plenty of water.

Keep Sodium, Potassium, Magnesium and Sugar in Balance

For about 30 percent of the population, reducing salt in the diet will help lower blood pressure naturally. Keep your salt intake moderate regardless, at 2,000 to 3,000 mg per day. Studies have shown that an extremely low-sodium diet causes more problems than it solves, so don't overdo it.

Reducing your salt intake won't be effective unless your potassium intake is also high, and yet people who take diuretic drugs to treat hypertension often become potassium-deficient. Signs of potassium deficiency include muscle cramps, weakness and an irregular heartbeat. Since potassium supplements may cause problems of their own, including diarrhea and nausea, eating a potassium-rich diet is the best way to maintain healthy potassium levels. Most fresh fruits and vegetables contain potassium. Those highest in potassium are bananas, apples, avocados, lima beans, oranges, potatoes, tomatoes, peaches, cantaloupes and apricots. Fish and meats also contain potassium.

Sufficient magnesium is essential for healthy blood pressure. It plays a key role, with sodium and potassium, in maintaining fluid balance in the cells and regulating how much water the cells hold. When your cells are holding onto water your blood pressure can go up. Just taking a magnesium supplement can significantly reduce blood pressure. Magnesium deficiency can cause a variety of heart problems, including irregular heartbeat, and it contributes to diabetes.

Cutting way back on sugar and refined carbohydrates such as white flour may be as important as cutting down on the salt. The insulin and adrenaline released when your blood sugar spikes cause the body to retain sodium and hold water, which raises blood pressure.

Coffee also stimulates the release of adrenal hormones and can cause a rise in blood pressure.

The Best Cure-All

One of the best ways to reduce blood pressure, which you may find hard to believe because it's so simple, is to drink plenty of clean water. Depending on your body size, you should be drinking six to 10 glasses of water per day.

Stress Hormones Raise Blood Pressure

If you do all of the above and your blood pressure is still high, take a good look at the stress in your life and take steps to manage it better or reduce it. The adrenal hormones released when you're under stress automatically raise blood pressure, so if you're chronically stressed you may have chronic hypertension.

Reducing stress may mean cutting down on your commitments, getting more sleep or making more time for recreation. Managing stress better may mean learning how to meditate, learning relaxation exercises or talking to a friend or therapist. Most of us know exactly what our life's stressors are. It's a matter of making your health and well-being important enough to make the needed changes.

CHOLESTEROL-LOWERING DRUGS AND THEIR NATURAL ALTERNATIVES

If you do a study of heart disease patients and cholesterol, you *will* find that cholesterol levels are higher in those with heart disease, and you will find cholesterol blocking the arteries of many people with heart disease. But to then assume that simply lowering cholesterol levels will make heart disease go away is a huge fallacy. High cholesterol does not cause heart disease, it is a symptom of heart disease! When you get a high cholesterol reading on a blood test, that can be an early warning system that you need to take better care of yourself, but it's certainly not a reason to take cholesterol-lowering drugs before you've given diet, exercise and supplements a good try.

Heart disease isn't the only disease that causes high levels of blood cholesterol. Diabetes, hypothyroidism, kidney disease and liver disease can also significantly raise cholesterol levels. Your doctor should first rule out these diseases as a cause of high cholesterol.

Debunking the Cholesterol Myths

Cholesterol is a fat-like material which is found in the brain, nerves, blood, bile and liver. Although it has been a victim of negative press, it is an essential component in the production of the steroid hormones and in nerve function as well as other essential body processes. When it is present in the blood in excess and in one of its destructive oxidated forms, it is one of *many* contributors to the development of hardening of the arteries or arteriosclerosis, better known as heart disease.

Let's examine some of the myths surrounding cholesterol. First, there is absolutely no evidence anywhere that normal cholesterol floating around in the blood does any harm. In fact, cholesterol is the building block for all your steroid hormones, which includes all the sex hormones and the cortisones. Even slightly low levels of cholesterol are associated with depression, suicide and lung cancer in older women. Not only that, a study in Britain found that low levels of cholesterol can even cause schizophrenia. What will harm you is oxidized cholesterol, but we'll talk about that in a minute.

How about the myth that eating high cholesterol foods raises cholesterol levels? This is only true for about 30 percent of the population. For most people, eating high cholesterol foods does *not* raise cholesterol. The body manufactures about 75 percent of its own cholesterol from the breakdown products of foods we eat. The rest we get directly from what we eat. If we eat more cholesterol, the body makes less or it is broken down by the liver and excreted. People who eat extremely excessive amounts of cholesterol-containing foods so that the body is unable to keep up with the elimination process, or whose livers are not functioning properly, may have high cholesterol due to their eating habits, but this is an exception, not the rule.

If you want to find out if you are one of the 30 percent for whom eating cholesterol does raise blood levels, try this. Have your HDL and LDL cholesterol levels measured, then cut way down on high-cholesterol foods for three months. Then go back and have your cholesterol levels measured again. If your cholesterol count is influenced by your cholesterol intake, your LDL (bad) cholesterol level should have dropped and your HDL levels should stay the same or rise.

If Cholesterol Doesn't Cause Heart Disease, What Does?

Heart disease has multiple causes which most Americans are very familiar with by now. The most familiar is diet. But why is diet so important? Why do people who eat lots of vegetables and less red meat have healthier hearts? Vegetables are high in antioxidants, your body's natural artery roto-rooters that disarm harmful oxidized cholesterol and keep it from clogging arteries.

Another potent risk factor for heart disease is low glutathione levels, which interferes with the body's ability to clear out harmful types of cholesterol and toxins that damage arteries.

Some villains in the heart disease drama directly harm artery walls. One of these villains is high homocysteine levels, often caused by a deficiency of B vitamins. Another such villain is rancid oil, such as unsaturated vegetable oils teeming with unstable molecules. The partially hydrogenated vegetable oils are equally if not more toxic to the heart.

Low magnesium levels do damage by weakening the heart muscles and interfering with nerve impulses and heartbeat.

And we all know by now that lack of exercise, depression, and high levels of chronic, unresolved stress are potent risk factors for heart disease.

Why Does Cholesterol Accumulate in the Arteries?

Drug company advertising for cholesterol-lowering drugs gives the impression that excessive cholesterol in the blood simply deposits itself on the artery walls, and that lowering cholesterol levels stops that process. It would be nice if it was that simple, but once again the magic pill theory falls short.

High cholesterol is a symptom of an underlying nutritional deficiency and/or toxicity (such as those mentioned above) that damages the arteries. Cholesterol takes on many forms, and some forms act as a component in the repair glue that the body calls on to repair damaged artery walls. If the cholesterol called in to do repair work is oxidized, the artery continues to get the message that it's damaged, and more cholesterol gets piled on. In a kind of double whammy, the same nutritional deficiencies and toxins that allow cholesterol to become oxidized, also impair the ability of the liver and other organs to do their clean-up work to eliminate harmful fatty acids in the blood. One of the ways cholesterol becomes oxidized is when you don't have high enough levels of antioxidants in your body to neutralize the harmful cholesterol.

The Myth of the Cholesterol Count

Another cholesterol myth perpetuated by the drug companies is that everyone with a total cholesterol count over 200 mg/dL should be concerned. This is blatantly false. Our individual biochemistry allows for a wide range of cholesterol levels. Your *relative levels* of HDL and LDL cholesterol are more important than your total cholesterol. A very high level of LDL "bad" cholesterol probably indicates that your body is not efficiently removing cholesterol from your blood, but that inefficiency, and the heart disease that may accompany it, is most likely caused by poor nutrition and a sedentary lifestyle.

What is more important is that your HDL "good" cholesterol levels stay high and your LDL "bad" cholesterol levels stay low relative to each other. However, keep your focus on high levels of HDL. A recent study in China found that people with low counts of LDL and low counts of HDL still have high coronary risk. We'll give specific suggestions later in the chapter for raising HDL levels.

The best way to evaluate your cholesterol status using the measurements given in most blood chemistry panels is to measure the ratio of your total cholesterol to your HDL count. For example, if you are a man and your total cholesterol count is 250 and your HDL is 85, you divide 250 by 85 and your ratio will be 2.9. When you calculate your ratio, compare it to these numbers: The average ratio for women is 4.4. For men, it is 5.0. If your ratio number is low, that's a fair indicator that your cholesterol balance is healthy.

Here's a general rule for total cholesterol levels: If your cholesterol level is under 200, consider this a green light. Don't worry, be happy! If your cholesterol levels are over 200, be aware that this *might* be an indication of some damage to your arteries. If you're leading a healthy lifestyle, don't be overly concerned, but be watchful. Consider this a yellow light. If your cholesterol levels are over 300, your body is trying to tell you something: "Help! You're plugging up my arteries!" Consider this a red light. You need to seriously evaluate your diet and lifestyle.

No matter what category you fall into, please *do not* try to totally eliminate cholesterol from your diet. It is the fundamental building block of all your sex hormones and the adrenal hormones, and plays an important part in the excretion of fats. Cholesterol is also found in high amounts in the brain and nervous system, where hormones play a critical part in balancing all bodily systems. We all need some cholesterol in our diet. If your cholesterol levels are high, your answer probably lies in overall diet and lifestyle changes.

Drugs Often Do More Harm Than Good

While a cholesterol-lowering drug will usually do a very good job of lowering your cholesterol, there's scant, if any, evidence that it will help you live longer or reduce your risk of a heart attack unless you are extremely ill or have just suffered from a heart attack. There are no studies that show that women benefit from these drugs—all the studies showing even marginal benefits have been done on men. Nor are there any studies showing that they reduce heart attacks or death in men aged 65 to 75. Since heart disease takes decades to develop, it's highly unlikely that cholesterol-lowering drugs will help anyone over the age of 75. That leaves men aged 35 to 55, but even here the evidence of benefit is slim, and the possible side effects are huge.

If the American public had even a clue of how destructive these drugs are, they wouldn't touch them except in an emergency. And don't think this is a revolutionary statement. There is complete consensus (or should we say lip service) among drug companies, physicians, and organizations such as the American Heart Association, that the first step in lowering cholesterol should be a *"vigorous"* attempt to improve diet and increase exercise. Sadly, few physicians are following this advice and drug company advertising and marketing certainly doesn't reflect it. But it's well-known that these drugs can cause severe side effects, and that long term follow up studies are sadly lacking. The studies that do exist juggle numbers and play with statistics to the point where the information becomes meaningless.

Every information sheet on the most commonly prescribed cholesterol-lowering drugs will tell you that they cause cancer in rodents when taken long term in relatively normal doses. It's also well-known that they can cause severe emotional imbalances in men, along with a wide array of life-threatening side effects. A study done at the Henry Ford Medical Center in Detroit showed that men taking cholesterol-lowering drugs had a higher risk of suffering from depression, crying spells, anxiety, worry and suicidal thoughts. Yet physicians routinely prescribe these drugs indefinitely for their older patients.

The wisest course of action is to avoid these drugs unless you are in imminent danger of a heart attack due to clogged arteries. If that's the case, it's important to do everything possible to reverse your heart disease using the cholesterol-lowering plan outlined here, and to get off the drugs as soon as possible. These drugs have ominous side effects especially when used on a long term basis. If you are taking these drugs, be sure to take supplements accordingly.

CHOLESTEROL-LOWERING DRUGS

Bile Acid Sequestrants

CHOLESTRYAMINE (Questran, Prevalite)

COLESTIPOL HCl (Colestid)

The bile acid sequestrants, also known as "bile-blockers" such as cholestyramine (Questran) and colestipol HCl (Colestid) are resins, often taken in powder form, that block the production of bile. Cholesterol is the building block of bile, a substance normally released via the liver to break down fats in the intestines and enhance their absorption. Then it is reabsorbed back into the liver. The bile-blockers bind to bile in the intestines so they can't be reabsorbed, and are instead excreted in the feces. This forces the liver to take up more cholesterol from the blood to produce more bile, in effect lowering cholesterol levels (and making your liver work a lot harder).

Seems like a neat solution, but the bile-blockers also bind to the fat soluble vitamins such as A, E, D and K, so that instead of absorbing these vitamins you excrete them. (Sound familiar? Olestra, the new fake fat, does the same thing.) Ironically, a shortage of vitamin E can be a direct cause of heart disease, which is what the drugs are meant to prevent in the first place. There is some evidence that along with blocking cholesterol absorption these drugs are blocking the absorption of the important EFA oils (essential fatty acids) that are essential to good health. Bile-blocking resins also lower folate (folic acid) levels, which will raise homocysteine levels, another potent risk factor for heart disease.

Here's a medical maze for you. Physicians prescribing bile-blockers will read on the drug information sheet that anticoagulant, blood-thinning drugs such as warfarin or Coumadin can become less effective when prescribed along with a bile blocker. And yet, long-term use of a bile blocker can cause a deficiency of vitamin K, which will *increase* the tendency to bleed, making the drugs *more* effective. In other words, what will happen when you combine these two types of drugs is truly unpredictable, and that is very dangerous.

WHAT DO THEY DO IN YOUR BODY?

Lower cholesterol by blocking the production of bile.

WHAT ARE THEY PRESCRIBED FOR?

Lowering cholesterol levels.

WHAT ARE THE POSSIBLE SIDE EFFECTS?

Constipation occurs in up to 50 percent of all patients who use these drugs! Constipation can be severe, especially if you already have a problem with constipation or hemorrhoids.

Chronic use of resins can lead to excessive bleeding or poor clotting from Vitamin K deficiency. Vitamin D deficiencies can also be a problem resulting in rashes and irritations on skin, tongue and anus as well as poor bone formation.

In addition, osteoporosis, liver dysfunction and disturbances of the acid base balance of the body are side effects of these drugs.

They can raise triglyceride levels. High triglyceride levels increase the risk of heart disease.

Most alarming, however, is the research that reports cancer as a possible side effect. Several studies stated that some rats who were given bile acid sequestrants, particularly Questran and Prevalite, grew cancerous intestinal tumors.

CAUTION: THINK TWICE ABOUT TAKING THESE TYPES OF DRUGS IF . . .

- You have severe constipation and especially if you are over 60 years of age with severe constipation.
- You have blood clotting problems, osteoporosis or severe vitamin deficiencies.
- You have a gallbladder obstruction (bile duct obstruction).
- You have phenylketonuria, a genetic disease; hypothyroidism; diabetes; kidney and blood vessel disorders; dysproteinemia; or obstructive liver disease or ischemic heart disease.

WHAT ARE THE INTERACTIONS WITH OTHER DRUGS?

Because bile acid sequestrants may delay or reduce the absorption of other drugs you take with them, it's best to take other medication at least one hour before or four to six hours after taking bile acid sequestrants.

The following drugs may be reduced in potency or decreased in the amount of time they are effective when taken with bile acid sequestrants:

↓ Anticoagulants
Aspirin
Chloroquine
Clindamycin
Clofibrate
Clorothiazide
Diclofenac
Digitalis glycosides
Digoxin
Diuretics, thiazide
Furosemide
Gemfibrozil
Glipizide
Hydrochlorothiazide
Hydrocortisone
Imipramine
Iron
Iopanoic acid

Methyldopa
Methotrexate (chemotherapy)
Metronidazole
Mycophenolate
Nicotinic acid (niacin)
Penicillin G
Phenytoin
Phosphate supplements
Piroxicam
Propranolol
Tenoxicam
Tetracyclines
Thyroid hormones
Tolbutamide
Ursodiol
Valproic acid
Warfarin*

WHAT ARE THE INTERACTIONS WITH FOOD?

These drugs decrease the absorption of nutrients you get from your foods such as sugars, fats, vitamins and minerals.

---

* Potentially dangerous interaction.

WHAT NUTRIENTS DO THEY DEPLETE OR THROW OUT OF BALANCE?

Calcium, carotene, electrolytes, folic acid, iron and the fat-soluble vitamins A, B12, D, E and K.

WHAT ELSE TO TAKE IF YOU TAKE THESE DRUGS

Take supplements of vitamins A, B12, D, E and K as well as folic acid, iron, electrolytes, beta-carotene and calcium.

To reduce constipation drink at least eight glasses of water every day and eat foods high in fiber like whole grains, vegetables and fruit.

OTHER TIPS ON THESE DRUGS

Because of the absorbing mechanism of these drugs, take other medications or supplements at least one hour before or four to six hours after a bile acid sequestrant.

HMG-CoA Reductase Inhibitors (Statins)

ATORVASTATIN (Lipitor)

FLUVASTATIN (Lescol)

LOVASTATIN (Mevacor)

PRAVASTATIN (Pravachol)

SIMVASTATIN (Zocor)

These drugs are known as the cholesterol-blockers or statins. They directly block an enzyme needed to make cholesterol in the body. Here's a question for the FDA—where are the long-term studies on these drugs? They didn't exist when the drugs were approved. How could that happen to a drug being enthusiastically pushed on millions of older Americans that profoundly affects health and well-being?

The biggest danger and most common side effect of taking these drugs is liver damage. It's frightening to imagine what's happening to a liver subjected to, say, a dose of Mevacor, a couple of alcohol drinks, and a Tylenol, all of which compromise liver function. This type of triple whammy could be enough to cause serious problems in someone already ill or weak, yet few physicians would think to mention this to their patients.

Remember, cholesterol is the basic building block for the cortisones, testosterone, estrogen, progesterone and DHEA. Is it any wonder that people taking cholesterol-blocking statins suffer from steroid hormone-related complaints, such as men growing breasts and being impotent, women becoming bald and both suffering from insomnia and fatigue?

But perhaps even more serious than the above side effects is the fact that the same mechanism that blocks cholesterol production also blocks the production of coenzyme Q10, a substance essential to a healthy heart and muscles. Your physician may tell you that you'll never have a shortage of CoQ10, but this is not borne out by the facts. The truth is that heart disease patients are consistently found to have low levels of coenzyme Q10. About one out of every 200 people who use the statins have side effects of muscle pain and weakness, which can be a sign of even more serious problems leading to kidney failure and even death. All indications are that the cause of these symptoms is a deficiency of CoQ10. So once again, we have a cholesterol-lowering drug supposedly given to reverse heart disease, causing a deficiency of a substance crucial to a strong and healthy heart.

The Zocor Story

Here's a story about Zocor, but it could probably apply to any of the statins, which have more similarities than differences. Consider this a cautionary tale that could apply to any drug.

A couple of years ago newspaper headlines trumpeted the results of a five-year study on a drug called Zocor showing that the drug reduced death from heart disease and other causes by lowering cholesterol. Reading the headlines and listening to the news reports, you'd think everyone in America should take this drug. The study was paid for by Merck, the maker of the drug. This alone makes the results questionable. Now Merck is allowed to advertise the drug as "life-saving." This is an advertising ploy for a very expensive drug: $150 for 90 capsules. Here are some facts on Zocor:

The Merck study on Zocor contradicts years of studies on very similar drugs which showed no benefit. The study was only done on people who already had heart disease, so it showed nothing about Zocor's ability to protect healthy people by lowering their cholesterol. Although "cardiac events" were reduced in women taking Zocor, compared to a placebo, mortality (death rate) was not reduced. The effect of the drug on people over the age of 60 was very reduced, and yet the majority of people likely to be prescribed the drug are over 60.

WHAT DO THEY DO IN THE BODY?

These drugs directly block an enzyme needed to make cholesterol in the body.

WHAT ARE THEY PRESCRIBED FOR?

Lowering cholesterol levels.

WHAT ARE THE POSSIBLE SIDE EFFECTS?

The most serious side effects of these drugs are stomach ulcers and a dangerous disease called rhabdomyolysis that actually destroys muscle tissue.

Other side effects include: back pain, insomnia, heartburn, greater susceptibility to upper sinus infections, alteration of taste, dizziness, memory loss, numbness in the extremities, tremors, loss of libido, impotence, enlarged thyroid and skin conditions such as bumps and rashes. They also tend to increase the formation of cataracts, and they cause cancer and birth defects in rodents and dogs. Some patients have experienced steroid hormone-related complaints such as impotence, insomnia and fatigue.

In addition, statins may cause severe liver damage. So be on the lookout for signs of jaundice or hepatitis such as yellow eyes and skin, dark-colored urine, and light-colored stools.

Statins also can cause kidney disease.

Caution: Think Twice About Taking These Drugs If . . .

- You have a stomach ulcer.
- You have the following conditions: an acute infection, a suppressed immune system, hypertension, are traumatized, experience uncontrollable seizures, have severe endocrine or electrolyte disorders. These drugs can cause kidney failure in patients with these conditions.
- You have liver disease, have poor liver function, kidney disease, poor kidney function or drink substantial amounts of alcohol. They can damage your liver and kidneys significantly.
- You are scheduled soon for surgery. Ask your physician how you can safely discontinue using these drugs.
- You have any disease that contributes to increased blood cholesterol such as hypothyroidism, diabetes, kidney and blood vessel disorders, liver disease or dysproteinemia.

What Are the Interactions with Other Drugs?

Statins may raise levels or prolong the effects of these drugs:

↑ Digoxin
  Oral contraceptives
  Warfarin

These drugs may increase the effects or prolong the action of statins:

↑ Alcohol   Gemfibrozil
  Cyclosporine   Itraconazole
  Erythromycin

These drugs may reduce the effects of statins:

↓ Antacids   Isradipine
  Bile acid sequestrants   Propanolol
    (Colestipol)   Rifampin

WHAT ARE THE INTERACTIONS WITH FOOD?

Take lovastatin and fluvastatin with meals. Pravastatin and simvastatin are taken without regard to food.

WHAT NUTRIENTS DO THEY DEPLETE OR THROW OUT OF BALANCE?

Coenzyme Q10.

WHAT ELSE TO TAKE IF YOU TAKE THIS DRUG

Coenzyme CoQ10, 30 to 60 mg daily of the gel capsules or 90 mg daily of the powder form. To support your liver, you can take the herb silymarin (milk thistle), the supplement alpha lipoic acid and NAC (N-acetyl cysteine).

OTHER TIPS ABOUT THESE DRUGS

Because of the real threat of muscle destruction, contact your physician immediately if you notice muscle pain, tenderness or weakness, particularly if a fever accompanies these symptoms.

In addition, your physician should monitor your liver and kidney functions regularly when you are taking these drugs.

OTHER CHOLESTEROL-LOWERING DRUGS

DEXTROTHYROXINE SODIUM (Choloxin)

WHAT DOES IT DO IN THE BODY?

Reduces cholesterol levels by stimulating the liver to excrete it faster.

WHAT IS IT PRESCRIBED FOR?

Lowering cholesterol levels.

WHAT ARE THE POSSIBLE SIDE EFFECTS?

This drug stresses the heart tremendously. It can cause heart attacks and increase the size of the heart.

This drug can also cause nausea, vomiting, constipation, diarrhea, gallstones, jaundice, hair loss, rashes, itching, menstrual irregularities, water retention, muscle pain, tremors, nervousness and dizziness.

CAUTION: THINK TWICE ABOUT TAKING THIS DRUG IF . . .

- You are scheduled for surgery in the next two weeks. Avoid it.
- You have liver or kidney disease.
- You have asthma.
- You have a heart condition.
- You are severely overweight.

Please think twice about taking this drug, period. It's too hard on the heart, the liver and the kidneys, and there are too many other safer alternatives available.

WHAT ARE THE INTERACTIONS WITH OTHER DRUGS?

Dextrothyroxines may raise levels or prolong the effects of these drugs:

↑ Anticoagulants
   Antidepressants (tricyclic)
   Thyroid hormones

The following drugs may be reduced in potency or decreased in the amount of time they are effective when combined with dextrothyroxines:

↓ Antidiabetic agents
   Beta-blockers
   Digitalis glycosides

This drug may reduce the effects of dextrothyroxine sodium drugs:

↓ Cholestryramine

CLOFIBRATE (Atromid-S)

WHAT DOES IT DO IN THE BODY?

Lowers triglycerides and very low-density lipoprotein cholesterol (VLDL) levels. It does not predictably lower LDL levels.

WHAT IS IT PRESCRIBED FOR?

Lowering high triglyceride levels.

WHAT ARE THE POSSIBLE SIDE EFFECTS?

This drug can cause anemia, liver and kidney dysfunction, gallbladder problems, peptic ulcers, abnormal heartbeat, and flu-like symptoms.

Liver cancer is also a possible side effect of this drug. It produced tumors in the livers of rodents and humans in published research.

CAUTION: THINK TWICE ABOUT USING THIS DRUG IF . . .

- You have a peptic ulcer.
- You have liver or kidney disease.
- You have a gallbladder obstruction.

You should think twice about taking this drug, especially if you haven't tried diet and exercise changes first. There are too many serious side effects, and it is a poorly studied drug.

WHAT ARE THE INTERACTIONS WITH OTHER DRUGS?

Clofibrate may raise levels or prolong the effects of these drugs:

↑ Anticoagulants   Insulin
  Dantrolene   Sulfonylureas
  Furosemide

This drug may be reduced in potency or decreased in the amount of time it is effective when combined with clofibrate drugs:

↓ Ursodiol

This drug may increase the effects or prolong the action of clofibrate:

↑ Warfarin

These drugs may reduce the effects of clofibrate:

↓ Oral contraceptives
 Probenecid

WHAT NUTRIENTS DOES IT DEPLETE OR THROW OUT OF BALANCE?

Minerals, carotenes, fats, iron, sugars, vitamins A, B12, D, E and K.

WHAT ELSE TO TAKE WITH THIS DRUG

Supplements which replenish the above vitamins, minerals and nutrients.

GEMFIBROZIL (Lopid, Novo-Gemfibrozil, Apo-Gemfibrozil)

WHAT DOES IT DO IN THE BODY?

Its major effect is to lower triglycerides and VLDL (very low-density lipoprotein), but it may also lower LDL levels, and it may raise HDL levels.

WHAT IS IT PRESCRIBED FOR?

Reducing triglycerides.

What Are the Possible Side Effects?

As is true with most of the other cholesterol-lowering drugs, this drug is essentially toxic and therefore stresses your liver and kidneys. As a result, liver dysfunction, hyperglycemia and kidney failure are possible side effects of this drug.

Other side effects include muscle pain, eczema, fatigue, drowsiness, vertigo, convulsions, appendicitis, abdominal pain, upset stomach, taste perversion, water retention, lupus-like syndrome, jaundice, pancreatitis, muscle pain, anemia, impotence, vitamin deficiencies and irregular heartbeat.

Liver cancer and cataracts occurred in rats tested with this drug.

Caution: Think Twice About Using This Drug If . . .

- You have an underactive thyroid or diabetes.
- You have liver, kidney or gallbladder disease.
- You have poor liver or kidney function.

What Are the Interactions with Other Drugs?

Gemfibrozil may raise the levels or prolong the effects of these drugs:

↑ Anticoagulants
HMG-COA reductase inhibitors*
Warfarin

This drug may be reduced in potency or decreased in the amount of time it is effective when combined with gemfibrozil:

↓ Glyburide

What Are the Interactions with Food?

Absorption of nutrients from food is reduced.

---

*Potentially dangerous interaction.

WHAT NUTRIENTS DOES IT DEPLETE OR THROW OUT OF BALANCE?

Vitamins A, B12, D, E, K, calcium, iron, magnesium and potassium.

WHAT ELSE TO TAKE IF YOU TAKE THIS DRUG

Vitamins A, B12, D, E, K, calcium, iron, magnesium and potassium.

OTHER TIPS ON THIS DRUG

Be especially cautious when driving or doing any activity that requires alertness, coordination or physical dexterity. This drug can make it difficult to focus and concentrate.

NATURAL ALTERNATIVES TO CHOLESTEROL-LOWERING DRUGS

It is so easy for nearly everyone to significantly lower LDL cholesterol and raise HDL levels with diet, exercise and supplements, that it seems extreme for physicians to prescribe cholesterol-lowering drugs until other, simpler measures have been taken and failed. The exception to this would be if you are in imminent danger of having a heart attack and need to take extreme measures.

Niacin Is a Potent Cholesterol Buster

Taking niacin (vitamin B3) is one of the safest and most effective ways to lower LDL or "bad" cholesterol and raise HDL or "good" cholesterol. It's at least as effective as the cholesterol-lowering drugs, and much less expensive. However, there are some down sides to niacin.

Niacin is a *vasodilator*, meaning it expands the blood vessels, bringing more blood into the upper part of the body. In large doses it can cause a "niacin flush" around the head, neck and shoulders. The skin becomes flushed and red, and this is accompanied by a burning or tingling sensation, which most people find uncomfortable and annoying. While a niacin flush is harmless, in high doses niacin can cause stomach cramps, diarrhea and nausea, and high doses taken for

EIGHT STEPS YOU CAN TAKE TO LOWER YOUR CHOLESTEROL NATURALLY

1. Eat more fiber. Studies show that fiber has a direct and dramatic cholesterol-lowering effect. You can get plenty of fiber by eating fresh, whole unprocessed foods and a plant-based diet. Pectin, a soluble form of fiber found in apples, blueberries and grapefruit, particularly helps reduce cholesterol. If you want to add more fiber, take 1 tsp. a day of psyllium with 8 oz. of water or juice. Psyllium is the active ingredient in Metamucil, but they also add sugar, preservatives and food colorings. Stick to the plain psyllium found in your health food store—it's cheaper, too.

2. Make olive oil and fish oil your predominant dietary fats. They both can actually lower LDL cholesterol. However, don't entirely neglect the other fats: keep your nutrition in balance.

3. Add garlic to your diet. Garlic is a powerful cholesterol-lowering substance, and lowers blood pressure too. Add it liberally to your diet and take it in capsules.

4. Have a glass of red wine with dinner or a cup of green tea, or take a bioflavonoid supplement such as grapeseed extract and/or green tea daily. Both are known to have a cholesterol-lowering effect. However, too much alcohol (more than two drinks per day) will raise cholesterol levels.

5. Take niacin.

6. Take your cholesterol-busting supplements.

7. Eat your cholesterol-busting foods.

8. Exercise will directly raise HDL cholesterol. It's a must for healthy arteries.

an extended period of time may adversely affect the liver. People with ischemic heart disease should be cautious with niacin. For these people, niacin can cause abnormal heartbeats.

The key to taking niacin successfully to lower cholesterol levels is to start with a small amount, 50 mg twice a day, and gradually work up to 400 mg three times a day over a period of two to three months. It's also important to take a "no-flush" niacin formula that delivers all of the benefits of niacin without the unpleasant side effects. These formulas are made with inositol hexanicotinate. If your doctor prescribes nicotinic acid, tell him or her about inositol hexanicotinate. It's the same thing in a safer form. If you stick to a healthy lifestyle, you shouldn't have to take the niacin for more than a year at the most. Please remember to taper it off gradually.

If your physician has you on cholesterol-lowering drugs, don't stop taking them without supervision.

Estrogen Lowers Cholesterol: Fact or Fiction?

That estrogen protects against heart disease has become an accepted "fact" in conventional medicine, but in reality there is little evidence to support this claim. Just for starters, a large percentage of the women in the study were taking a synthetic progesterone (a progestin) with the estrogen, and we don't know what effect that had. Women who aren't taking a progestin usually have had a hysterectomy (taking estrogen alone raises your risk of some types of cancer), and we don't know what effect that would have on cholesterol levels.

We do know that estrogen can slightly raise HDL cholesterol and lower LDL cholesterol, but at the same time it often dramatically raises triglyceride levels and significantly raises the risk of some types of stroke. If you're over the age of 40 and contemplating hormone replacement therapy, do yourself a big favor and first read the book that Virginia Hopkins co-authored with John Lee, M.D., *What Your Doctor May Not Tell You About Menopause: The Breakthrough Book on Natural Progesterone* (Warner Books, 1996). Dr. Lee is the world's leading expert on the use of natural progesterone, and this book is an excellent guide for all premenopausal and menopausal women.

Do Fish Oil Supplements Really Lower Cholesterol?

Fish oil is excellent not only for reducing overall cholesterol, but also for increasing your HDL or "good" cholesterol. The best source of fish oil is to eat fish during your daily meals. There has been a lot of speculation that taking a fish oil supplement can give you the same benefits as eating fish, but the data published from several studies indicate that it just isn't true. In fact, taking a supplement of fish oils may make your cholesterol worse! It's possible that fish oil supplements are rancid by the time they get to our refrigerators. Some studies done with fish oil preserved with vitamin E are encouraging, but your best bet is to eat fish (and not deep fried!) at least twice a week.

Cholesterol-Busting Supplements

If your cholesterol is over 300, you'll want to add the following vitamins and minerals to the Six Core Principles for Optimal Health for six months. Most of these essential nutrients are antioxidants which help lower your LDL or "bad" cholesterol levels:

Vitamin C: 1,000 mg three times daily. If this high a dose gives you diarrhea, back off the dose until it goes away.

Magnesium: 300 mg daily

Calcium: 200 mg daily

Copper: 2 to 3 mg

Vitamin E: 400 IU (total 800 IU daily). In one study, ingesting this amount daily brought a 26 percent reduction in LDL or "bad" cholesterol production.

Psyllium: 1 to 2 teaspoons a day. Be sure to drink eight glasses of water a day too.

N-acetyl cysteine (NAC): 500 mg three times a day. This will help raise your glutathione levels, which will support your liver so it can more efficiently excrete cholesterol.

Green tea: The active beneficial ingredients in green tea are called polyphenols, substances that act as antioxidants, neutralize harmful fats and oils, strengthen the liver and lower LDL cholesterol while increasing HDL levels. You can either drink green tea, or take it in a concentrated form as a supplement.

PCOs or proanthocyanidins: PCOs (grapeseed extract, for example) work specifically to stop "bad" cholesterol from forming and sticking to artery walls.

Cayenne: This spice lowers cholesterol. Take a daily supplement of cayenne in capsules, or use it liberally on your food.

Curry: Another spice that lowers cholesterol.

Guggul: Taking this is a new but old way to lower cholesterol. Ayurvedic medicine is an ancient form of healing from India that relies largely on dividing people into body and personality types, and then prescribing a variety of treatments that include plant medicines. Lately we've been learning more about the large number of safe, effective medicines Ayurveda has in its pharmacy, and scientific research is following. One of the best known Ayurvedic medicines is called guggul, a plant traditionally used mainly to treat arthritis and obesity.

Studies have shown that guggul significantly reduces cholesterol levels without side effects. One study used an active component of guggul called guggulipid, which participants took for 12 weeks. In 80 percent of the patients serum cholesterol was lowered by an average of 24 percent and serum triglycerides were lowered by an average of 23 percent, which is comparable to the prescription drugs. Of these, 60 percent showed an increase in their HDL (good) cholesterol. When guggulipid was compared to the drug clofibrate (Atromid-S), it came out about the same, without the side effects.

WHAT BOOSTS GOOD (HDL) CHOLESTEROL

Carnitine, an amino acid
Fish
Guggulipid
Yams

YOUR TOP CHOLESTEROL-BUSTING FOODS

Apples
Alfalfa sprouts
Berries, especially blueberries and raspberries
Brewer's yeast
Carrots (raw)
Fenugreek (an herb)
Fish, especially salmon, mackerel, herring, sardines, cod, tuna, trout
Eggplant
Garlic
Grapefruit
Legumes

Oat bran
Onions
Prunes
Soy products such as miso, tempeh and tofu
Whole grains including rice, barley, millet, oats, wheat and rye
Yogurt

A NATURAL BLOOD PRESSURE-LOWERING PROGRAM

Maintain a healthy weight.

Get some moderate exercise at least 30 minutes every day or 45 minutes three to four times a week.

Eat a low-fat, low-sodium, low-sugar diet emphasizing whole, fresh foods, especially vegetables, grains and plenty of fiber.

Avoid refined, packaged and processed foods.

Limit alcohol consumption to two drinks per day or less.

Avoid coffee.

Stop smoking.

Avoid drugs that raise blood pressure.

Drink plenty of water.

DAILY VITAMINS

(Add to the Vitamin Plan found in Chapter 8)

Vitamin C, 1,000 to 2,000 mg
Vitamin E, 400 IU daily (800 IU total)
Magnesium, 500 to 800 mg
Calcium, up to 500 mg

Zinc, 10 mg daily
Carnitine, up to 1,000 mg, three to four times daily between meals
Coenzyme Q10, 30 to 90 mg daily

HERBS

You can take these herbs alone or in a formula that combines them. They come as tablets, capsules or in a liquid tincture.

Cayenne
Dandelion (acts as a diuretic)
Dong Quai

Garlic (eat fresh or take the odorless pills three times a day)
Gingko biloba (improves blood flow to the extremities)
Ginseng
Hawthorn (strengthens the heart)

FOODS

Fresh fruits and vegetables
Fresh celery (four stalks a day has been known to significantly reduce blood pressure—try drinking a carrot/celery juice mix daily)

Cold water, deep sea fish (cod, mackerel, sardines, salmon, herring)
Olive oil (instead of vegetable oils or butter)
Onions

CHAPTER 10

Drugs for the Digestive Tract and Their Natural Alternatives

A HEALTHY DIGESTIVE TRACT is an essential cog in the wheel of a healthy body. If you're serious about living a long, healthy, vibrant life, your digestive system needs to be able to break down and assimilate your food efficiently and effectively. The millions upon millions of cells that make up your body wouldn't know what to do with a whole piece of fruit. They can only use the simplest breakdown products of food to fuel their activities and can only use the vitamins and minerals locked away in that juicy apple once they are released in their simplest form.

Digestion begins in the mouth. As soon as you take a bite of food, enzymes and mucins in your saliva begin to break it down and lubricate it for a trip down the esophagus. Meanwhile, down in the stomach, the taste, smell or even the thought of food stimulates the secretion of hydrochloric acid and the enzyme pepsin, which digests protein. Enzymes from the gallbladder and pancreas are also stimulated by the smell and taste of food.

Chewing is another potent trigger of acid and enzyme secretion. Your mother was absolutely right when she reminded you to chew your food thoroughly. The longer you chew, the more time the rest of your digestive tract has to prepare for its role in the process. Smaller particles of well-chewed food are, for practical purposes, predigested. This helps to insure optimal breakdown and absorption of what you eat.

STOMACH ACID, HEARTBURN AND ULCERS

In the stomach, muscular contractions thoroughly mix food with hydrochloric acid. Stomach acid—powerful enough to strip paint—is a vital part of good digestion. A thick mucous layer protects the stomach walls from harm as the acid kills bacteria and parasites and frees up minerals (such as magnesium and potassium) and the B vitamins folate and B12 so that they can be absorbed in the small intestine.

If sufficient stomach acid isn't produced, digestion suffers. The passage of food out of the stomach into the small intestine is delayed, which can lead to heartburn as the stomach pushes food mixed with acid back into the esophagus. Burning is caused by acid coming in contact with the lining of the esophagus, which isn't protected by a mucous layer like the stomach is.

Heavy, fatty meals, large meals, eating on the run or while under stress, lying down just after a meal, or eating just after heavy exercise also set the stage for heartburn.

Contrary to what the huge drug companies that make antacids and H2 blocker drugs such as Tagamet and Zantac say, excessive acid production is almost never the reason for heartburn or ulcers. In fact it is now estimated that up to one-third of all bleeding ulcers are caused by taking NSAID drugs such as aspirin and ibuprofen. In many cases, the antacids and H2 blockers given to alleviate the symptoms of stomach pain mask the symptoms until the problem is life-threatening.

Antacids and H2 blockers alleviate symptoms for a short while by buffering acid and decreasing acid secretion, but can actually aggravate the underlying problem: too *little* acid in the stomach. With chronic use of these medications, digestion is compromised and decreased absorption of some vitamins and minerals can result. Once the food finally makes its way into the intestines, it isn't broken down enough for it to be properly absorbed.

There are other factors that contribute to low secretion of stomach acid. Drinking icy cold liquids with meals can suppress it and stomach acid levels decline with age. A large percentage of people over 50 make too little stomach acid for thorough digestion of food.

A few years ago, if you asked your physician what causes ulcers, he or she would promptly reply that too much stomach acid was to blame. Now we know that a spiral-shaped bacteria called *Helicobacter pylori* (*H. pylori* for short) is the primary culprit. It suppresses acid production and creates holes in the stomach's protective mucous layer, allowing acid to seep through and burn holes in the delicate tissue underneath. An *H. pylori* infection can also cause symptoms of indigestion and heartburn.

THE SMALL INTESTINE AND ITS ENZYMES

Food leaving the stomach is squirted in small amounts into the duodenum, which is the first part of the small intestine. The pancreas and small intestine secrete the enzymes amylase (to digest starches), protease (to digest proteins) and lipase (to digest fats) when they detect food in the duodenum. These enzymes break food down into parts your body can use, including carbohydrates, amino acids, free fatty acids, vitamins and minerals. The pancreas also makes bicarbonate that buffers acid so that the food won't burn holes in the small intestine. Bile which has been made in the liver and stored in the gallbladder to emulsify fats is released into the duodenum as food passes through.

Enzymes play a major role in all of the body's functions. Digestive enzymes are only one variety of these important catalysts of biological reactions, which are named for the substance they break down. For example, the enzyme that breaks down sucrose (table sugar) is called sucrase; cellulose (plant starch) is broken down by cellulase. The absence or shortage of a single digestive enzyme can have serious consequences. Abdominal cramping and diarrhea after drinking milk are the symptoms of a deficiency of lactase, the enzyme responsible for the digestion of the sugars in milk (lactose).

Digestive enzymes are built from amino acids and vitamin or mineral cofactors or *coenzymes*. Zinc and magnesium are two of the most common digestive enzyme cofactors. The B vitamins thiamin, riboflavin, pantothenic acid and biotin, as well as the minerals molybdenum, manganese, copper, iron and selenium, play the role of coenzymes as well. Each time the enzyme does its job, it uses up its coenzyme, which then needs to be replaced. Eating foods rich in vitamins and minerals will insure that your digestive enzymes will be able to quickly reactivate. Raw foods contain their own enzymes that help your digestive tract do its job.

The surface of the small intestine is designed to absorb the nutrients your body has worked so hard to extract from your food and turn them over to the bloodstream and liver for processing. Your small intestine is 22 feet long, with an inside surface lined with tiny finger-like protuberances called *villi*. These protrusions greatly increase the available surface area for absorption of nutrients to a whopping 2,000 square feet—a little bigger than half of a football field.

LEAKY GUT SYNDROME AND FOOD ALLERGIES

Your small intestine is vulnerable to harm due to poor diet, certain drugs or disease. If the villi are damaged, food isn't well-absorbed and what is known as "leaky gut syndrome" can result. In a healthy intestine, nutrients are "tagged" by specialized immune cells so that the body will recognize them as safe. Without these tags, needed nutrients are treated as foreign invaders and your immune system creates antibodies to destroy them. In a damaged gut your tagging mechanism is not up to par and food allergy results. The symptoms of food allergy can be as diverse as fatigue, a chronic rash, headaches and arthritis.

Food allergy is created in a damaged gut when microscopic holes in the intestinal lining allow undigested food molecules to escape into the bloodstream. The immune system can't recognize these molecules and so it sends out its battalions in an effort to destroy them. An immune system that's working overtime will definitely keep you from feeling your best, as anyone with allergies knows from experience. Food allergies have been implicated in a wide variety of digestive problems including constipation, diarrhea, Crohn's disease and irritable bowel syndrome.

If you think you might have leaky gut syndrome, you can ask a health professional to give you what's called the lactulose/mannitol absorption test. Levels of lactulose, a large molecule that shouldn't be passed into the bloodstream, are measured. Elevated levels are a good indication that your gut is leaky. Medical testing for delayed food allergies can be done by your doctor; the ELISA/ACT test, cytotoxic testing, ALCAT testing and the IgA test are specific tests you can ask about.

Even as conventional physicians deny the existence of delayed food allergies, they can't cure many of the chronic digestive diseases such as Crohn's disease, irritable bowel syndrome (IBS), arthritis and auto-immune diseases, and yet health-care professionals such as naturo-pathic doctors who are treating these diseases as symptoms of food allergies are having success in treating them.

The causes and effects of food allergies are hard to separate. If your secretions of digestive juices aren't adequate, more undigested food particles pass into the small intestine and then potentially into the bloodstream through the damaged gut lining. Some damage may be done to the intestines by foods you have become allergic to. Some people are more susceptible to food allergy than others; if you weren't breastfed and were introduced to difficult-to-digest foods like grains or cow's milk too soon, you probably have some leaky gut and food allergy problems. When a child's delicate digestive system isn't ready to assimilate a food, it's quickly labeled as potentially harmful by the immune system. Immediate reactions such as diarrhea or vomiting can result, or there may be inflammatory responses like asthma and eczema.

For adults, some of the causes of food allergy can be chronic stress, drugs that knock the secretion of digestive juices out of balance, poor diet or overindulgence in alcohol. Any number of environmental tox-ins including pesticides, food additives, intestinal parasites and heavy metals can bring on delayed food allergy in adults.

THE LARGE INTESTINE AND PROBIOTICS

Once your meal has passed through the twists and turns of the small intestine, the nutrients available for absorption have been drawn into the bloodstream. In the lower part of the small intestine, where it meets the large intestine, the vitamins B12, A, D and E are absorbed. A sphincter called the *ileocecal valve* controls the flow of waste into the large intestine. If your digestion isn't good, there is probably some undigested food remaining as well, which can cause gas and bloating as colon bacteria break it down by fermenting it. Irritable bowel syndrome is what physicians often diagnose in people with this complaint and a wide variety of other gastrointestinal complaints including constipation, diarrhea and abdominal cramping.

As waste moves through the colon, water and minerals are pulled from it back into the body. A solid mass of feces is formed and is eventually excreted through the rectum and anus during a bowel movement.

The bacteria that reside in your colon are indispensable for good digestive health. Generically known as *probiotics*, these friendly bacteria are also found in the urinary tract, the mouth and the vagina. In the intestines probiotics have a variety of jobs. They do battle with foreign bacteria that might otherwise cause infection; they manufacture some vitamins, such as vitamin K; and they keep the growth of a fungal yeast called *Candida albicans* under control. All told, we play host to 100 trillion friendly bacteria belonging to at least 400 different species.

Prescription drugs like antibiotics and steroids, undue stress and nutritional imbalances all contribute to the demise of good bacteria. When their numbers are low, bad bacteria and Candida albicans become overgrown. Yeast overgrowth in particular can cause many unpleasant symptoms. If you suffer from bloating, gas, unusual fatigue, diarrhea, constipation, skin problems, headaches, mental fogginess, joint pains or environmental allergies, yeast overgrowth could be a culprit. This problem is especially common during and following treatment with antibiotics, so you should always follow a course of antibiotics with two weeks or more of probiotic supplementation.

You can buy refrigerated capsules containing acidophilus, bifidus and other friendly strains of bacteria in your local health food store. Fructooligosaccharides (FOS), a kind of sugar found plentifully in bananas that enhances the growth of probiotics, are another ingredient you should look for in a probiotic supplement.

YOU CAN PREVENT COLON CANCER

Living a lifestyle that maintains a healthy colon will protect you against colon cancer, a disease that strikes about 160,000 people each year and kills more than 57,000 people each year. It is estimated that 68 percent of colon cancers could be prevented and the evidence is piling up. A genetic predisposition in some people can't be discounted, but no matter what your genes are programmed for, you can reduce your risk by doing a few simple things to prevent constipation and to keep the bowel from being exposed to toxins day in and day out.

Your first step towards good colon health is to eat more fiber and avoid constipation. Fiber is an effective sponge that absorbs cancer-causing toxins and sweeps them out of the body in the feces. Hard, difficult-to-pass stools sit in the colon for too long. Toxins that should have been passed out of the body unabsorbed are more likely to seep back into the bloodstream or to cause damage to the colon itself.

The trace mineral selenium is your top colon health supplement. People who live in areas where the soil is high in selenium have dramatically lower rates of colon cancer.

The other biggest known risk factors for colon cancer are folic acid deficiency and high alcohol consumption (which interferes with folic acid synthesis). In fact, a folic acid deficiency is associated with many types of cancer, and supplementing it has repeatedly been shown to reverse cervical dysplasia, a precancerous growth in the cervix. A small but pioneering study done some 10 years ago showed that supplementation with folic acid significantly decreased precancerous lung cells in smokers.

Folic acid is a B vitamin found in fresh, leafy, dark green vegetables such as spinach and kale, turnips, endive, asparagus, wheat bran, yeasts and liver. It plays an important role in the synthesis of RNA and DNA, and thus in the process of cell division and growth. Chromosomes are more likely to have breaks if the cell is deficient in folic acid, creating the cell changes associated with cancers.

People who take aspirin regularly have been found to have lower rates of colon cancer, but aspirin may be acting as a stand-in for folic acid. Aspirin and folic acid compete for some of the same receptor sites in cells. If you're concerned about preventing colon cancer, be sure to take a daily folic acid supplement and save the aspirin for occasional use only.

If you're taking the recommended dosages of daily vitamins (see Chapter 8), you're getting all the folic acid you need. If you have had colon cancer or are at a high risk for colon cancer, you can take an additional 400 mcg of folic acid daily as a preventive measure, as well as 1,000 mcg daily of sublingual or intranasal vitamin B12, which works hand-in-hand with folic acid. You can find both vitamins at your health food store.

PRESCRIPTION AND OVER-THE-COUNTER DRUGS FOR THE DIGESTIVE SYSTEM

H2 Blockers

CIMETIDINE (Tagamet)

FAMOTIDINE (Pepcid)

NIZATIDINE (Axid)

RANITIDINE (Zantac)

WHAT DO THEY DO IN THE BODY?

H2 blockers block acid production in the stomach. They make up a class of drugs which block the stomach's response to acid stimulators such as food, caffeine, insulin and histamine. The H2 blockers, once sold as anti-ulcer drugs, are now being marketed as antiheartburn agents, sold over the counter. They are different enough so that even though they are in the same class of drugs, we'll cover each drug and its effects separately.

You know from the first few pages of this chapter that ulcers aren't caused by excessive stomach acid production, but by bacteria. Most adults actually produce too little stomach acid. When ulcers are already established, it may help in the healing process to further reduce acid production, but in the long run this strategy can be counterproductive and doesn't deal with the root of the problem, which is probably *H. pylori* infection. Some of these drugs are used as part of an *H. pylori* eradication regime.

H2 blockers can cause mineral imbalances in the body. Calcium, phosphorus and magnesium levels are affected. Vitamin B12 isn't absorbed well by people using H2 blockers. If you have an allergy to one of the H2 blockers, you shouldn't use any of them. If you are using H2 blockers over the counter, don't use the maximum dose for more than two weeks at a time without consulting with your physician. If you have symptoms like difficulty swallowing or persistent abdominal pain, you should think twice about using H2 blockers over the counter.

Any acid-blocking medication interacts with the food you eat. Inadequate acid production in the stomach means that your ability to digest what you eat is impaired and your body may not be able to absorb nutrients properly. The valve that must open to allow food to pass from the stomach into the small intestine is triggered by the acidity of the stomach's contents and heartburn can result if acid levels are low and food sits too long in the stomach.

If you are using an acid-reducing medication for more than a week, be sure to use an intranasal or sublingual vitamin B12 supplement in addition to your multivitamin.

RANITIDINE (Zantac)

WHAT IS IT USED FOR?

Treatment of duodenal or gastric ulcer, gastroesophageal reflux disease (heartburn), erosive esophagitis, heartburn, *H. pylori* eradication, treatment of Zollinger-Ellison syndrome (a condition that causes oversecretion of stomach acid), prevention of damage of the gastrointestinal lining that can result from long-term use of nonsteroidal anti-inflammatory drugs (NSAIDs), prevention of stress ulcers, control of upper gastrointestinal bleeding.

WHAT ARE THE POSSIBLE SIDE EFFECTS/ADVERSE REACTIONS?

Zantac adversely affects the liver's ability to detoxify other drugs you may be taking. That could mean that other drugs will have magnified effects on your body. Other possible side effects include severe headache, sleepiness or fatigue, diarrhea, stomach pain and itching. Very rarely there may be a decrease in the number of blood cells, vertigo, blurred vision and blood pressure and liver function changes.

CAUTION! THINK TWICE ABOUT TAKING THIS DRUG IF . . .

- You have any of a group of disorders known as *porphyria*.
- You have kidney or liver problems.
- You are under 16 years of age.

WHAT ARE THE INTERACTIONS WITH OTHER DRUGS?

Ranitidine may raise levels or prolong the effects of:

↑ Ethanol (alcohol)
  Procainamide
  Sulfonylureas (used for adult-onset diabetes)
  Theophyllines
  Warfarin

Ranitidine may cause the following drugs to be reduced in potency or decreased in the amount of time they are effective:

↓ Diazepam
  Ketoconazole (an antifungal drug)

These drugs may reduce the effects of ranitidine:

↓ Antacids
  Gastrointestinal anticholinergics used to treat irritable bowel
    syndrome

FAMOTIDINE (Pepcid, Pepcid AC)

WHAT IS IT USED FOR?

Duodenal and stomach ulcer, heartburn, acid indigestion, sour stomach, Zollinger-Ellison syndrome (a condition that causes oversecretion of stomach acid).

WHAT ARE THE POSSIBLE SIDE EFFECTS/ADVERSE REACTIONS?

Headache, sleepiness, fatigue, dizziness, confusion, diarrhea, growth of breasts in males (gynecomastia), kidney or liver impairment, impotence, loss of appetite, dry mouth, musculoskeletal pain, numbness, acne, dry or peeling skin, flushing, ringing in the ears, changes in sense of taste, fever, heart palpitations and itching.

CAUTION! THINK TWICE ABOUT TAKING THIS DRUG IF . . .

• You have kidney or liver problems.

HOW DOES THIS DRUG INTERACT WITH FOOD?

Food increases the absorption of famotidine.

NIZATIDINE (Axid)

WHAT IS IT USED FOR?

Duodenal and stomach ulcer, heartburn, acid indigestion, sour stomach, erosive esophagitis, gastroesophageal reflux disease, prevention of upper gastrointestinal bleeding.

WHAT ARE THE POSSIBLE SIDE EFFECTS/ADVERSE REACTIONS?

Sleepiness, fatigue, dizziness, diarrhea, constipation, sweating, heart rhythm irregularities, a rise in uric acid levels in the bloodstream, changes in blood cell counts, fever.

WHAT ARE THE INTERACTIONS WITH OTHER DRUGS?

Nizatidine increases blood levels of salicylates (aspirin).
It can make alcohol's effects on you more pronounced.
If you are using antacids, they can make nizatidine less effective.

CIMETIDINE (Tagamet, Tagamet HB)

WHAT DOES IT DO IN THE BODY?

Cimetidine blocks acid production in the stomach.

WHAT IS IT USED FOR?

Duodenal and stomach ulcer, heartburn, acid indigestion, sour stomach, erosive esophagitis, gastroesophageal reflux disease, Zollinger-Ellison syndrome, prevention of upper gastrointestinal bleeding. It has also been used to treat hyperparathyroidism, chronic viral warts in children, prevention of stress ulcers, herpes virus infections, excessive body hair growth in women and dyspepsia (general symptoms of stomach upset, heartburn, nausea, lack of appetite).

WHAT ARE THE POSSIBLE SIDE EFFECTS/ADVERSE REACTIONS?

Headache, sleepiness, fatigue, dizziness, confusion, hallucinations, diarrhea, breast development in males (gynecomastia), impotence. Rarely, side effects can include inflammation of the pancreas, effects on the liver, changes in blood cell counts or immune function, skin problems, cardiac arrhythmias or arrest, joint pain and hypersensitivity reactions.

In people with arthritis, cimetidine may aggravate joint symptoms; stopping the drug reverses this effect. Severely ill people, especially those with compromised liver or kidney function, may experience mental confusion, agitation, psychosis, anxiety or disorientation when given this drug (which is reversible when the drug is discontinued).

There is some evidence that cimetidine may impair male fertility.

CAUTION! THINK TWICE ABOUT TAKING THIS DRUG IF . . .

- You have impaired kidney or liver function. People with liver or kidney disease can't clear the drug from their systems as rapidly as others and so blood concentrations may be too high. This is a common concern for elderly people.

WHAT ARE THE INTERACTIONS WITH OTHER DRUGS?

Cimetidine may raise levels or prolong the effects of these drugs:

↑ Antiarrhythmic drugs like amiodarone, procainamide and quinidine
Benzodiazepines
Beta-blocker drugs like labetalol
Caffeine
Calcium channel blockers (nifedipine)
Carbamazepine
Carmustine,* a chemotherapy drug; increased bone marrow suppression may result
Chloroquine
Coumadin*
Ethanol (alcohol)
Flecainide
Fluorouracil
Lidocaine
Metoprolol

Metronidazole
Moricizine
Narcotic analgesics*
Pentoxifylline
Phenytoin
Procainamide
Propafenone
Propranolol
Quinine
Succinylcholine*
Sulfonylureas
Tacrine
Terfenadine
Theophyllines*
Triamterene
Tricyclic antidepressants
Valproic acid
Warfarin

Cimetidine may cause the following drugs to be reduced in potency or decreased in the amount of time they are effective:

↓ Digoxin
Ferrous salts
Fluconazole
Indomethacin

Ketoconazole
Tetracyclines
Tocainide

These drugs may decrease the effects of cimetidine:

↓ Antacids
Anticholinergics

Metoclopramide

*Potentially dangerous interaction.

WHAT ARE THE INTERACTIONS WITH FOOD?

Tyramine-rich foods like Bovril and English cheddar cheese can cause severe headache and can temporarily raise your blood pressure. Food delays the absorption of cimetidine.

Proton Pump Inhibitors

OMEPRAZOLE (Prilosec)

LANSOPRAZOLE (Prevacid)

Omeprazole (Prilosec) and lansoprazole (Prevacid) are proton pump inhibitors. They suppress stomach acid production by inhibiting the cellular mechanism that pumps acid into the stomach.

OMEPRAZOLE (Prilosec)

WHAT DOES IT DO IN THE BODY?

Suppresses stomach acid production. It is much more powerful than the H2 blockers in this respect.

WHAT IS IT USED FOR?

Gastric or duodenal ulcer, gastroesophageal reflux disease (heartburn), to maintain healing of erosive esophagitis, with antibiotics for eradication of *H. pylori*, treatment of Zollinger-Ellison syndrome (a condition that causes oversecretion of stomach acid).

WHAT ARE POSSIBLE SIDE EFFECTS/ADVERSE REACTIONS?

Headache, dizziness, weakness, diarrhea, abdominal pain, nausea, vomiting, constipation, upper respiratory infection, rash, cough, back pain, constipation.

Combination therapy with the antibiotic clarithromycin may cause your sense of taste to change, or may result in tongue discoloration, runny nose, inflammation of the pharynx, or flu-like symptoms.

Dozens of other cardiovascular, nervous system, gastrointestinal, urinary, metabolic, musculoskeletal and respiratory symptoms have been reported, but are rare. Severe rash (Stevens-Johnson syndrome), changes in blood cell counts, liver function, hearing and taste are other rarely observed side effects.

WHAT ARE THE INTERACTIONS WITH OTHER DRUGS?

Omeprazole may raise levels or prolong the effects of these drugs:

↑ Clarithromycin   Phenytoin
  Diazepam   Warfarin

The following drug may increase the effects or prolong the action of omeprazole:

↑ Clarithromycin

LANSOPRAZOLE (Prevacid)

WHAT DOES IT DO IN THE BODY?

Suppresses stomach acid production. It is much more powerful than the H2 blockers in this respect.

WHAT IS IT USED FOR?

Duodenal ulcer, healing and maintenance of erosive esophagitis, Zollinger-Ellison syndrome (a condition that causes oversecretion of stomach acid).

WHAT ARE THE POSSIBLE SIDE EFFECTS/ADVERSE REACTIONS?

Diarrhea, abdominal pain, nausea, headache.

CAUTION! THINK TWICE ABOUT TAKING THIS DRUG IF . . .

- You are elderly.

WHAT ARE THE INTERACTIONS WITH OTHER DRUGS?

Because of its profound, long-lasting inhibition of stomach acid secretion, lansoprazole can interfere with drugs that require a specific pH for absorption. The effects of the antifungal drug ketoconazole, the antibiotic ampicillin, iron salts and the heart drug digoxin can be decreased if given with lansoprazole.

If you are taking theophylline, lansoprazole can increase blood levels of this asthma drug.

The acid-reducing medication sucralfate can decrease levels of lansoprazole.

WHAT ARE THE INTERACTIONS WITH FOODS?

If taken after meals, the drug's effects are minimized. Take lansoprazole on an empty stomach.

MISCELLANEOUS DRUGS FOR HEARTBURN AND OTHER STOMACH DISORDERS

SUCRALFATE (Carafate)

WHAT DOES IT DO IN YOUR BODY?

It creates a sticky gel in your stomach or small intestine which binds to ulcers, protecting them from further burning and ulceration by stomach acid.

WHAT IS IT USED FOR?

Treatment of stomach and duodenal ulcers

WHAT ARE THE POSSIBLE SIDE EFFECTS?

Constipation, dry mouth, diarrhea, nausea, stomachache, gas, indigestion, headache, insomnia, sleepiness, dizziness or back pain.

CAUTION!

- If you develop a rash, swelling, or have trouble breathing, you may be allergic to sucralfate.
- Those with kidney problems should not take this drug with aluminum-containing antacids. Sucralfate contains aluminum and the two combined could bring too much of the mineral into the body at once for weakened kidneys to handle.
- This drug should be used with caution if you have kidney failure or need dialysis.
- Because of its high aluminum content, there doesn't seem to be any good reason to use this drug.

WHAT ARE THE INTERACTIONS WITH OTHER DRUGS?

The following drugs may be reduced in potency or decreased in the amount of time they are effective when taken with sucralfate:

↓ Cimetidine (Tagamet)   Phenytoin
Ciprofloxacin   Ranitidine (Zantac)
Digoxin   Tetracycline
Ketoconazole   Theophylline

WHAT ARE THE INTERACTIONS WITH FOOD?

Take this drug on an empty stomach, at least one hour before meals.

CISAPRIDE (Propulsid)

WHAT DOES IT DO IN THE BODY?

Cisapride increases the contractions of the stomach and small intestine that propel food along the digestive tract.

WHAT IS IT USED FOR?

Treatment of nighttime heartburn.

WHAT ARE THE POSSIBLE SIDE EFFECTS/ADVERSE REACTIONS?

Diarrhea, abdominal pain, nausea, constipation, flatulence, stomach discomfort, runny nose, sinus congestion, upper respiratory infection, coughing, urinary tract infection, frequent urination, pain, fever, headache, insomnia, anxiety, rash, increased susceptibility to infection.

CAUTION! DON'T TAKE THIS DRUG IF . . .

- You have gastrointestinal hemorrhage, obstruction or perforation.
- This drug interacts dangerously with so many other drugs that there doesn't seem to be any good reason to use it unless absolutely nothing else works.

WHAT ARE THE INTERACTIONS WITH OTHER DRUGS?

Cisapride may raise levels or prolong the effects of these drugs:

↑ Anticoagulants*

These drugs may reduce the effects of cisapride:

↓ Anticholinergic drugs

These drugs may increase or prolong the action of cisapride:

↑ Azole antifungals*
 H2 blockers (for ulcer treatment), especially cimetidine (Tagamet), ranitidine (Zantac)
 Macrolide antibiotics*

WHAT ARE THE INTERACTIONS WITH FOOD?

Because food is moved more quickly through the digestive tract, there may be alterations in the way your body absorbs nutrients and water. Your body may not get the nutrients it needs.

---

*Potentially dangerous interaction.

DICYCLOMINE (Bentyl, Byclomine, Di-Spaz, Antispas, Dibent, Dilomine, Or-Tyl)

WHAT DOES IT DO IN THE BODY?

Decreases the muscular contractions of the gastrointestinal tract. It also has this effect on the gallbladder and urinary tract.

WHAT IS IT USED FOR?

Treatment of irritable bowel syndrome (IBS), which can have a wide variety of symptoms including constipation, diarrhea, gas and abdominal cramping. Your physician may also refer to the problem as irritable colon or spastic colon. This drug is also used in the treatment of mucous colitis.

WHAT ARE THE POSSIBLE SIDE EFFECTS/ADVERSE REACTIONS?

Dicyclomine may cause drowsiness, blurred vision and dizziness. Use caution while driving.

Other possible side effects include dry mouth, altered taste, nausea, vomiting, difficulty swallowing, heartburn, constipation, a bloated feeling, intestinal obstruction, difficulty urinating, impotence, blurred vision, abnormal dilation of the pupils, increased sensitivity to light (photophobia), paralysis of the muscles that dilate the pupils, increased pressure of the fluid within the eyes, heart rhythm irregularities, headache, flushing, nervousness, drowsiness, weakness, dizziness, confusion, insomnia, fever (especially in children), mental confusion or overexcitement (especially in the elderly), rash, itching, nasal congestion, decreased sweating, suppression of milk production in nursing mothers.

CAUTION!

This drug is potentially harmful in such a wide variety of situations that its use does not seem justified unless absolutely nothing else works. Don't take this drug if . . .

- You have narrow-angle glaucoma, severe heart problems, any kind of obstructive gastrointestinal disease, chronic constriction of intestinal walls (achalasia), blockage between the stomach and small intestine, cardiospasm (where the muscles in your esophagus and intestines contract and won't relax, blocking the passage of food), paralytic ileus (where the intestinal walls don't contract), severe ulcerative colitis, toxic megacolon (an extremely dilated colon, a complication of ulcerative colitis), kidney disease, myasthenia gravis, or liver disease.
- You are elderly or debilitated and have a condition called intestinal atony (reduced muscle tone in your intestines).
- You have trouble urinating, which may be due to an enlarged prostate gland.

Dicyclomine HCl should not be given to infants under six months of age.

This drug should be used cautiously in people with the following conditions: open-angle glaucoma, ulcerative colitis, hiatal hernia, enlarged prostate, coronary artery disease, heart failure, heart arrhythmias, high blood pressure, chronic respiratory disease (dicyclomine reduces bronchial secretions, which can lead to plugging of bronchial tubes) such as asthma or allergy, autonomic neuropathy and hyperthyroidism.

If you are sensitive to either tartrazine or sulfites, you should know that these are contained in some gastrointestinal antispasmodic drugs. People who are sensitive to aspirin are often also sensitive to tartrazine. Asthma symptoms or anaphylaxis, a life-threatening allergic reaction, may result from sulfite sensitivity.

WHAT ARE THE INTERACTIONS WITH OTHER DRUGS?

The high blood pressure drug atenolol and the heart drug digoxin increase dicyclomine's pharmacologic effects.

Amantadine and tricyclic antidepressants may worsen side effects such as dry mouth, constipation and difficulty urinating.

WHAT ARE THE INTERACTIONS WITH FOODS?

You should take dicyclomine on an empty stomach, one-half to one hour before a meal.

Antacids

ALUMINUM CARBONATE GEL (Basaljel)

ALUMINUM HYDROXIDE GEL (Amphojel, Alu-tab, Alu-Cap, Dialume)

CALCIUM CARBONATE (Amitone, Mallamint, Dicarbosil, Equilet, Tums, Chooz, Maalox Antacid Caplets, Mylanta)

MAGNESIUM HYDROXIDE (Phillips' Chewable, Milk of Magnesia)

MAGNESIUM OXIDE (Mag-Ox 400, Maox 420, Uro-Mag)

MAGALDRATE (Riopan, Iosopan)

SODIUM BICARBONATE (Bell/ans)

SODIUM CITRATE (Citra pH)

Antacids are some of the biggest selling over-the-counter drugs in pharmacies. But these drugs not only don't treat the underlying problem, they may actually make the symptoms worse. Although antacids such as Mylanta, Rolaids and Tums can temporarily suppress the symptoms of heartburn, in the long run they'll do you more harm than good. You may even become dependent upon them. These over-the-counter medications help neutralize the acid in your stomach for up to an hour. That's fine for the moment, but your stomach may respond an hour later by producing even more acid to make up for what was neutralized, causing you to reach for more antacids. They also contain aluminum, silicone, sugar and a long list of dyes and preservatives. Your stomach acid is one of your front-line defenses against harmful bacteria. Suppress it and the rest of your systems have to work overtime to protect you.

WHAT DO THEY DO IN YOUR BODY?

Antacids neutralize stomach acid. By increasing the pH of the stomach and duodenum (the first part of the small intestine), they also inhibit the action of the enzyme pepsin, which breaks down proteins. Antacids also increase the tone of the sphincter between the esophagus and the stomach, which decreases the likelihood of gastroesophageal reflux (heartburn).

WHAT ARE THEY USED FOR?

Relief of upset stomach, heartburn, acid indigestion and sour stomach. Aluminum- and magnesium-based antacids are also used to prevent stress ulcer bleeding and antacids are often used in the treatment of ulcers.

WHAT ARE THE POSSIBLE SIDE EFFECTS?

Magnesium-containing antacids may cause diarrhea.

Aluminum-containing antacids can cause constipation, intestinal blockage or dangerously high body levels of aluminum. There is no conceivable reason to use aluminum-containing antacids.

Antacids may cause rebound acid production, where acid levels rise above normal once the antacid wears off.

Use of high doses of calcium carbonate and sodium bicarbonate at the same time can lead to *milk-alkali* syndrome. Symptoms are headache, nausea, irritability, weakness, electrolyte imbalances and kidney damage.

Long-term use of aluminum-containing antacids can lead to phosphate depletion (hypophosphatemia) if intake of this mineral isn't adequate. Hypophosphatemia can lead to loss of appetite, exhaustion, weakness and bone problems.

Antacids can deplete calcium levels. Using antacids such as Tums as a source of calcium is not useful, since at best it will replace what the antacid is blocking.

CAUTION! THINK TWICE ABOUT USING THESE TYPES OF DRUGS IF . . .

- You have hypertension, congestive heart failure, kidney failure or if you are on a low-sodium diet. Most antacids are very high in sodium, so look for a low-sodium version.
- You are undergoing dialysis. Avoid aluminum-containing antacids. (I recommend avoiding aluminum-containing antacids, period.)
- You have had recent gastrointestinal hemorrhage. Use aluminum hydroxide with care.

WHAT ARE THE INTERACTIONS WITH OTHER DRUGS?

Aluminum antacids may cause the following drugs to be reduced in potency or decreased in the amount of time they are effective:

↓ Allopurinol   Iron
  Chloroquine   Isoniazid
  Corticosteroids   Penicillamine
  Diflusinal   Phenothiazines
  Digoxin   Tetracyclines
  Ethambutol   Thyroid hormones
  H2 blockers   Ticlopidine

Calcium antacids may cause the following drugs to be reduced in potency or decreased in the amount of time they are effective:

↓ Fluoroquinolones   Salicylates (aspirin)
  Hydantoins   Tetracyclines
  Iron

Magnesium antacids may cause the following drugs to be reduced in potency or decreased in the amount of time they are effective:

↓ Benzodiazepines   Iron
  Chloroquine   Nitrofurantoin
  Corticosteroids   Penicillamine
  Digoxin   Phenothiazines
  H2 blockers   Tetracyclines
  Hydantoins   Ticlopidine

Sodium bicarbonate antacids may cause the following drugs to be reduced in potency or decreased in the amount of time they are effective:

↓ Benzodiazepines
  Iron
  Ketoconazole
  Levodopa
  Lithium

  Methenamine
  Methotrexate
  Salicylates
  Sulfonylureas
  Tetracyclines

Magnesium-aluminum antacids may cause the following drugs to be reduced in potency or decreased in the amount of time they are effective:

↓ Benzodiazepines
  Captopril
  Corticosteroids
  Fluoroquinolones
  H2 blockers
  Hydantoins
  Iron

  Ketoconazole
  Penicillamine
  Phenothiazines
  Salicylates
  Tetracyclines
  Ticlopidine

Aluminum antacids may raise levels or prolong the action of:

↑ Benzodiazepines

Calcium antacids may raise levels or prolong the action of:

↑ Quinidine

Magnesium antacids may raise levels or prolong the action of the following drugs:

↑ Dicumarol
  Quinidine
  Sulfonylureas

Sodium bicarbonate antacids may raise levels or prolong the actions of:

↑ Amphetamines   Quinidine
  Flecainide   Sympathomimetics

Magnesium-aluminum combinations may raise levels or prolong the actions of:

↑ Levodopa   Sulfonylureas
  Quinidine   Valproic acid

How Do Antacids Interact with Nutrients?

Aluminum- and magnesium-containing antacids can bind with phosphate and deplete the body of calcium, resulting in weakening of bones. Phosphate depletion can cause muscle weakness.

Vitamins A, B1(thiamin) and D are not well-absorbed or are destroyed if antacids are in your system.

Antacids in general block the action of stomach acid, reducing the absorption of nutrients.

Anti-Diarrhea Drugs

DIFENOXIN WITH ATROPINE SULFATE

DIPHENOXYLATE WITH ATROPINE SULFATE

LOPERAMIDE

BISMUTH SUBSALICYLATE

Diarrhea is your body's way of getting rid of substances that are harmful to your body. When you have diarrhea, food containing bacteria or viruses can be flushed out of the body quickly. You may also have diarrhea when you eat certain foods that don't agree with you. If diarrhea goes on for more than five days, you may have a medical problem that needs attention. Severe diarrhea in infants, children or the elderly should get medical attention within three days, since they can rapidly become dangerously dehydrated.

DIFENOXIN WITH ATROPINE SULFATE (Motofen)

WHAT DOES IT DO IN YOUR BODY?

Slows the contractions of the intestines so that their contents move through more slowly.

WHAT IS IT USED FOR?

Treatment of diarrhea.

WHAT ARE THE POSSIBLE SIDE EFFECTS/ADVERSE EFFECTS?

Nausea, vomiting, dry mouth, upset stomach, constipation, dizziness, lightheadedness, drowsiness, headache, burning eyes, blurred vision.

In some people, especially children, atropine (an ingredient of this drug) may cause skin and mucous membrane dryness, flushing, low body temperature, fast heartbeat and difficulty urinating.

CAUTION! DON'T USE THIS DRUG IF . . .

- Your diarrhea could be caused by bacteria such as *E. coli*, salmonella or shigella.
- You have been taking broad-spectrum antibiotics.
- You have colitis.
- You have jaundice.
- You have narrow-angle glaucoma or adhesions between the iris and lens of the eye.
- You have a heart condition such as rapid heartbeat or angina, gastrointestinal obstructive disease, urinary problems or myasthenia gravis.
- You have liver or kidney disease. Use difenoxin with caution.

DIPHENOXYLATE WITH ATROPINE SULFATE (Logen, Lomotil, Lonox, Lomanate)

WHAT DOES IT DO IN YOUR BODY?

It has a constipating effect, making feces more solid.

WHAT IS IT USED FOR?

Treatment of diarrhea.

WHAT ARE THE POSSIBLE SIDE EFFECTS/ADVERSE EFFECTS?

If you are hypersensitive to diphenoxylate, you may experience rash, swelling in the gums and elsewhere, or a life-threatening allergic reaction called anaphylaxis.

Other potential side effects include dizziness, drowsiness, sedation, headache, general feeling of not being well, lethargy, euphoria, depression, confusion, numbness of the extremities, loss of appetite, vomiting, abdominal discomfort, problems with the natural movements of the intestines, or inflammation of the pancreas.

CAUTION! DON'T USE THIS DRUG IF . . .

- Your diarrhea could be caused by bacteria such as *E. coli*, salmonella or shigella, if you have been taking broad-spectrum antibiotics or have colitis.
- You have liver or kidney disease. Use diphenoxylate with caution.

WHAT ARE THE INTERACTIONS WITH OTHER DRUGS?

If used with monoamine oxidase (MAO) inhibitors, blood pressure can shoot up suddenly.

If used with barbiturates, tranquilizers or alcohol, the depressant action of these drugs can be increased.

LOPERAMIDE (Diar-Aid, Imodium A-D, Kaopectate, Maalox, Neo-Diaral, Pepto Diarrhea Control)

WHAT DOES IT DO IN YOUR BODY?

Decreases the movement of the intestines and slows water and electrolyte transfer into the bowel.

WHAT IS IT USED FOR?

Treatment of diarrhea.

WHAT ARE THE POSSIBLE SIDE EFFECTS/ADVERSE EFFECTS?

Usually minor, they include abdominal pain, distention or discomfort, constipation, dry mouth, nausea, vomiting, tiredness, dizziness or skin rash.

CAUTION! DON'T USE THIS DRUG IF . . .

- You have a disease that would be worsened by constipation.
- You have bloody diarrhea or a fever above 101°F.
- Your diarrhea could be caused by bacteria such as *E. coli*, salmonella or shigella.
- You have been taking broad-spectrum antibiotics.
- You have acute ulcerative colitis. Loperamide can cause your colon to become very distended and unable to do its job properly.

Use with caution if you have kidney problems.

BISMUTH SUBSALICYLATE (Bismatrol, Pepto-Bismol)

WHAT DOES IT DO IN YOUR BODY?

It suppresses secretions into the intestines, decreases inflammation and has some antimicrobial effects.

WHAT IS IT USED FOR?

Treatment of diarrhea, nausea, indigestion, abdominal cramps. It is also used with antibiotics to treat *H. pylori* infection.

WHAT ARE THE POSSIBLE SIDE EFFECTS/ADVERSE EFFECTS?

Severe constipation can occur in debilitated people and infants. Feces may temporarily be gray or black.

CAUTION! DON'T USE THIS DRUG IF . . .

- Diarrhea is accompanied by high fever or continues for more than two days.

WHAT ARE THE INTERACTIONS WITH OTHER DRUGS?

This drug can increase the potency of aspirin. It can also decrease the absorption of tetracyclines.

CAUTION! THINK TWICE ABOUT USING THIS DRUG IF . . .

- Constipation is not relieved with laxatives.
- There is rectal bleeding, muscle cramps, weakness or dizziness. Call your health professional.
- You are on a salt-restricted diet. Look for low-sodium versions of these antidiarrheal drugs.
- You have congestive heart failure or kidney disease. Dangerous electrolyte imbalances can occur.

DRUGS FOR CONSTIPATION

SALINE LAXATIVES

IRRITANTS/STIMULANTS

BULK-PRODUCING LAXATIVES

LUBRICANTS

SURFACTANTS

Drugs for constipation fall into several categories, all with different mechanisms of action for bringing about a bowel movement. Some are taken orally while others can be used as suppositories or enemas. Any of these laxatives can result in dependency if used for too long. Your digestive system essentially "forgets" how to have a bowel movement without them.

SALINE LAXATIVES (Epsom salts, Milk of Magnesia, Citrate of Magnesium, Fleet Phospho-Soda, Sodium Phosphates)

WHAT DO THEY DO IN YOUR BODY?

Draw water and electrolytes into the intestines to make feces softer.

WHAT ARE THE POTENTIAL SIDE EFFECTS/ADVERSE EFFECTS?

May alter the body's fluid and electrolyte balance.

WHAT ELSE TO DO WHEN TAKING THESE DRUGS

Drink plenty of water and use a mineral supplement containing magnesium and potassium.

IRRITANTS/STIMULANTS (cascara sagrada, phenolphthalein, senna, bisacodyl, castor oil; brand names include Ex-Lax, Espotabs, Feen-A-Mint, Modane, Evac-U-Gen, Medilax, Senexon, Senolax, Senokot, Dulcagen, Dulcolax, Fleet Laxative, Bisco-Lux)

WHAT DO THEY DO IN YOUR BODY?

Stimulate the intestinal walls to move feces through the intestinal tract. They also alter water and electrolyte secretion into the gut. Evacuation is rapid and complete, so these drugs are often used before surgery or in very severe cases of constipation.

WHAT ARE THE POSSIBLE SIDE EFFECTS/ADVERSE EFFECTS?

Too-frequent use results in loss of electrolytes (especially potassium) and dehydration; the colon may become unable to contract on its own. Cascara sagrada, phenolphthalein and senna can discolor feces.

BULK-PRODUCING LAXATIVES (methylcellulose, psyllium, polycarbophil; brand names include Citrucel, Unifiber, Maltsupex, FiberCon, Equalactin, Mitrolan, FiberNorm, FiberLax, Fiberall, Genfiber, Hydrocil, Konsyl, Maalox Daily Fiber, Metamucil, Mylanta Natural Fiber, Reguloid, Restore, Serutan, Syllact, Modane Bulk, V-Lax)

WHAT DO THEY DO IN YOUR BODY?

These drugs are basically fiber which holds water in feces to make them softer and easier to evacuate, and gives them bulk.

WHAT ARE THEY USED FOR?

Psyllium is useful in irritable bowel syndrome, spastic colon and hemorrhoids. LDL cholesterol can be lowered up to 20 percent with psyllium.

Polycarbophil also is used to treat irritable bowel syndrome and diverticulosis.

WHAT ARE THE POSSIBLE SIDE EFFECTS/ADVERSE EFFECTS?

Bulk-forming agents are the safest method to use for relief of constipation. Excessive bowel activity (diarrhea, nausea, vomiting), anal irritation, bloating, flatulence, abdominal cramping, weakness, dizziness, fainting, sweating, or palpitations happen rarely.

Esophageal, stomach, small intestinal and rectal obstruction have been reported with bulk laxatives. Be sure to take them with plenty of water.

LUBRICANTS (castor oil, mineral oil; brand names include Fleet Flavored Castor Oil, Purge, Neoloid, Neo-Cuetol, Milkinol)

WHAT DO THEY DO IN YOUR BODY?

These oils don't allow water from the feces to be absorbed back into the body through the walls of the colon, so that bowel contents don't dry out.

WHAT ARE THE POSSIBLE SIDE EFFECTS/ADVERSE EFFECTS?

Large doses of mineral oil can cause leakage from the anus, anal itching, irritation, hemorrhoids and general anal discomfort.

WHAT ARE THE INTERACTIONS WITH FOOD?

Lubricants may decrease the absorption of fat-soluble vitamins such as A, D and E.

SURFACTANTS (Docusate; brand names include Dialose, Regutol, Colace, Disonate, DOK, DOS Softgel, Regulax, Dioeze, Correctol, Sulfalax Calcium, Diocto-K)

WHAT DO THEY DO IN YOUR BODY?

Surfactants help to mix fats with the contents of the colon, which makes stools softer and bowel movements easier.

WHAT ARE THEY USED FOR?

Treatment of diarrhea, or in conditions like anal fissure or hemorrhoids where passing firm stool is painful.

Miscellaneous Laxatives

Glycerin suppositories draw extra water into the colon and cause slight irritation of the colon walls, stimulating contractions.

Lactulose (Chronulac, Constilac, Dulphalac) brings more water and electrolytes into the colon. Diabetics shouldn't use lactulose. It can cause flatulence, belching, abdominal cramping, nausea and vomiting.

NATURAL ALTERNATIVES FOR TREATING DIARRHEA

Although it's uncomfortable and inconvenient to have diarrhea, your best bet is to let nature take its course. Allow your body to cleanse itself unless the diarrhea is severe or lasts for more than a day or two. Drink at least eight large glasses of water a day while you have diarrhea. You can try a sports drink that contains replacement electrolytes. Stay away from caffeine, soft drinks and sugary foods. As soon as you feel well enough, eat foods like rice, cereal, bananas and potatoes which are rich in carbohydrates and gentle on your stomach.

If you have chronic diarrhea, try to figure out if foods are causing it. Lactose intolerance, an allergy to milk sugars, can cause diarrhea when dairy products are eaten.

Use probiotics or yogurt to help put your body back into balance after a bout of diarrhea. A mineral supplement containing magnesium and potassium will restore your body's depleted electrolyte stores.

NATURAL ALTERNATIVES TO ULCER DRUGS

The bacteria *H. pylori* is found in 90 percent of duodenal ulcer and 70 percent of stomach ulcer patients. This bacteria increases your risk of insufficient acid secretion (atrophic gastritis), ulcer and stomach cancer. Your doctor can give you a *Helicobacter pylori* IgG antibody blood test to see if this nasty little bacteria is at the root of your problem. If it is, you'll be put on a course of antibiotics and a bismuth preparation (you know it as Pepto-Bismol) for a week. This is one instance in which conventional medicines may be your best bet. Quick eradication of *H. pylori* is important for healing of ulcers. There are some herbal remedies you can try first, however, if you want to avoid antibiotics.

Licorice extract (deglycyrrizinated licorice or DGL) is a wonderful herbal healing aid for ulcers. It increases the production of protective mucus in the stomach. Use 300 mg four to six times a day. Unripe banana also has anti-ulcer effects, as do the herbs slippery elm (*Ulmus fulva*; take 200 mg four to six times a day), marshmallow root (*Althaea officinalis*; take 200 mg four to six times a day) and the juice of raw cabbage. You can buy extract of unripe plantain banana (*Musa paradisiaca*); take 150 mg four to six times a day.

If you have any type of ulcer, be sure to eliminate gastrointestinal irritants such as tobacco, NSAIDs, coffee and alcohol.

Once your ulcer has healed, try taking steps to enhance your body's secretion of digestive acids and enzymes to prevent a recurrence.

NATURAL ALTERNATIVES FOR TREATING HEARTBURN AND INSUFFICIENT ACID SECRETION

If you have chronic heartburn you probably know exactly what triggers it. If you don't, here are the most common culprits: overeating, or too much fat and/or fried food; processed meats with nitrates or nitrites in them; too much sugar, alcohol, chocolate, drugs, stress; clothes that fit tightly around the waist, obesity and pregnancy. Obesity, tight clothes and pregnancy put excess pressure on the esophageal muscle. Pregnancy also stimulates the release of hormones that relax the muscles so they will stretch to accommodate the growing baby—the esophagus muscles relax along with all the other ones.

Eating a balanced diet of unprocessed, organic whole foods is your foundation for a healthy stomach. Eat a green salad or raw vegetables at least once a day. Sprouted legumes and seeds are excellent sources of enzymes. Chew your food thoroughly.

Drinking cold or hot liquids with meals decreases stomach acid production. To help increase stomach acid, you can drink a glass of room temperature water a half-hour before eating. If that doesn't help, you can add a tablespoon of apple cider vinegar. If neither of those

10 GOOD REASONS TO THROW AWAY YOUR ANTACIDS

1. Rebound acid.
2. They block action of aspirin.
3. They block action of antibiotics.
4. They block action of quinidine.
5. They decrease iron and calcium absorption.
6. Metoclopramide (Reglan, Maxolon) increases absorption of alcohol.
7. An overly alkaline environment causes imbalances of intestinal flora, stresses kidneys and causes urinary tract infections.
8. Aluminum may be connected to Alzheimer's disease and slows digestion.
9. May cause diarrhea or constipation.
10. High sodium content.

DRUGS THAT CAN CAUSE HEARTBURN

Many prescription and over-the-counter drugs can cause or aggravate heartburn. Drugs that specifically relax the esophageal sphincter muscle, allowing stomach acid to reflux up, include: anticholinergics (such as drugs to treat Parkinson's), calcium channel blockers (heart disease drugs), nicotine and beta-blockers (to lower blood pressure and prevent spasms in the heart muscle).

Here is a list of other common offenders:

Antacids (can cause acid rebound and dependency)
Antibiotics
Antidepressants (fluoxetine, buspirone)
Asthma drugs (aminophylline, theophylline)
Chemotherapy drugs
Corticosteroids (prednisone)
Drugs that affect the heart and blood vessels, including drugs for lowering cholesterol and blood pressure, diuretics and beta-blockers.
Painkillers/narcotics (aspirin, acetaminophen, ibuprofen, naproxen, codeine, piroxicam, indomethacin)
Synthetic estrogens and progestins (Premarin, Provera)
Tranquilizers/barbiturates
Ulcer drugs (sulfasalazine, sucralfate, misoprostol)

solutions work, try taking a betaine hydrochloride supplement (HCl) *with* your meal. Follow the directions on the bottle, starting with the smallest dose and increasing it if needed. Do not take HCl supplements when you have an ulcer. Since stomach acid production declines as we age, HCl supplementation can be a good anti-aging strategy.

Natural heartburn therapies include deglycyrrhizinated licorice extract or DGL. Try one or two 380-mg tablets chewed and swallowed on an empty stomach, three to four times a day. A glass of room temperature water, raw cabbage or potato juice, or herbal teas such as fenugreek, slippery elm, comfrey, licorice and meadowsweet (lukewarm, no lemon) can bring quick relief. Fresh papaya or banana can help as well.

If you do need to lower your stomach acidity you can use a form of organic sulfur called MSM (methylsulfonylmethane) in supplement form, 1,000 mg daily. Don't eat a lot of fat, either, as fat slows the emptying of the stomach. Use alcohol and chocolate in moderation. Eat several small meals a day so that you don't overeat at any one meal. Don't eat on the run or right before exercising. Don't lie down after eating. Reduce stress with exercise and meditation.

NATURAL ALTERNATIVES FOR CONSTIPATION

Bulk laxatives like psyllium are your best bet for safe, quick relief. Once you're moving again, it's up to you to change your habits to prevent a recurrence. Here are some guidelines to follow to avoid constipation:

- One of the simplest and most effective things you can do to banish constipation is to drink more water. If you aren't getting enough water your stools will be hard and dry and straining to pass them can result in hemorrhoids or anal tears and bleeding.
- Eat more fiber. Fresh vegetables are full of fiber, as are fruit, legumes and whole grains. These foods should make up a generous portion of your diet. Use extra bran or nibble on prunes if you don't feel your bowels are moving regularly and easily. (If you have irritable bowel syndrome, bran might not be the best solution for you, as it tends to worsen bloating and gas for people with this problem.)
- If you're having trouble getting enough fiber in your diet, use psyllium in the morning before breakfast. Use one to three teaspoons in at least eight ounces of water or juice. Drink it immediately after you stir the psyllium in.
- Go when the urge strikes you. If you habitually hold back bowel movements, constipation can result.
- Get some exercise. Moving your whole body keeps things moving in the digestive tract.
- Check your medicine cabinet for drugs that cause constipation. Diuretics, painkillers, tranquilizers, antidepressants, antihistamines, narcotics and decongestants are potential culprits. The overuse of over-the-counter laxatives can cause dependency, as the colon is cleaned out so completely with one use that it may take a couple of days for another bowel movement to happen naturally. If you don't realize this you might take another dose

too soon, thinking that you are constipated again. Damage to the lining of the large intestine and loss of the bowel's ability to do the work of moving the bowel contents often result from overuse of laxatives.

- Sitting for hours on planes or in cars, changes in quality of water and food, and change from your ordinary routine can make you "irregular." When you travel pack natural remedies like prunes, psyllium or bran.
- Herbal remedies that contain cascara sagrada or senna stimulate contractions in the large intestine and rectum, moving the contents of the bowel. Don't use them more than once in a while, because you can quickly develop a dependency on them.
- Supplementation of magnesium at 600 to 900 mg a day helps to relieve constipation by drawing water into the contents of the large intestine and by relaxing irritated, constricted intestinal walls. Many vegetables are good sources of magnesium and herbs such as gotu kola, skullcap, horsetail, alfalfa, nettle, hawthorn berry and wild oat seed are also rich in this essential mineral.
- If you're on a very low-fat diet, you may want to try adding a tablespoon of olive or avocado oil a day. A little extra oil may be what's needed to make transit through the bowel smooth and easy.
- Probiotic supplements containing acidophilus should help with constipation and gas. Use a refrigerated supplement from your health food store.
- If you're constipated and really uncomfortable and don't feel like swallowing anything, try an Epsom salts bath. You can buy Epsom salts (magnesium salts) in your local market or drugstore. Dump an entire box into a bath and sit in it for 20 minutes and within a couple of hours you'll have a bowel movement.

BEAT IRRITABLE BOWEL SYNDROME AND TREAT FOOD ALLERGIES NATURALLY

Identification and treatment of food allergies is the most important step you can take to cure yourself of irritable bowel syndrome. How do you know whether you have food allergies? There is some controversy about this subject, but let's keep it simple. Think of negative reactions to foods as either immediate or delayed. If you respond to a food by sneezing, itching, wheezing, breaking out in hives, watering and itchy eyes, runny nose, or even a life-threatening reaction called anaphylaxis (this involves sudden swelling of the throat that can close off the airways), you have an immediate allergy to that food. Most of the immediate allergic reactions to foods happen in children and are outgrown. Strawberries, seafood, beans and milk products are the most common culprits.

Delayed allergies are much more difficult to pinpoint. Because symptoms may not occur until days after the food is eaten, the exact cause is not always obvious. Symptoms can include headache, other allergies such as hay fever, stiff achy joints, indigestion and fatigue. If allowed to progress, food allergy can lead to impaired digestion and general symptoms of malnutrition including dry skin, dull hair and increased susceptibility to illness. Most problems caused by food allergies aren't quite serious enough to stop people from getting through their days, but they have little energy and don't look healthy.

Digestive disturbances, rashes, minor aches and pains and vague health problems that can't be attributed to anything specific are common complaints of those with delayed food allergies. These unfortunate individuals may simply decide that it's an inevitable part of growing older. Don't let yourself fall into this way of thinking! The difference between feeling like you're sick all the time and feeling great might be one or two of the foods in your diet.

Start to keep a record of the foods you eat. Look for the most common triggers of delayed food allergies: wheat, corn, dairy products, soy, citrus fruit, nightshade vegetables (tomatoes, potatoes, eggplant, red and green peppers, cayenne pepper), peanuts (usually due to *aflatoxin*, a fungus found in most peanuts), eggs, beef and coffee. Ironically, foods that you feel you "must" have every day are most often the culprits. The release of the offending foods into your bloodstream causes the body to release adrenal hormones that give you a temporary surge of energy.

Irritable bowel syndrome is often a result of allergy to dairy products. People with celiac sprue, which is an allergy to gluten, are allergic to wheat, rye, barley, oats and all other gluten-containing grains. Food additives and colorings such as BHT, BHA, MSG, benzoates, nitrates, sulfites and red and yellow food dyes cause delayed allergic reactions in many people, especially children.

Watch out for antibiotics and NSAIDs (nonsteroidal anti-inflammatory drugs such as aspirin and ibuprofen) which are very hard on the stomach. Just a few ibuprofen a month can cause a chronically upset stomach.

Medical testing for delayed food allergy is tricky business. The existing tests vary in reliability and can be very expensive. Fortunately, self-diagnosis can be done with what is known as an elimination diet.

How to Do an Elimination Diet

You can do an elimination diet with the support of a health care professional if you don't feel able to tackle it on your own. A terrific resource on food allergy and elimination diets is *Optimal Wellness*, a book by Ralph Golan, M.D. (Ballantine Books, 1995). Precede the two-week period with 10 days of eating your normal diet, keeping careful track of everything you eat or drink and of any symptoms. Then make a list of the foods you eat every day and a list of the foods you eat more than five times during your record-keeping. After you finish your 10-day period of eating your regular diet, eliminate all of the foods on your "everyday foods" list and "more than five times in 10 days" list, as well as any other suspected allergens, for two weeks. Continue to record everything you eat and how you're feeling. Be very careful to eliminate all potential sources of allergenic foods. Vitamins contain fillers and fibers that may be allergens. Common food allergens like wheat, corn, dairy products and eggs are hidden in many processed foods. Be careful not to get into a pattern of eating some other food frequently during this time, or you may set yourself up for sensitivity to yet another food. Vary what you eat throughout the day and from day to day.

At the end of the two weeks, reintroduce foods one at a time. No more than one food should be reintroduced every 24 hours. Your response to foods you have allergies to will be pronounced. Continue to record all symptoms you experience. If you are allergic to a food you have avoided for two weeks you may experience rapid or uneven heart rhythms, sudden sleepiness, stomach cramps, bloating, gas, diarrhea, constipation, headache, chills, sweats, flushing and achiness.

If you notice that you are feeling very good on the limited diet, this is an important piece of feedback that you're on the right track. Your intestinal wall is shed and regenerated completely every three days, so that healing of a leaky gut happens quickly.

While you're on an elimination diet you can take some supplements to aid in healing your intestines. Glutamine is an amino acid essential for healthy gut mucosa; take 500 mg three times a day. Essential fatty acids, found in borage and evening primrose oils, help prevent inflammatory reactions in the gut and throughout the body. The B vitamin pantothenic acid (B5) is an important building block of the intestinal walls. Use 500 mg twice a day.

During an elimination diet, keep drinking the six to eight glasses of clean water every day that is recommended in the Six Core Principles for Optimal Health, and take supplements to help heal your small intestine.

If you've suffered for many years from chronic, low grade health problems caused by food allergy and leaky gut, you may be dealing with other problems such as nasal allergy, sinus infection, arthritis, autoimmune disease or candida overgrowth.

Once you've pinpointed problem foods, omit them from your diet for two months. Try reintroducing them again, one at a time, at that point. If you still have a reaction, wait six months and try again. You should eventually be able to reintroduce food allergens into your diet and enjoy them *occasionally*, but chances are that if you start eating them every day again you'll become sensitive to them again.

Children generally outgrow food allergies, but it can be frustrating for the family to deal with a child's sensitivity to common foods like wheat or dairy products. However, the improvement in health should be well worth a few months of deprivation.

CHAPTER 11

Cold, Cough, Asthma and Allergy Drugs and Their Natural Alternatives

It used to be that when we got a cold or flu we would attribute it to "catching" the germs from someone else and then our physicians would try to blast the germs away with antibiotics. Now we know that antibiotics generally don't help and most people with a cold or flu can tell you exactly how they brought it upon themselves:

"I was tired but I went out and partied anyway."

"I went to the office party and pigged out on cookies and punch."

"I was starting to get a sore throat but I ignored it and went skating."

These days we know that stress, a weakened immune system and poor nutrition can all tip the scales in favor of coming down with a cold or flu. Pay attention to your body's signals. It will tell you, in no uncertain terms, when it is fighting off a cold or flu. If you ignore the signals, the cold or flu bug will win. You already know the signals. Your sinuses may be painful when you wake up in the morning. You may feel especially tired and achy after work. A sore throat and fatigue are two of the hallmarks of impending illness. For some people it's a headache or achy muscles. For others it's sneezing or chills. If you act as soon as you get these signals, you have a good chance of staying healthy.

Natural cold/flu recommendations have a lot to do with prevention, and they will be covered in detail at the end of this chapter. You can go to your pharmacy and find lots of ways to suppress the symptoms, but that usually doesn't help much. The best strategy is to go on the offensive and go after the bugs before they go after you.

Physicians are adamantly pushing flu shots to everyone these days, but there is very little good evidence that they are an effective form of prevention. If you take a close look at the studies on flu shots, they appear to be just another way for physicians and pharmaceutical companies to rake in more money.

IS IT A COLD OR AN ALLERGY?

When we start sniffling and sneezing in the spring, it can be hard to tell whether it's a cold or an allergy. Although the symptoms of nasal congestion may be very similar and the underlying causes have to do with a malfunctioning immune system, what precipitates a cold or an allergy is very different.

In the case of a cold, a weakened immune system allows a cold virus to take hold. Cold viruses are always in our environment, and whether you "catch" a cold is a function of how healthy you are. Cold symptoms are caused when a cold virus attacks and kills cells, which then release substances that cause inflammation, mucus production and infection. You may also have a slight fever during a cold. In the vast majority of cases, a cold will resolve itself within five to seven days. If you take care of yourself by getting plenty of rest and warm fluids, taking vitamin C and the immune-stimulating herb echinacea, a cold can resolve itself within three days.

The influenza or flu virus tends to sweep into an area and cause widespread illness. Symptoms tend to be more severe with a flu, including a higher fever, aches and chills, and nausea.

Neither a cold nor flu can be effectively treated with an antibiotic. Antibiotics kill bacteria and colds and flus are caused by viruses. While a cold or flu can cause a bacterial infection, you are best off allowing your own body to fight it off and heal it unless a doctor determines that you are at risk for pneumonia or some other serious infectious disease.

Allergy symptoms, on the other hand, are caused when the immune system overreacts to an irritant such as dust mites, pollen, perfumes, air pollutants, pet dander or food. When the immune system mistakes these harmless invaders for deadly enemies, it sends out the histamines to attack, which in turn cause inflammation.

Inflammation caused by allergy can occur almost anywhere in the body. The most common sites are the mucus membranes of the nose, eyes, ears and throat. However, inflammation in the joints (arthritis), the brain (headaches, confusion, fatigue), lungs (asthma, cough), gastrointestinal system (cramps, indigestion, diarrhea) and skin (hives, rash) can also be caused by allergies.

What we're most often concerned about in the spring is known as allergic rhinitis or hay fever, which usually consists of a runny, itchy nose and watery eyes. About 20 percent of the population of the U.S. suffers from hay fever and the incidence is rising. Thirty years ago estimates were that under 100,000 people suffered from hay fever. Today the number has risen to more than 40 million. According to W. Steven Pray, Ph.D., a pharmacist and professor at Southwestern Oklahoma State University College of Pharmacy and a specialist in allergy treatment, the growing number of chemicals in the environment, combined with growing air pollution, is causing the steep rise in hay fever. And, he says, it's only going to get worse. Pray says these chemicals appear in our foods, clothes, cosmetics, soaps and an almost endless list of other consumer products.

Allergies are also on the rise because children's immune systems are under attack from vaccinations, antibiotics and the constant use of medicines such as Tylenol which harm the liver, our most important organ of detoxification. Then they are fed foods devoid of nutrition but loaded with additives, dyes, preservatives, pesticides and hormones. Children with an unrecognized sensitivity to dairy products, wheat or sugar, for example, who have also had their immune systems and intestinal systems compromised by constant antibiotics, are primed for a lifetime of allergies and other environmental sensitivities. Adults are in the same boat, but to a less sensitive degree. But let's get back to hay fever.

Spring is a big season for hay fever because that's when trees pollinate. In the late spring and summer, grasses pollinate. In the fall, weeds are the culprits. But there are plenty of nonseasonal indoor causes of allergies, including food, dust mites, cigarette smoke, aerosol sprays, room deodorizers, insecticides, cleaning products, fresh paint or varnish, mold, fungi and pets. Some experts even think that the thousands of artificial additives found in processed foods are partially to blame for the rising number of allergy cases.

How can you tell if your runny nose is being caused by hay fever? According to Dr. Pray, some of the differences between a cold and an allergy are:

- A runny nose caused by allergies is usually clear, while a cold causes a yellow discharge within a few days, indicating infection. Chronic, long-term allergies can eventually cause a sinus infection, but in general discharge from the nose will be clear.
- The nose is itchy in hay fever, usually not with a cold.
- Sneezes comes in groups during a hay fever attack, sometimes as many as 10 or 20 sneezes one right after another. Sneezes caused by a cold generally come on one at a time.
- Watery, itchy eyes tend to be a sign of hay fever rather than a cold.

The ears are often involved in an allergy, causing hearing problems, popping and sometimes ringing in the ears. Older children and adults who get a cold don't often get an ear infection with it.

A classic sign of chronic allergies and particularly food allergies has been dubbed the "allergic shiner," a semi-circular area below the eyes that is dark or bluish in color. Long-term blocked nasal passages interfere with the ability of blood to flow away from below the eyes, resulting in an accumulation of blood in that area and a darkening under the skin that makes it look bruised. The person with dark circles under his eyes isn't usually suffering from lack of sleep, he is more likely to have an allergy.

Chronic allergies can cause many side effects, especially in children, that may go unrecognized. Some of these side effects include fatigue, headaches, irritability, a poor sense of smell and taste, hearing problems, fatigue in the morning, snoring and eye, ear, nose and throat infections. More than 80 percent of people who suffer from frequent ear infections have allergies as well. In children, permanent facial changes can be a result of chronic allergies.

Let's explore why we get allergies to pollen. The body's reaction of sinus congestion and sneezing is the first sign that our immune system is reacting or sensitive to something in the environment that is actually harmless. It's helpful (if not pleasant!) when our bodies fight off a *real* invader such as a virus or bacteria with an immune reaction, which we call a cold or flu. But when we react to pollens, it's annoying and can interfere with our enjoyment of life.

Once our immune system decides that a particular type of pollen is a hostile invader, it becomes "sensitized" to it and can react with allergy symptoms for years and perhaps a lifetime. When spring arrives and the pollen begins to fly, our sensitized bodies release histamines, designed to fight the enemy pollen. In the process of attacking the invaders, the histamines cause inflammation and even damage tissues, causing sinus irritation, itchy eyes and often lung irritation as well. Some people may even develop rashes, eczema or hives.

The often accompanying headaches and mental fogginess are caused by sinus congestion. Sneezing is caused by irritated sinuses. Sore throats are caused by the mucus that runs down the back of the throat. Asthma can be triggered by an overload of irritants and mucus. If the body tries to rid itself of the invaders via the skin, rashes, eczema and hives may result.

Allergy drugs work to suppress symptoms rather than treat the cause of the allergy. The consequences of this type of treatment are generally unpleasant side effects and often a rebound effect where the symptom is worse if the medication starts to wear off or treatment is stopped.

TREATING ASTHMA

More than 15 million Americans have asthma, a potentially life-threatening lung disorder. The symptoms of asthma can include wheezing, coughing, labored breathing and coughing up mucus from the lungs. While most asthma attacks are precipitated by an allergen such as dust, mold or pollens, they can also be caused by emotional stress, exercise and infections. Asthma attacks are ordinarily no more than an unpleasant, uncomfortable and inconvenient wheezing and labored breathing, but if the lungs continue to constrict and fill with mucus, asthma can kill.

Asthma constricts the bronchial tubes leading to the lungs, which reduces the flow of air in and out of the lungs. Severe attacks can happen suddenly, but more often the asthma sufferer's condition deteriorates slowly, so that he delays getting medical help. Please don't make this mistake. You can do a lot to naturally relieve asthma symptoms, but if you have any suspicion that you might be in trouble, take whatever actions are necessary to open up your airways.

Asthma Medications: Is the Cure Worse than the Disease?

When you're having an asthma attack, each breath becomes an effort, and a deep breath is impossible. If you have ever been around somebody with asthma, you're well aware that it's a scary, severely limiting illness that can be life-threatening. The number of people in the U.S. with asthma has risen steadily since the 1970s, with a 50 percent increase just since 1990. Deaths from asthma have also risen steeply, with a 40 percent rise in the number of young people dying from asthma in the past decade.

Although asthma medications have saved many lives, it's likely that improper use of them has probably taken just as many. They temporarily stop symptoms without addressing underlying problems. This can be a lifesaver if you're having an acute asthma attack, but I'd rather see asthma sufferers work with prevention and not rely on these drugs so much, all of which have negative side effects when used long term. Most physicians treat asthma with bronchodilators that open up the air passageways in the lungs, or treat the underlying inflammation of the lungs with corticosteroids. The list of dangerous side effects of these two types of drugs is as long as your arm. It's especially tragic to see children condemned to taking these types of drugs.

Just as with flu shots, the alarming rise in the number of people getting asthma and dying from it are a very good indication that these medications aren't working, and may be doing more harm than good. In fact, a Johns Hopkins study recently published in the *Journal of Epidemiology* suggests a link between beta-agonists, a very popular type of asthma drug, and an increased rate of heart disease.

There are lots of theories as to why the rate of asthma is rising so fast, ranging from long-term side effects of childhood vaccinations to increased consumption of polyunsaturated and hydrogenated oils, to increased levels of air pollution and radiation. One of the most plausible theories is the increased numbers of people living, working and

DRUGS THAT CAN CAUSE OR AGGRAVATE ASTHMA

Antiarrhythmia drugs for the heart such as the beta-blockers (e.g., propranolol, timolol) and moricizine

The anti-nausea drug dimenhydrinate (Dramamine, Dimetabs)

Anti-Parkinson's drugs

Antipsychotic drugs such as the phenothiazines and lithium

Antiviral drugs mainly used to treat HIV such as cidofovir and protease inhibitors

Barbiturates

The benzodiazepines, anti-anxiety drugs (Valium, Dalmane)

Cephalosporin, sulfonamide antibiotics

Cholinesterase inhibitors used to treat Alzheimer's

Drugs to lower blood pressure such as guanethidine (Ismelin)

The ibuprofen-related family of NSAIDs (nonsteroidal anti-inflammatory drugs).

Narcotics

Over-the-counter sleeping pills such as diphenhydramine (Nytol, Sleep-Eze, Sominex, Tylenol PM)

The SSRIs (selective serotonin reuptake inhibitors), antidepressants such as fluoxetine (Prozac), fluvoxamine (Luvox) and paroxetine (Paxil)

The tricyclic antidepressants

Weight-loss drugs such as dexfenfluramine

going to school in airtight buildings that are energy efficient but which trap asthma-triggering allergens such as dust mites and mold, and harmful vapors emitted by carpeting, plastics and fiberboards.

Tartrazine (yellow dye no. 5) is a yellow food coloring used in some 60 percent of prescription and over-the-counter drugs, as well as in hundreds of processed foods such as cakes, cookies, cereals, soft drinks, ice cream, gelatin, pudding and pasta. It is well-known to be a potent allergen in many people, commonly provoking breathing difficulties and asthma attacks. If you are allergic to aspirin you are probably allergic to tartrazine. Children are especially susceptible to tartrazine, and there's a good chance it's responsible for many cases of childhood asthma in homes where processed foods are a dietary staple. This is a classic case where consumer groups have tried for years to have tartrazine banned from food and drugs, but the food industry lobbyists won. Efforts to remove tartrazine from asthma and allergy drugs have also been unsuccessful.

Some of the cough, cold and allergy drugs that contain tartrazine

ARE YOU SENSITIVE TO TARTRAZINE?

Tartrazine (yellow dye no. 5) is a yellow food coloring used in 60 percent of prescription and over-the-counter drugs, as well as in hundreds of processed foods such as cakes, cookies, cereals, soft drinks, ice cream, gelatin, pudding, butter and pasta. It is a well-known and potent allergen for many people, commonly provoking breathing difficulties and asthma attacks. If you are allergic to aspirin you are probably allergic to tartrazine. Children are especially susceptible to tartrazine, and it's very likely responsible for many cases of childhood asthma in homes where processed foods are a dietary staple. This is a classic case where consumer groups have tried for years to have tartrazine banned from food and drugs, but the food industry lobbyists won. Efforts to remove tartrazine from asthma and allergy drugs have also been unsuccessful.

Some of the cough, cold and allergy drugs that contain tartrazine include Spec-T, Vicks Cough Silencers, NyQuil Nighttime, Genite Liquid, Rynatuss Pediatric Suspension and Covangesic Tablets. There doesn't seem to be any reason to take one of these drugs containing tartrazine for a respiratory problem when there are so many others available that do not contain tartrazine.

Another possible cause of allergic reactions are pills that have red coloring in them. Both red dyes and the iron oxides used to color some pills can cause allergic reactions.

include Spec-T, Vicks Cough Silencers, NyQuil Nighttime, Genite Liquid, Rynatuss Pediatric Suspension and Covangesic Tablets. There's no reason why you would ever want to take one of these drugs containing tartrazine for a respiratory problem when there are so many others available that do not contain tartrazine.

In adults, asthma is more common in women, which gives us a clue that some part of it is hormonally related. Excessive estrogen, especially when not balanced by progesterone (not the synthetic progestins), can aggravate an existing asthma problem or even bring it on. Although natural progesterone tends to improve asthma symptoms, the synthetic progestins can cause or aggravate asthma.

Many premenopausal women also suffer from tired adrenal glands, and are then unable to produce the necessary steroid hormones such as cortisols and adrenaline that the body would naturally produce to ward off asthma.

DRUGS FOR ASTHMA

Sympathomimetic Bronchodilators

ALBUTEROL

EPHEDRINE SULFATE

EPINEPHRINE

ETHYLNOREPINEPHRINE

ISOETHARINE

ISOPROTERENOL

METAPROTERENOL SULFATE

SALMETEROL

TERBUTALINE SULFATE

Bronchodilating inhalers are popular among asthma sufferers because they are very quick and effective at relieving the symptoms of an asthma attack and opening up the bronchial tubes for four to six hours. They work on the same receptor sites as the body's natural hormone adrenaline, a substance released when you are under severe stress. They increase heart rate and blood pressure, and can cause anxiety, restlessness and insomnia. Bronchodilators are meant to be used occasionally to relieve "mild acute" asthma attacks. The reality

---

USING AN INHALER FOR ASTHMA

If you are regularly using inhalers to control your asthma, it's very important that you keep track of your usage. If you find yourself needing to take it more and more frequently to feel like your symptoms are controlled, heed it as a warning. Many studies have shown that more frequent inhaler use leads to a downward spiral of worsening bronchoconstriction and possibly a life-threatening attack.

of how they are used is far different: Many asthmatics come to depend on them, using them many times a day. This is dangerous, because they become less effective over time, and the risk of serious side effects is increased. At a recent Annual Meeting of the American College of Allergy and Immunology, it was acknowledged that misuse of a type of bronchodilator called beta agonists may actually *worsen* asthma control and may even be responsible for the increase in asthma and asthma-related deaths. A large Canadian study confirmed this view.

The Beta Agonists

ALBUTEROL (Proventil, Ventolin, Repetabs, Volmax, Airet)

ISOETHARINE (Arm-a-Med Isoetharine, Beta-2, Bronkosol)

ISOPROTERENOL (Isuprel Glossets, Isuprel, Medihaler-Iso, Dispos-a-Med)

METAPROTERENOL SULFATE (Alupent, Metaprel)

TERBUTALINE SULFATE (Brethine, Bricanyl)

WHAT DO THEY DO IN THE BODY?

These bronchodilating drugs work by stimulating receptors that cause opening of the bronchial tubes that lead to the lungs. Beta agonists inhibit the release of histamine from mast cells in the airways and increase the movement of the tiny cilia that help to propel allergens out of the lungs.

WHAT ARE THEY USED FOR?

Beta agonists reverse the constriction of the bronchial tubes that occurs during an asthma attack, exercise-induced asthma, chronic bronchitis, emphysema and other chronic obstructive pulmonary diseases. They are used alone as needed as an inhaler for mild, well-controlled asthma. In more severe cases they may be taken as a pill or inhaler along with another anti-inflammatory drug such as theophylline or cromolyn sodium.

WHAT ARE THE POSSIBLE SIDE EFFECTS/ADVERSE REACTIONS?

Beta agonists stimulate the central nervous system, which can give you a case of the "jitters," as if you've had too much coffee. Mood swings, increased appetite, fatigue, nightmares and aggressive behavior are other possible side effects. Bronchitis, nasal congestion, increased secretion of saliva, nosebleed, muscle cramps, conjunctivitis or discoloration of the teeth may occur.

CAUTION! THINK TWICE ABOUT TAKING THIS DRUG IF . . .

- You have ever had any kind of dangerous cardiac arrhythmias or heart blockage.
- You have narrow-angle glaucoma.
- You are going to have surgery. Tell your physician that you use this drug. You won't want to have albuterol in your system while under general anesthesia.
- You have diabetes, high blood pressure, heart disease, history of stroke, congestive heart failure, hyperthyroidism, are elderly or have a history of seizures or psychoneurotic illness. Dosages may need to be adjusted.

Diabetics who use albuterol should be aware that the jittery feeling they get when blood sugar is too low is hard to distinguish from the side effects of the drug.

With repeated, excessive use of inhalers, your body may begin to respond with what's known as paradoxical bronchoconstriction. Instead of opening your airways, use of the inhaler causes them to constrict even further. If you think this is happening to you, discontinue use immediately and see a doctor as soon as possible.

Tolerance may occur; temporary discontinuation should bring back the drug's original potency. Lower doses may be required for elderly people because of heightened sensitivity to nervous system stimulation.

WHAT ARE THE INTERACTIONS WITH OTHER DRUGS?

The following drugs may raise levels or prolong the effects of beta agonists:

↑ Furazolidine   Rauwolfia alkaloids
  Guanethidine   Reserpine
  Lithium   Tricyclic antidepressants*
  Methyldopa

Beta agonists may reduce potency or decrease the amount of time the following drugs are effective:

↓ Guanethidine
  Digoxin

FOODS HIGH IN TYRAMINE

The following foods are high in tyramine, which may interfere with the sympathomimetic drugs used in many asthma inhalers, including albuterol, salmeterol and epinephrine. Any type of protein such as meat, fish or dairy product that has been sitting around for too long will start to form tyramines. Be cautious with leftovers more than a few days old, and check freshness dates when you buy fish, meat and dairy products. Any type of aged, pickled or fermented product such as aged cheeses, wine and pickles may contain tyramines.

Keeping track of tyramine-containing foods is especially important for parents of asthmatic children who are using sympathomimetic drugs. An inhaler dose that follows a bologna sandwich, for example, could cause a serious interaction.

Aged cheeses
Aged dairy products, especially sour
  cream
Avocado
Beef and chicken liver
Chocolate
Dried and pickled fish
Flavor enhancers such as hydrolyzed
  vegetable protein
Raisins
Sausages, pepperoni, salami,
  bologna
Soy products such as tofu, miso, soy
  sauce, teriyaki sauce
Tomatoes
Wine, beer, liqueurs, champagne
Yeast

*Potentially dangerous interaction.

WHAT ARE THE INTERACTIONS OF BETA AGONISTS WITH FOODS?

Foods rich in the amino acids tyrosine and tyramine such as aged cheeses, wine and chocolate, interfere with enzymes needed to metabolize sympathomimetic drugs such as beta agonists. Side effects of mixing these foods with beta agonists in sensitive people can include severe high blood pressure, intracranial bleeding, severe headache, chest pain, sweating, palpitations, changes in pulse rate, visual problems, breathing difficulties. In rare cases, coma can result.

SALMETEROL (Serevent)

WHAT DOES IT DO IN THE BODY?

Salmeterol stimulates receptors in the airways that help to keep them from constricting. It has a much longer duration of action than the other sympathomimetic drugs used to treat asthma.

WHAT IS IT USED FOR?

Long-term maintenance treatment of asthma and prevention of asthma attacks.

WHAT ARE THE POSSIBLE SIDE EFFECTS/ADVERSE EFFECTS?

The most common are shakiness, nervousness, tension, inflammation of the nasal passageways and throat, sinus problems and upper and lower respiratory tract infection. Others include palpitations, rapid heartbeat, chest tightness, angina (heart pains), tremor, dizziness, vertigo, headache, nausea, vomiting, diarrhea, joint and back pain, muscle cramping, generalized muscle aches, giddiness, susceptibility to flu virus and viral gastroenteritis, itching, dental pain, fatigue, rash, menstrual irregularities, nasal allergies, runny nose, laryngitis, bronchitis, dry mouth and cough.

CAUTION! THINK TWICE ABOUT TAKING THIS DRUG IF . . .

- You have ever had any kind of dangerous cardiac arrhythmias or heart blockage, especially if these were caused by high levels of the heart drug digitalis in your bloodstream.
- You have narrow-angle glaucoma.
- You have diabetes, high blood pressure, heart disease, a history of stroke, congestive heart failure or hyperthyroidism, are elderly or have a history of seizures or psychoneurotic illness. Use special caution while taking this drug.

Diabetics who use salmeterol should be aware that the jittery feeling they get when blood sugar is too low is hard to distinguish from the side effects of the drug.

WHAT ARE THE INTERACTIONS WITH FOODS?

Foods rich in the amino acid tyramine, such as aged cheeses, wine and chocolate, interfere with enzymes needed to metabolize sympathomimetic drugs such as salmeterol. Side effects of mixing these foods with salmeterol in sensitive people can include: severe high blood pressure, intracranial bleeding, severe headache, chest pain, sweating, palpitations, changes in pulse rate, visual problems, breathing difficulties and even coma.

WHAT ELSE TO DO WHILE TAKING THIS DRUG

Salmeterol is not for treatment of an acute asthma attack. It's meant to be taken twice a day on an ongoing basis. Increasing the dose on your own to try to alleviate worsening symptoms is definitely not a good idea either. Keep albuterol, epinephrine or another fast-acting inhaler with you to open airways during an attack.

The Epinephrines

EPINEPHRINE (Adrenalin Chloride, AsthmaNefrin, microNefrin, Nephron, S-2, Vaponefrin, AsthmaHaler Mist, Bronitin Mist, Primatene Mist, Bronkaid Mist, Sus-Phrine)

EPHEDRINE SULFATE

ETHYLNOREPINEPHRINE (Bronkephrine)

WHAT DO THEY DO IN THE BODY?

Like albuterol, the epinephrines are bronchodilating drugs that work quickly by stimulating receptors that cause opening of the bronchial tubes that lead to the lungs. They also work as a nasal decongestant when inhaled through the nose.

WHAT ARE THEY USED FOR?

Epinephrines are mainly used in inhalers, but may be used in an injection to offset a severe allergic reaction. Inhalers are useful for treatment of an acute asthma attack or nasal congestion, while the injectable form is only for emergency situations where there is threat of complete closure of the bronchial tubes due to asthma attack or anaphylaxis (a life-threatening allergic reaction that involves swelling of the airways).

WHAT ARE THE POTENTIAL SIDE EFFECTS/ADVERSE EFFECTS?

These are extremely potent stimulant drugs that can cause sharp increases in blood pressure and heart pains. Rupture of the blood vessels in the brain and rupture of blood vessels around the heart have been reported in people using epinephrines. Heartbeat irregularities develop in some people even with low doses. Epinephrines have caused permanent electrocardiogram changes in healthy people, indicating some very significant effects on the conduction system that keeps the heart beating.

Bronchial irritation, nervousness, restlessness and sleeplessness may be signs that you need to have your dosage of epinephrine reduced. If you do not feel your asthma symptoms have been relieved within 20 minutes after your usual dose, don't keep taking it. Seek medical assistance immediately.

- **Inhaled form:** palpitations, anxiety, fear.
- **Injected form:** cerebral hemorrhage caused by rapid rises in blood pressure, especially in elderly people with diseased arteries in the brain. Agitation, disorientation, memory impairment, assaultive behavior, panic, hallucinations, suicidal or homicidal tendencies, and other serious psychological disturbances can be a result of epinephrine injection. Children may faint after being injected. Fatal arrhythmias, spasm of the arteries that feed the retinas of the eyes and shock have also been reported.

Other side effects may include pain, itching, hemorrhage or raised red welt at injection site.

WHAT ARE THE INTERACTIONS WITH OTHER DRUGS?

The following drugs may increase levels or prolong the effects of epinephrines:

↑ Beta-blockers* Methyldopa
Furazolidine Rauwolfia alkaloids
Guanethidine Tricyclic antidepressants*

Epinephrines may decrease levels or prolong the effects of the following drugs:

↓ Diabetes drugs, oral or insulin
Guanethidine

---

*Potentially dangerous interaction.

The following drug may decrease levels or reduce the effects of epinephrines:

↓ Lithium

WHAT ARE THE INTERACTIONS WITH FOODS?

Foods rich in the amino acid tyramine, such as aged cheeses, wine and chocolate interfere with enzymes needed to metabolize sympatho-mimetic drugs such as epinephrines. Side effects of mixing these foods with epinephrines in sensitive people can include severe high blood pressure, intracranial bleeding, severe headache, chest pain, sweating, palpitations, changes in pulse rate, visual problems, breathing diffi-culties and even coma.

Xanthine Derivatives

AMINOPHYLLINE (Phyllocontin, Truphylline)

DYPHYLLINE (Dilor, Lufyllin)

OXTRIPHYLLINE (Choledyl)

THEOPHYLLINE (Theo-Dur, Slo-Phyllin, Theolair, Quibron-D Dividose, Bronko-dyl, Elixophyllin, Aquaphyllin, Theoclear, Theostat, Accurbron, Asmalix, Elixomin, Lanophyllin, Aerolate, Slo-bid Gyrocaps, Theo-24, Theospan-SR, Theovent, Theochron, Quibron-T/SR Dividose, Respbid, Sustaire, Theo-Sav, Theo-X, T-Phyl, Uni-Dur, Uniphyl)

WHAT DO THEY DO IN THE BODY?

These are a class of drugs known as the *xanthine derivatives* or *methyl-xanthines*, which relax the smooth muscle that lines the blood vessels of the bronchial tubes and lungs. These drugs also stimulate the cen-tral nervous and respiratory systems, induce water loss (diuresis), de-crease the tone of the lower esophageal sphincter and inhibit uterine contractions.

WHAT ARE THEY USED FOR?

Relief of symptoms and prevention of bronchial asthma or other bronchospasm associated with chronic obstructive pulmonary disease (COPD). Regular use may improve lung function and shortness of breath in COPD patients.

WHAT ARE THE POSSIBLE SIDE EFFECTS/ADVERSE EFFECTS?

If theophylline clearance from the body is reduced, harmful levels of the drug can accumulate in the body. Carefully consider any potential for interactions with other drugs and don't take anything over the counter without first consulting your physician or pharmacist.

At even slightly elevated blood levels of this drug, you're likely to experience nausea, vomiting, diarrhea, headache, insomnia and irritability. In some people, the first signs of dangerous levels of theophylline in the body may be more severe. Moderately high blood levels lead to high blood sugar, low blood pressure, irregular heart rhythms, seizures, brain damage and even death.

Other potential adverse effects at normal blood levels of theophyllines include: fever, flushing, high blood sugar, oversecretion of antidiuretic hormone (which can cause fluid and electrolyte imbalances), rash, hair loss, irritability, restlessness, headache, insomnia, overexcited reflexes, muscle twitching, convulsions, nausea, vomiting, stomach pains, vomiting of blood, diarrhea, heartburn (gastroesophageal reflux) during sleep, life-threatening heart rhythm abnormalities, circulatory failure, changes in breathing patterns, respiratory arrest, protein in the urine and rapid loss of fluid through the urine.

CAUTION! THINK TWICE ABOUT TAKING THESE DRUGS IF . . .

- You have peptic ulcer.
- You have an underlying seizure disorder that is not being treated with anticonvulsant medication.
- You have heart disease, low blood oxygen levels, liver disease, high blood pressure, congestive heart failure, are elderly or are or have ever been an alcoholic.
- You are a man over 55 years of age.

- You have chronic obstructive pulmonary disease.
- You have heart failure.
- You are suffering from a sustained high fever.

In an acute episode of asthma, don't rely on theophylline to open your airways. It doesn't work quickly enough. Keep albuterol or another fast-acting beta agonist inhaler around just in case.

WHAT ARE THE INTERACTIONS WITH OTHER DRUGS?

The following drugs may reduce potency or decrease the amount of time theophylline is effective:

↓ Aminoglutethimide Ketoconazole
  Barbiturates Loop diuretics
  Carbamazepine Rifampin
  Charcoal Smoking tobacco, marijuana
  Hydantoins Sulfinpyrazone
  Isoniazid Thioamines

The following drugs may raise levels or prolong the effects of theophylline:

↑ Allopurinol Isoniazid
  Beta-blockers Loop diuretics
  Calcium channel blockers Macrolides
  Carbamazepine Mexiletine
  Cimetidine (Tagamet)* Oral contraceptives
  Corticosteroids Probenecid (dyphylline only)
  Disulfiram Quinolones
  Ephedrine Ranitidine (rarely)
  Influenza virus vaccine Thiabendazole
  Interferon Thyroid hormones

---

*Potentially dangerous interaction.

Other Drug Interactions to Be Aware Of

- Benzodiazepines (sedatives such as Xanax) can be antagonized by theophylline, making them less effective.
- Halothane and theophylline used together may lead to heart rhythm irregularities.
- Ketamine and theophylline used together may lead to seizures.
- Blood levels of lithium (used for depression and manic-depression) may be reduced by theophylline.
- The action of some muscle relaxants can be reduced in the body by theophylline.
- The use of tetracycline along with theophylline increases the likelihood of side effects.

What Are the Interactions with Food?

Theophylline has a shorter duration of action when you eat a low-carbohydrate, high-protein diet.

Charcoal-broiled beef is high in polycyclic carbon, which also diminishes the effectiveness of theophylline. On the other hand, the drug stays in the body longer with a high-carbohydrate, low-protein diet.

Avoid large amounts of cocoa, tea, coffee or other caffeinated drinks. Be aware that chocolate contains caffeine too.

Hot pepper sauces, such as Tabasco sauce, can increase blood levels of theophylline, but this hasn't been demonstrated to be dangerous.

To avoid toxicity that can result when sustained-release capsules empty into the body too quickly, take theophylline on an empty stomach. If you aren't using sustained-release tablets, you can take them with food, but less of the drug may be absorbed.

Cruciferous vegetables such as broccoli, cauliflower, cabbage and Brussels sprouts, eaten in large amounts, increase the rate at which your body metabolizes theophylline.

Foods that acidify the urine cause the drug to be emptied more quickly from the bloodstream, while foods that alkalinize the urine have the opposite effect. Meat, chicken, fish, eggs and grains tend to acidify the urine. Vitamin C and cranberries also acidify the urine. Foods that alkalinize the urine include most fruits (exceptions are cranberries, plums and orange juice), dairy products (except cheese) and vegetables.

WHAT ELSE TO TAKE WHILE TAKING THESE DRUGS

Studies have shown that asthmatics tend to be deficient in the mineral magnesium and that the body's ability to cope with stressful situations is compromised when low on this mineral. Daily use of beta agonists like albuterol, salmeterol and epinephrine, as well as the use of theophylline, can further deplete the body's magnesium stores. Supplement magnesium citrate, gluconate or glycinate, 500 mg a day in divided doses.

Leukotriene Receptor Drugs

ZAFIRLUKAST (Accolate)

ZILEUTON (Zyflo)

WHAT DO THEY DO IN THE BODY?

These relatively new drugs block or inhibit leukotriene receptors. Leukotrienes are one of the inflammatory substances produced during an allergic reaction. Levels of leukotrienes shoot up during an allergic asthma attack and zafirlukast and zileuton block the swelling of the airways that results.

WHAT ARE THEY USED FOR?

Prevention and treatment of asthma in people above the age of 12. Not all asthmatics respond to this drug, but it is very effective in about half of those who try it.

WHAT ARE THE POSSIBLE SIDE EFFECTS/ADVERSE EFFECTS?

Zafirlukast: headache, dizziness, nausea, diarrhea, abdominal pain, vomiting, infection, generalized pain, weakness, muscle aches, fever, back pain and stomach discomfort.

Zileuton: headache, pain, abdominal pain, weakness, lowered white blood cell counts and muscle pain. Side effects frequently cause people to stop taking zileuton.

The most serious side effect that occurs with these drugs is elevation of liver enzymes, which indicates that there may be liver damage. Your physician should check your liver enzyme levels regularly, especially if you are 65 or older.

CAUTION! DON'T TAKE THESE DRUGS IF . . .

- You have liver disease or transaminase elevations that are three or more times the upper limit of normal. This is an indication that your liver cells are being damaged by something and you shouldn't risk further harm to this vital organ by taking these drugs. Leukotriene antagonists aren't cleared from the body as well when the liver isn't doing its work properly.

Zafirlukast isn't suitable for acute asthma attacks.

People over the age of 55 who took zafirlukast reported more frequent respiratory infections, especially when they also used corticosteroids.

WHAT ARE THE INTERACTIONS WITH FOOD AND OTHER DRUGS?

Zafirlukast:

The following drugs may reduce potency or decrease the amount of time zafirlukast is effective:

↓ Erythromycin   Theophylline
  Terfenadine

The following drug may raise levels of zafirlukast:

↑ Aspirin*

Zafirlukast may raise levels of:

↑ Warfarin

---

*Potentially dangerous interaction.

Zileuton:

Zileuton may raise levels or prolong the effects of the following drugs:

↑ Propranolol*   Theophylline*
  Terfenadine*   Warfarin*

Corticosteroid Inhalers

BECLOMETHASONE (Beclovent, Vanceril, Vancenase)

BUDESONIDE (Pulmicort, Rhinocort)

FLUNISOLIDE (AeroBid)

TRIAMCINOLONE (Azmacort)

WHAT DO THEY DO IN THE BODY?

These drugs belong to a class of drugs called corticosteroids. Steroid drugs are usually given to reduce inflammation. These inhaled corticosteroids minimize the systemic side effects commonly seen with versions taken in pill form.

WHAT ARE THEY USED FOR?

Control of asthma symptoms not adequately controlled by other means.

WHAT ARE THE POTENTIAL SIDE EFFECTS/ADVERSE EFFECTS?

There is evidence that inhaled corticosteroids can increase your risk of open-angle glaucoma, an eye disease that causes blindness, by up to 50 percent. This alone is a good reason to avoid using these drugs unless absolutely necessary.

Throat irritation or hoarseness which may be due to yeast (candida)

---

*Potentially dangerous interaction.

overgrowth in the throat; rash, wheezing and swelling of the face. Fungal infections of the throat are a common side effect of inhaled corticosteroid use.

Even inhaled steroids can cause side effects throughout the body. Dozens of side effects may occur, including weight gain, water retention, increased susceptibility to infection, high blood pressure, imbalances of minerals such as potassium and calcium and protein loss.

CAUTION! THINK TWICE ABOUT TAKING THESE DRUGS IF . . .

- You are having an acute attack of asthma. Corticosteroids don't work fast enough to help under these circumstances.
- You have any kind of systemic fungal infection, including candida, a very common problem that can be made much worse by taking steroid drugs.

USE CAUTION WITHDRAWING FROM STEROID DRUGS

A special warning is warranted for those with asthma who have been using systemic steroid medications, such as prednisone or hydrocortisone, and who replace these drugs with inhaled steroids like beclomethasone. A potentially dangerous side effect of taking large doses of steroids is that your adrenal glands may shut down or greatly decrease their production of these substances. If you have been taking steroids regularly for a long period of time, it can take several months for your endocrine system to recover. In older people the adrenal glands may never recover and they may be dependent on steroid drugs for life. If you have asthma, you are particularly vulnerable to a life-threatening asthma attack while you are withdrawing from steroids.

Anyone who is taking or has recently stopped taking oral corticosteroids or large doses of inhaled steroids over a long period of time should carry a warning card with this information on it. If you have an acute attack of asthma or are under a lot of stress, you should resume the systemic steroid immediately and see your doctor.

One way to minimize the risk of dependency on steroids is to use the smallest possible dose of hydrocortisone, the natural form of cortisone, rather than the more potent man-made drugs such as prednisone.

The long-term effects of inhaled corticosteroids are unknown. Although your physician will tell you that inhaled steroids are essentially free of the side effects of systemic versions, some who use them for extended periods may experience weight gain, mood swings or even adrenal suppression, and recent studies indicate that inhaled steroids may cause systemic side effects more quickly than anyone suspected, including osteoporosis.

WHAT ARE THE INTERACTIONS WITH FOODS AND OTHER DRUGS?

The following drugs may reduce potency or decrease the amount of time inhaled corticosteroids are effective:

↓ Barbiturates
  Hydantoins
  Rifampin

The following drugs may raise levels or prolong the effects of inhaled corticosteroids:

↑ Estrogen replacement therapy
  Ketoconazole
  Oral contraceptives

Inhaled corticosteroids may reduce potency or decrease the amount of time the following drugs are effective:

↓ Anticholinesterase drugs   Salicylates
  Isoniazid   Somatrem

Inhaled corticosteroids may raise levels or prolong the effects of the following drugs:

↑ Cyclosporine   Diuretics (this interaction may cause
  Digitalis*   depletion of potassium)

---

* Potentially dangerous interaction.

OTHER INTERACTIONS TO BE AWARE OF

- If you are taking oral anticoagulant drugs and corticosteroids, your physician may have to adjust the anticoagulant dose; conversely, in some cases, corticosteroids cause the anticoagulant to be less effective.
- Theophylline and corticosteroids used together may result in some alteration of the effects of either or both.
- Alcohol can add to stomach irritation that can be a side effect of corticosteroid use.
- Use salt in moderation if you are using a steroid drug. The two together can cause stomach irritation and fluid and sodium retention.

WHAT ELSE TO TAKE WHILE TAKING THIS DRUG

Corticosteroids cause increased excretion of potassium, calcium, zinc and magnesium and this can result in depletion of these important minerals. Use supplements of each mineral.

Your need for the vitamins B6, C and D is increased during corticosteroid therapy. A good multivitamin should supply enough B6 and D, but you should use extra vitamin C. Try 2,000 mg a day in divided doses.

Use extra probiotics to help maintain healthy intestinal flora and be sure to rinse your mouth thoroughly after each inhaled dose to prevent oral candida infection.

With oral administration of steroid drugs, high-fat meals cause increased drug absorption and foods in general are better absorbed so that weight gain can result. It isn't unheard of for the body to absorb enough of the inhaled form to cause these side effects.

Miscellaneous Asthma Drugs

IPRATROPIUM BROMIDE (Atrovent)

WHAT DOES IT DO IN THE BODY?

Inhibits the body's overreaction to asthma triggers by blocking the action of the excitatory neurotransmitter acetylcholine. It also has anti-secretory effects, helping to relieve the discomfort of a runny nose.

WHAT IS IT USED FOR?

Bronchial inhaler: Reversal of bronchospasm caused by asthma, emphysema or other cardio-pulmonary diseases.

   Nasal inhaler: Relief from nasal allergies and common cold symptoms.

WHAT ARE POSSIBLE SIDE EFFECTS/ADVERSE EFFECTS?

Headache, pain, nausea, flu-like symptoms, back and chest pain, dizziness, dry mouth, nausea, constipation, coughing, shortness of breath, bronchitis, paradoxical bronchospasm, increased production of sputum, upper respiratory infection, inflammation of the pharynx, runny nose and inflammation of the sinuses.

CAUTION! DON'T USE THIS DRUG IF . . .

- You are sensitive to the drug atropine, soy lecithin (commonly found in processed foods), soybeans or peanuts.
- You are trying to treat an acute asthmatic episode; it won't work quickly enough.

Use caution if you have narrow-angle glaucoma, enlarged prostate or bladder neck obstruction.

When using Atrovent, be very careful not to get it in your eyes.

WHAT ARE THE INTERACTIONS WITH OTHER DRUGS?

No dangerous interactions have been reported. You can safely use a beta agonist inhaler as needed during long-term therapy with ipratropium bromide.

DRUGS FOR ALLERGIES

Antihistamines

AZATADINE MALEATE (Optimine)

AZELASTINE (Astelin)

BROMPHENIRAMINE MALEATE (Dimetapp)

CETIRIZINE

CHLORPHENIRAMINE (Chlor-Trimeton, Aller-Chlor)

CLEMASTINE FUMARATE (Antihist-1, Tavist)

CYPROHEPTADINE (Periactin)

DEXCHLORPHENIRAMINE MALEATE (Polarmine)

DIPHENHYDRAMINE (AllerMax, Benadryl, Banophen, Diphenhist)

FEXOFENADINE (Allegra)

LORATADINE (Claritin)

PHENINDAMINE (Nolahist)

PROMETHAZINE (Phenergan, Allergan)

TRIPELENNAMINE (PBZ)

There are dozens of prescription and over-the-counter varieties of antihistamines. Because histamine is only one of many substances that cause allergy symptoms, these drugs work only 40 to 60 percent of the time. They are most effective at relieving sneezing and itching, but don't have much effect on nasal congestion.

All antihistamines have the potential to adversely affect heart rhythms; terfenadine (Seldane) and astemizole (Hismanal), which were finally pulled off the market, can cause a very rare and potentially fatal arrhythmia. If you still have these drugs in your medicine cabinet, please throw them away.

A new drug called fexofenadine (Allegra) is chemically similar to terfenadine but reportedly doesn't have the dangerous side effects. The smart choice is to adopt a wait-and-see attitude about this drug and avoid being a guinea pig.

Ethylenediamines (pyrilamine maleate, tripelennamine, tripelennamine citrate and hydrochloride) are associated with more digestive system side effects than other antihistamines and cyproheptadine (Periactin) appears to cause more pronounced increases in appetite and weight gain than other drugs in this class.

Most antihistamines cause drowsiness and other sedating drugs will have an additive effect, so don't combine them with alcohol or anti-anxiety drugs such as Ativan, Librium, Xanax or Valium.

Fiorinal, a drug for tension headaches, tricyclic antidepressants, antiseizure drugs, prescription pain relievers and muscle relaxants also will knock you out when taken with most antihistamines.

Don't use any antihistamine without a doctor's supervision if you have high blood pressure, cardiovascular disease, diabetes, enlarged prostate or hyperthyroidism.

Most antihistamines are combined with one or more of the following: a decongestant such as pseudoephedrine, an analgesic (painkiller) such as acetaminophen, an expectorant such as guaifenesin, and an antitussive (anti-cough) such as menthol, codeine or dextromethorphan. Well-known brand names of such combinations include Actifed, Advil Cold & Sinus, Alka-Seltzer Plus, Naldecon, Benylin, Chlor-Trimeton, Comtrex, Robitussin, Sudafed, Contac, Vicks, Dimetapp, Tylenol and Dristan.

WHAT DO THEY DO IN THE BODY?

These drugs compete with histamines at specific receptor sites, blocking allergic symptoms.

WHAT ARE THEY USED FOR?

Relief of symptoms associated with seasonal allergies or the common cold, including runny nose, watery, itchy eyes, sneezing and itchy rash. Claritin and Allegra don't cause drowsiness.

WHAT ARE THE POSSIBLE SIDE EFFECTS/ADVERSE EFFECTS?

Fexofenadine (Allegra) is a relatively new drug so there isn't much information on its side effects. In drug-approval studies it did not show the dangerous interactions with antifungal drugs that its relative terfenadine (Seldane) did.

Some people are allergic to antihistamines. Fluid retention (edema) in the extremities, throat or even around the heart can occur. Other signs of allergy to antihistamines include dermatitis, asthma, lupus-like symptoms, rash, increased sensitivity to light or even life-threatening anaphylaxis.

Other side effects that have been observed include precipitous dips in blood pressure when moving from sitting to standing or from lying down to standing, palpitations, heart rhythm irregularities (ranging from merely uncomfortable to life-threatening), faintness, blood pressure changes and changes on electrocardiogram (ECG) readings.

Drowsiness, sedation, dizziness, disturbances in coordination, headache, irritability and a host of other psychological effects have been reported.

Also reported: Stomach distress, anorexia, weight gain, nausea, vomiting, diarrhea, constipation, urinary problems (difficulty urinating or too-frequent urination), breast development in males (gynecomastia), lactation in women, decreased libido, impotence, thickening of bronchial secretions, chest tightness, wheezing, nasal stuffiness, dry or sore mouth, nose or throat, depressed respiratory function, tingling, feeling of heaviness, weakness of hands, easy bruising, jaundice, skin redness, stomach inflammation, high or prolonged glucose tolerance curves, increased levels of glucose in the urine (a symptom of diabetes), changes in blood cell and spinal fluid protein counts, increased blood cholesterol levels, excessive perspiration, chills, hair loss, visual disturbances, cough, spontaneous lactation and menstrual disturbances, nightmares, moderate to mild transaminase elevations (indicating liver damage) and anemia.

CAUTION! THINK TWICE ABOUT USING THESE DRUGS IF . . .

- You are taking MAO inhibitors.

Taking the drugs erythromycin, ketoconazole or itraconazole can prompt life-threatening arrhythmias if taken with Claritin.

Don't use these drugs if you have narrow-angle glaucoma, stenosing peptic ulcer, symptomatic enlarged prostate, bladder neck obstruction, pyloric (stomach) or duodenal (small intestine) obstruction or liver disease.

People over the age of 60 are more likely to experience dizziness, sedation, fainting, confusion and dipping blood pressure.

Children using these drugs may become less mentally alert or become very excited. Overdoses in children can lead to hallucinations, convulsions or even death.

It's a good idea to stay out of the sun while taking loratadine. It can make you more sensitive to ultraviolet light.

These drugs won't work to reverse the bronchospasm that occurs during an acute asthma attack.

WHAT ARE THE INTERACTIONS WITH OTHER DRUGS?

The following drugs may raise levels or prolong the effects of loratadine:

↑ Azole antifungals* (ketoconazole, fluconazole, itraconazole)
Macrolide antibiotics* (erythromycin, clarithromycin, troleandomycin and azithromycin)

The following drugs may raise or prolong the effects of antihistamines.

↑ Monoamine oxidase inhibitors (MAO inhibitors)

---

*Potentially dangerous interaction.

The following drugs may interact with antihistamines to raise blood levels and cause toxicity, but this hasn't been proven in clinical studies yet. Be wary.

↑ Anti-arrhythmia drugs   Haloperidol*
Probucol*   Thioridazine*

OTHER INTERACTIONS TO BE AWARE OF

Alcohol and other central nervous system depressant drugs can have an additive effect when taken with antihistamines. Your ability to drive may be impaired by very small amounts of alcohol when you take antihistamines.

WHAT ARE THE INTERACTIONS WITH FOOD?

Citrus and other acidic juices can cause decreased drug activity when mixed with antihistamines. Vitamin C helps your kidneys more quickly clear antihistamines from the body.

DRUGS FOR COLDS, COUGHS AND ALLERGIES

Expectorants

GUAIFENESIN (Guiatuss, Anti-Tuss, Genatuss, Glyate, Halotussin, Mytussin, Robitussin, Siltussin, Scot-Tussin Expectorant, Tusibron, Uni-Tussin, Diabetic Tussin EX, Organidin NR, Naldecon Senior Ex, Breonesin, GG-Cen, Hytuss 2X, Gee-Gee, Glytuss, Duratuss-G, Guaifenex LA, Fenesin, Humibid LA, Liquibid, Monafed, Muco-Fen-LA, Pneumomist, Respa-GF, Sinumist-SR Capulets, Tonro EX)

WHAT DOES IT DO IN THE BODY?

Guaifenesin is an expectorant. It enhances the output of lubricating fluid in the respiratory tract so that mucus is easier to expel by coughing. Coughs are less frequent and more productive.

What Is It Used For?

Relief of dry, nonproductive cough and respiratory conditions where mucus is present.

What Are the Possible Side Effects/Adverse Effects?

Nausea, vomiting, dizziness, headache or rash.

Caution! Don't Use This Drug If . . .

- Your cough is caused by asthma, smoking or emphysema or you have excessive mucus in your respiratory tract.

A cough that won't go away may be an indication of a serious medical condition. If it persists for more than one week or if you seem to have recurrences frequently, see a health professional for evaluation. If the cough is accompanied by a rash or a headache that won't go away, you should also consult with your doctor.

Decongestants

EPHEDRINE (Pretz-D, Kondon's Nasal)

EPINEPHRINE (Adrenalin Chloride)

NAPHAZOLINE (Privine)

OXYMETAZOLINE (Afrin, Allerest, Dristan 12-Hour Nasal)

PHENYLEPHRINE (Alconefrin, Neo-Synephrine, Rhinall, Sinex)

PHENYLPROPANOLAMINE (Propagest)

PSEUDOEPHEDRINE (Afrin, Drixoral Non-Drowsy, Congestion Relief, Genaphed, Halofed, Pseudo-Gest, Sendotabs, Sudafed, Sudex, Cenafed, DeFed-60, Efidac/24, Allermed, Triaminic AM, Decofed Syrup, Cenafed Syrup, PediaCare Infants')

This class of drugs works by constricting blood vessels. Decreased blood flow to the nasal passageways and sinuses helps to reduce swelling and mucous congestion. They are often used along with anti-histamines and are available in oral and topical (nasal spray and eye drop) versions.

After three to five days' use of topical decongestants, rebound congestion often occurs. Despite repeated use, nasal congestion is no longer relieved with the drug. If this happens to you, gradually wean yourself from the medication and allow one to two weeks for things to get back to normal.

When taken orally, decongestants cause central nervous system stimulation. Nervousness, irritability, insomnia, elevations in blood pressure and heart rate, irregular heartbeats, headache, pupil dilation and palpitations can result. If you use a beta agonist asthma medication (albuterol, salmeterol) and add a decongestant, the two drugs can have additive effects, making you feel as though you'd had a few too many cups of coffee. This effect can be dangerous in people with high blood pressure and other types of heart disease.

What Do They Do in the Body?

Swollen mucous membranes in the nose and eyes are a hallmark of seasonal allergies, colds and flu. These over-the-counter drugs counter this inflammation by causing constriction of mucous membranes.

What Are They Used For?

Hay fever, nasal allergies, sinusitis, common cold symptoms and relief of congestion in the middle ear caused by infection. Inhaled through the nose, some can work directly on nasal inflammation or relieve ear blockage and pressure during air travel.

Pseudoephedrine and phenylpropanolamine are mixed-acting agents, which means they have a more generalized effect on the body, while epinephrine is a direct-acting agent with very specific effects on the airways.

WHAT ARE THE POTENTIAL SIDE EFFECTS/ADVERSE EFFECTS?

With topical use as a nasal spray: burning, stinging, sneezing, dryness, local irritation, rebound congestion after stopping the drug.

When taken internally: fear, anxiety, tension, restlessness, headache, lightheadedness, dizziness, drowsiness, tremors, insomnia, hallucinations, psychological disturbances, convulsions, central nervous system depression, weakness, heart rhythm abnormalities, low blood pressure connected with cardiovascular collapse, transient high blood pressure, nausea, vomiting, paleness, difficulty breathing, loss of tone in the muscles of the face and mouth, sweating, urinary problems, twitching of the eyelids (blepharospasm), eye irritation or tearing, heightened sensitivity to the sun (photosensitivity).

CAUTION! THINK TWICE ABOUT TAKING THESE DRUGS IF . . .

- You are taking monoamine oxidase inhibitors (MAO inhibitors).
- You are hypersensitive to stimulating drugs. Some people's bodies respond very strongly to small doses. If you are experiencing dizziness, weakness, tremor and heart arrhythmias you may be getting too high a dose.
- You have glaucoma or if you are using the ophthalmic decongestant naphazoline, don't use nasal sprays containing these drugs.

Powerful stimulation of the central nervous system by these medications can lead to convulsions or cardiovascular collapse.

Don't take internally if you have severe hypertension or heart disease.

Use with caution if you have any of the following conditions: hyperthyroidism, diabetes, any kind of cardiovascular disease, elevated intraocular pressure (often a warning sign of glaucoma in its early stages) or enlarged prostate. Consult with your doctor if you have high blood pressure and want to use an over-the-counter decongestant.

There is some potential for addiction to phenylpropanolamine and pseudoephedrine. Only use when necessary and discontinue as soon as you can.

In elderly people, long-term, high-dose therapy can lead to toxicity and psychosis more easily than in young people.

Beware of rebound congestion, particularly with nasal sprays. Don't fall into a pattern of increasing doses to compensate. Even the nasal inhaler can deliver enough drug to your system to cause toxicity.

WHAT ARE THE INTERACTIONS WITH OTHER DRUGS?

Pseudoephedrine and/or phenylpropanolamine may reduce potency or decrease the amount of time the following drugs are effective:

↓ Insulin
  Oral diabetes drugs

Pseudoephedrine, epinephrine and/or phenylpropanolamine may increase potency or prolong the actions of the following drugs:

↑ Bromocriptine*   Nardil
  Caffeine   Parnate

The following drugs may reduce potency or decrease the amount of time that pseudoephedrine, epinephrine and/or phenylpropanolamine are effective:

↓ Guanethidine   Tricyclic antidepressants
  Phenothiazines   Urinary acidifiers
  Rauwolfia alkaloids (pseudoe-
    phedrine and phenylpropa-
    nolamine only)

The following drugs may increase potency or prolong the actions of pseudoephedrine, epinephrine and/or phenylpropanolamine:

↑ Furazolidone   MAO inhibitors*
  Guanethidine   Rauwolfia alkaloids
  Indomethacin   Tricyclic antidepressants
  Methyldopa   Urinary alkalinizers

---

* Potentially dangerous interaction.

OTHER INTERACTIONS TO BE AWARE OF

Theophylline* and nasal decongestants taken together can lead to theophylline toxicity. Dangerous heart arrhythmias can result.

Beta-blockers increase levels of epinephrine in the bloodstream when they are taken together. A hypertensive episode followed by slowed heartbeat can result.

Diabetics may need to use higher doses of insulin or oral hypoglycemic drugs while using epinephrine.

Steroid Nasal Decongestants

BECLOMETHASONE DIPROPIONATE (Beconase AQ)

FLUTICASONE PROPIONATE (Flonase)

WHAT DO THEY DO IN THE BODY?

When inhaled through the nose, these steroid preparations have an anti-inflammatory effect on nasal mucous membranes. As with the steroid inhalers used for asthma, inhalation somewhat decreases the risk of the adverse effects commonly seen with steroid medications.

WHAT ARE THEY USED FOR?

Relief of symptoms of nasal allergies.

WHAT ARE THE POTENTIAL SIDE EFFECTS/ADVERSE EFFECTS?

Mild inflammation of the nose and throat, burning, stinging, dryness and headache are most common. More rarely: lightheadedness, nausea, nosebleed, bloody mucus, rebound congestion, bronchial asthma symptoms, occasional sneezing attacks, decreased sense of smell, loss of or unpleasant taste in the mouth, throat discomfort, ulceration or deterioration of the mucosa that lines the nasal passages, watery eyes, sore throat, vomiting, *Candida albicans* infection in the nose and/or

---

* Potentially dangerous interaction.

throat, wearing through of the septum that separates the nostrils, raised intraocular pressure (which can lead to glaucoma), or signs of hypercorticism (known as Cushing's syndrome) including swelling of the face, weight gain around the middle of the body and osteoporosis.

Caution! Think Twice About Using These Drugs If . . .

- You have an untreated infection of the nasal mucous lining. Don't use intranasal steroids.
- You are already using systemic steroid drugs such as prednisone. Adding a nasal steroid inhaler can increase the likelihood of suppression of the body's natural production of steroid hormones. If your doctor is weaning you off of systemic steroids and onto inhaled versions, look out for signs of adrenal insufficiency (joint and muscle pain, lack of energy, depression).
- You are using intranasal steroids long term. You should have regular exams to be sure your nasal passages don't suffer permanent damage.

Some people who are sensitive to these medications may develop acne, menstrual irregularities, swelling of the face, weight gain or other symptoms of elevated levels of steroid hormones.

Use these drugs cautiously if you have tuberculosis, an untreated fungal, bacterial or systemic viral infection or herpes of the eye or if you are recovering from an ulcerated nasal septum, nasal surgery or trauma, as healing is slowed by steroid drugs.

Avoid exposure to chicken pox or measles while using these drugs.

What Are the Interactions with Other Drugs?

See page 246 on inhaled steroids for asthma.

Other Things to Do While Taking These Drugs

If your nose is very runny, you may want to use a topical nasal decongestant for the first couple of days you use intranasal steroids.

This will dry things up a bit so that the nasal steroid isn't simply flushed out of your nose without being absorbed.

Cough Suppressants

CODEINE (Codeine Sulfate)

WHAT DOES IT DO IN THE BODY?

Suppresses cough (at low doses); blocks pain response (at higher doses).

WHAT IS IT USED FOR?

Relief of symptoms of cough caused by respiratory tract irritation or relief of mild to moderate pain.

WHAT ARE THE POTENTIAL SIDE EFFECTS/ADVERSE EFFECTS?

Codeine is an addictive narcotic and should not be used unless absolutely necessary. There are other nonaddicting drugs with similar actions, so the use of codeine seems unnecessary.

Nausea, vomiting, sedation, dizziness and constipation are the most common side effects. Other side effects can include allergic reactions, central nervous system depression, lightheadedness, euphoria, restlessness, weakness, headache, hallucinations, disorientation, visual disturbances, convulsions, biliary tract spasm, heart rhythm irregularities, fainting, decreased urinary output and other urinary problems, water retention and rapid blood pressure changes when moving from lying to sitting or from sitting to standing.

CAUTION! THINK TWICE ABOUT USING THIS DRUG IF . . .

- You have recently had a head injury or if you have known intracranial lesions or elevated pressure of the fluid surrounding the brain and spinal cord. Codeine is more likely to have dangerous side effects in these cases. Drowsiness, dizziness and other symptoms of head injury are also side effects of codeine, so you should avoid taking any medications containing this drug until you've been thoroughly evaluated. The same goes for acute abdominal conditions.

- You have asthma or other chronic obstructive pulmonary diseases. Codeine can depress respiratory function.
- You are prone to drug dependency. Addiction can occur. Use only when absolutely necessary. Don't use this drug for more than a few days at a time.

WHAT ARE THE INTERACTIONS WITH OTHER DRUGS?

Central nervous system depressants (opiates, general anesthetics, phenothiazines, tricyclic antidepressants, tranquilizers and alcohol) and codeine have additive effects, meaning they increase the effects of the other drugs, and can impair your ability to drive or perform other tasks.

HYDROCODONE COMBINATIONS

WHAT DOES IT DO IN THE BODY?

Hydrocodone is a narcotic cough suppressant and analgesic (pain reliever) that works by blocking receptors that transmit pain impulses, and by suppressing the cough reflex. It causes euphoria, sedation and general physical depression. It is used in combination with other pain-killer drugs such as acetaminophen and the ibuprofen-type drugs.

WHAT IS IT USED FOR?

Relief of moderate to severe pain, and for relief of cough. It is also used before and during surgery to enhance the effects of anesthesia. Dozens of over-the-counter drugs contain hydrocodone in very small amounts. It's a very potent narcotic analgesic, it's addictive, and it's one of the top 10 most-prescribed drugs in the U.S. If anybody at the FDA was paying attention, it might occur to them that when an addictive drug is found among the top 10 prescribed drugs in the country, we must have an abuse problem with that drug on a national scale.

WHAT ARE THE POTENTIAL SIDE EFFECTS/ADVERSE EFFECTS?

Most frequent: lightheadedness, dizziness, sedation, nausea, vomiting, sweating.

Also: respiratory depression or arrest, apnea (irregular breathing), circulatory depression, coma, shock, cardiac arrest, drastic mood swings, delirium, insomnia, agitation, disorientation, drowsiness, sedation, lethargy, physical impairment, headache, mental cloudiness, visual changes, increased intracranial pressure, pupil dilation, cramps, abdominal pain, taste alterations, dry mouth, loss of appetite, constipation, spasm of the biliary tube (where bile passes from the gallbladder into the intestines), facial flushing, chills, faintness, heart rhythm irregularities, dramatic blood pressure fluctuations, urinary problems, reduced libido.

Those who are hypersensitive to narcotic analgesics may have rash, itching, profuse sweating, spasm of the larynx or fluid retention.

Other possible side effects include bronchospasm, depression of the cough reflex (although hydrocodone may be administered for this purpose, complete suppression of coughing may do more harm than good), interference with the body's ability to regulate its temperature, muscular rigidity and tingling in the extremities.

CAUTION! DON'T TAKE THIS DRUG IF . . .

- You are hypersensitive to narcotics.
- You are having an asthma attack.
- You have diarrhea caused by poisoning. The toxic material should be eliminated from the system completely before you use any narcotic-containing drug.
- You are prone to depression or addiction. Stay away from this drug completely. Hydrocodone is addicting.
- You have had a head injury, or have a brain tumor or any other kind of brain lesions. Don't take hydrocodone.

Use any narcotic-containing drug with extreme caution if you are elderly or debilitated. Those with cardiovascular disease, convulsive disorders, raised eye pressure (which can lead to glaucoma), alcoholism, delirium tremens, hardening of the arteries in the brain, ulcerative colitis, fever, emphysema, severe obesity, hypothyroidism, Addison's disease, enlarged prostate, urinary problems, gallbladder disease or recent gastrointestinal or urinary tract surgery are at special risk when using narcotics.

Those with asthma or other chronic obstructive pulmonary diseases should use extreme caution when taking this drug. It significantly depresses respiratory function, decreasing both the depth and frequency of breaths.

If you are prone to low blood pressure, you should know that hydrocodone can cause blood pressure to dip further.

Kidney and/or liver impairment can cause this drug to accumulate in the bloodstream, making adverse effects more likely.

This drug may cause you to become constipated. Those with ulcerative colitis should be aware that narcotics can cause diarrhea or toxic dilation of the colon.

WHAT ARE THE INTERACTIONS WITH FOODS AND OTHER DRUGS?

The following drugs may prolong effects or increase potency of hydrocodone:

↑ Alcohol
  Barbiturate anesthetics

Chlorpromazine
Cimetidine (adverse effects more likely)

NATURAL ALTERNATIVES FOR COLDS AND ALLERGIES

Prevention is by far the easiest way to deal with colds, flus and allergies. The Six Core Principles for Optimal Health provide the groundwork for prevention and there are other steps you can take as well, which will be covered in this chapter.

Preventing Allergies

To prevent allergies it's important to take the necessary steps to allergy-proof your home, car and workplace, to consciously manage the stress in your life, and to get plenty of rest, good nourishment and exercise.

You can find out what you're allergic to by noticing when you sneeze and wheeze. Is it when you dust or clean out your closets? Is your asthma at its worst when you wake up in the morning with your face buried in your pillow? When you hug your beloved cat, dog or rabbit are you rewarded with several sneezes in succession or tightening in your bronchial tubes? Does the heavily perfumed woman in the elevator make your nose run and your eyes itch? Does mowing the lawn give you itchy eyes and a rash? If so, you probably are one of the scores of people who react to dust mites, pollens, pet danders, molds, synthetic perfumes and other airborne allergens.

If you fall into this category, environmental controls are the first step you need to take to control allergy symptoms. If you're allergic to dust, try to keep closets, carpets, shelves and drapes as dust-free as possible, and wear a dust mask while you do housework. Buy dust mite-proof covers for pillows and mattresses and wash bedding in hot water once a week.

If you're allergic to your pets but can't bring yourself to give them away, keep them well-groomed and don't let them sleep on your furniture or in your bedroom.

If you're allergic to pollens, learn what times of day pollen counts are high in your area and stay indoors during those times.

If you're allergic to perfumes, be sure to buy unscented laundry detergents and fabric softeners, which are loaded with synthetic odors. Don't use the so-called air fresheners (maybe they should be called air polluters), and avoid buying cheap perfumes, which are usually the culprits.

If you find yourself sniffling and sneezing when you're driving, try to determine whether it's caused by car exhaust from other cars or something inside your own car. Many plastic fabrics give off fumes that can be allergenic. If you find you're allergic to car exhaust, set up your life so that you don't have to be in it every day. People running or bicycling for exercise along streets with heavy traffic, inhaling toxins with every breath, aren't being smart. If you live in the city, go to a gym to work out.

Of course, you should do your best to avoid being anywhere near cigarette smoke—especially if you have asthma. As we're finding out, secondhand smoke can be a nose, throat and lung irritant and carcinogen even if you're not allergic to it.

CHECK YOUR VENTILATION SYSTEM

Is air conditioning giving you allergies or summer colds? Most of us who live in hot and humid summertime climates wouldn't think of going without our air conditioning. Not only can it bring relief from stifling heat and humidity, it can filter out the summer pollens that give one in 13 Americans hay fever. But if you're suffering from lung and sinus-related illnesses in spite of being snug in your AC'd house or office, be sure your cooling system is putting out clean air. Studies have shown that cooling systems can either make bronchial and sinus problems such as asthma, bronchitis, allergies and summer colds better or they can make them worse, depending on whether the air is clean.

Let's take air conditioning first. The good news about air conditioning is that it reduces humidity, making a less friendly environment for unfriendly microorganisms. There are two primary causes of air conditioner air pollution. One is a dirty filter and the other is standing water. There are a variety of air conditioning filters, some more effective than others. Predictably the more effective filters, called electrostatic filters, are more expensive, in the range of $50 to $125. However, if you keep the less expensive filters clean, they can work just fine. Here is a very sophisticated way for you to check your air conditioning filter—pull it out and look at it. If it looks dirty, wash it or vacuum it, depending on the type. (Follow directions on the package.) Check your filter at least once a month during the summer or simply vacuum it off when you're vacuuming the rest of the house.

All air conditioners create drops of water condensation which should drip somewhere *outside* the house, but which often drip inside and collect in a puddle. This puddle will quickly grow mold, fungus and bacteria, which will be picked up by your air conditioner and blown into the rest of your house. This is a primary cause of air conditioning-related lung problems. If your air conditioner drips inside the house, put a plate or shallow pan underneath and clean it well with soap and hot water at least once a week.

If you have a forced air cooling and ventilation system, pay attention to whether the ducts are clean, where the outside air source is, whether the air is recycled, and where the intake duct is. Be sure your air sources are clean. If your ducts need cleaning, be aware that an expensive professional cleaning won't do you any good if the whole house isn't cleaned immediately afterwards. A duct cleaning stirs up dust and mold, spreading it through the house. If you don't clean your house at the same time, it will just end up back in the ducts.

Another factor in the summertime quest for clean indoor air is how well your house or office is sealed and insulated. Well-sealed buildings, while more energy efficient, can suffer from what is known as "sick building syndrome." Dozens of household and office products, from furniture to cleaning products, emit vapors that can be harmful if they aren't ventilated out. Some examples are carpet and carpet backing, particle board, plastic furniture and copy machines that use toner. Even your gas heater and stove emit fumes which are harmless in an open environment, but harmful in a closed one. An air conditioner filter will make little impact on these types of fumes and forced air systems often just concentrate and recycle them. You can solve this problem by leaving windows open a crack to let in fresh air from the outside or by having an air purifier.

If you have taken all of the above steps and are still suffering from lung and sinus problems, it would be smart to invest in an air purifier. They can be particularly helpful in office buildings and in bedrooms where dust mites tend to concentrate. The best air purifiers have the HEPA (High Efficiency Particulate Arresting) filter that captures pretty much everything of any consequence in the air within 1500 square feet. It has maximum efficiency, is a real work horse that will go for three to five years on one filter and produces no byproducts such as positive ions or ozone, which are generated by the other types of filters. You can also buy vacuum cleaners equipped with HEPA filtration systems. This is a big investment, but it will most likely pay for itself by saving you the cost of doctor's bills and prescription medicines if your air is making you sick. This air purifier can make a big difference for children with asthma.

Negative ion generators send out negative ions, which soothe the sinus and respiratory tract membranes. Keeping one at your bedside or in other places you spend many hours each day can alleviate allergy symptoms somewhat.

And don't forget about the air conditioning unit in your car. These filters can also become dirty and moldy. Have your mechanic show you where your air conditioning filter is and how to clean it. When you turn on the air conditioning in your car, keep the windows rolled down for a few minutes so new, fresh air will be circulated in. When you're on a busy freeway or stopped at a light, recirculate the air inside the car rather than pulling in the air around you, which will contain concentrated car exhaust.

Natural Allergy Remedies

Treating allergies with antihistamines is a temporary stopgap measure that doesn't address the underlying problem and shouldn't be used for more than a few weeks at a time. If you want to avoid commercial antihistamines, you can try drinking ephedra tea or taking ephedra in capsule form. (Find it at your health food store.) The ephedrine found in ephedra tea is the natural form of the pseudoephedrine found in many antihistamine remedies.

If you've tried everything and your allergy symptoms are still affecting the quality of your life, look into desensitization. Minuscule amounts of allergens are injected in gradually increasing amounts so that your body can learn not to respond with an allergic reaction. Treatment can be expensive and take up to three years, but it doesn't work for everyone.

Some cases of hay fever or allergic sinusitis can be greatly improved when food allergens are identified and eliminated. Decreasing the total allergic load the body has to cope with helps you to become less sensitive to allergens in general. Refer to pages 220–223 to find out how to identify foods that might be causing problems for you.

Elimination of white flour, refined sugar and any foods containing chemicals (additives, preservatives and dyes) is another simple but helpful step you can take before deciding you need drugs to get through hay fever season. Tartrazine, or yellow dye no. 5, is well-known to provoke allergic responses, and for some people just cutting out the processed foods that contain yellow dye is enough to control their allergy problems. Tartrazine is contained in some 60 percent of commercial medications as well as the majority of processed foods. See page 231 for more details on tartrazine.

VITAMIN C

Vitamin C is your number-one natural remedy for allergies. This essential vitamin, which most Americans aren't getting in optimal amounts, directly lowers histamine levels in the body, supports the adrenal glands that produce allergy-fighting hormones and supports the immune system in many ways. The Six Core Principles for Optimal Health recommend 2,000 mg of vitamin C for everyone as part of a daily regimen. During allergy season, you can take an additional 1,000 mg to 2,000 mg throughout the day. If your symptoms continue or worsen, increase the dosage to 1,000 mg every two or three hours. If you get diarrhea, back off the dose until it stops. Your tolerance for vitamin C can increase dramatically when you have allergies, a cold or a flu.

THE DEFENSIVE HERBS

We have many herbs at our disposal that effectively strengthen and support the immune system without encouraging it to overreact. You can try a regimen of two weeks of the herb echinacea followed by two weeks of the herb astragalus. For some people, stinging nettle (*Urtica dioica*) works wonders to alleviate allergy symptoms. Follow directions on the container.

ADDITIONAL ANTIOXIDANT POWER

Quercetin is a powerful antioxidant flavonoid (from buckwheat, citrus or eucalyptus) that for some people is highly effective in preventing allergy symptoms.

PANTOTHENIC ACID (Vitamin B5)

Pantothenic acid can be helpful in treating allergies, especially when they are aggravated by fatigue, exhaustion or stress. Try taking one gram (1,000 mg) twice daily.

ESSENTIAL FATTY ACIDS (EFAs)

Unsaturated fatty acids such as those found in flaxseed, fish, evening primrose, borage and black currant oils may help diminish allergic inflammation. There's a current nutritional fad that says everyone should be taking a lot of essential fatty acid supplements such as flaxseed oil all the time, but this isn't a good idea because they are highly unstable, unsaturated oils that we only need in tiny amounts, and overdoing it is just asking for another imbalance in the body. However, they can be very useful for temporarily treating inflammatory conditions such as allergies. Normally you can get all the EFAs you need from eating plenty of fresh fruits, vegetables and whole grains and fish a few times a week.

BEE REMEDIES

Bee pollen may give some people relief, but try just a little bit first in case you are one of the few who are allergic to it. If you can buy fresh local honey at the farmer's market or health food store, you can try that instead. The local pollens in the honey can desensitize your hay fever reactions.

Carry allergy-fighting supplements with you so that as soon as you feel an allergic reaction coming on you can nip it in the bud. You can travel with packets of Emergen-C, which contains 1,000 to 2,000 mg of vitamin C and smaller amounts of a handful of other immune-supportive vitamins. The bioflavonoids found in grapeseed extract (proanthocyanidins) and green tea are especially powerful and effective for treating allergies.

Alternative Approaches to Treating Asthma

There are a number of good studies showing that homeopathy can work very well to control asthma. If this appeals to you, work with a certified homeopath.

Yoga exercises that include deep breathing and deep relaxation techniques have been found to be very effective in reducing the number and severity of asthma attacks.

WHAT SETS OFF AN ASTHMA ATTACK?

Once a person is predisposed to have asthma, all kinds of things can set it off. Here is a list of the best-known culprits:

Airborne allergens such as pollen

Animal dander

Carbon dioxide released by cooking or heating with gas

Drugs such as aspirin and beta blockers

Emotional stress

Exercise

Food additives such as:

   Food dyes (especially yellow dye #5)

   Preservatives such as sulfites and benzoates

   Flavorings such as salicylates, aspartame and MSG (often disguised as "natural flavors," and hydrolyzed vegetable protein)

   Stabilizers and emulsifiers such as carageenan and vegetable gums

Food allergies (most commonly eggs, wheat, citrus)

Fresh paint

Room deodorizers and household cleaners

Strong odors from cooking

Tobacco smoke

There is also a substantial body of research showing that acupuncture can help with asthma.

Although sudden bouts of exercise can trigger an asthma attack, for many, regular aerobic exercise is very helpful because it increases the capacity of the lungs to take in oxygen, and strengthens the heart.

Drs. Jonathan Wright and Alan Gaby, two pioneering M.D.s in the use of nutrition to prevent and cure illness, swear by intramuscular vitamin B12 injections (1,000 mcg) for childhood asthma. Talk to your doctor—he or she should be happy to try B12 for any child dependent upon asthma drugs.

Some studies show that vitamin B6 is useful in treating asthma. You can try 50 mg of vitamin B6 twice daily taken with food.

We have a growing body of evidence that there is a hormonal link to asthma. Women are four times as likely to have an asthma attack when they are premenstrual, and hormone replacement therapy that uses estrogens can aggravate asthma. The hormonal culprit is most likely what Dr. John Lee has termed "estrogen dominance," meaning even though estrogen levels may be low premenstrually, there is little or no progesterone in the body to balance or oppose it, causing symptoms of estrogen excess. It is very common for premenstrual asthma to clear up with the use of natural progesterone cream. (The synthetic progestins are apt to aggravate asthma.) See Chapter 18 for details on using natural progesterone.

Another intriguing theory appears in the book *Your Body's Many Cries for Water* by F. Batmanghelidj, M.D. (Global Health Solutions, 1995). Dr. Batmanghelidj's theory is based on the fact that part of the physical response the body has prior to and during an asthma attack is the release of histamines, which cause inflammation. Histamine plays an important role in the regulation of water distribution in the body. He explains that when concentrated blood (due to dehydration) enters the lungs, the body's response is to release histamines, which causes constriction of the airways in the lungs, thus reducing the need for water. Batmanghelidj also believes that long-term dehydration can cause an up-regulating of the immune system, causing it to overreact to allergens.

This theory makes a lot of sense. If you feel an asthma attack coming on, you can try drinking three or four eight-ounce glasses of water and see if that helps.

THE EMOTIONAL STRESS FACTOR IN ASTHMA

Although people don't like to talk about this, asthma has a very clear and definite link to chronic emotional stress. People who tend to hold in their emotions, and even deny to themselves that they are feeling sad, angry or scared (for example), and suffer anxiety as a result, tend to get asthma more often than those who are able to acknowledge and express their emotions and relieve their anxiety. One woman almost entirely eliminated her asthma by learning to yell. First, when she began to feel that "wheezy" sensation that all asthmatics dread, she learned to ask herself what she was feeling. She let her asthma be her guide that something was up emotionally. Then she would get in her car and roll up the windows, get on the freeway, and yell. Even when she couldn't do that, she found that simply admitting to herself that she was angry or sad or scared was very helpful in warding off her asthma attacks.

Asthma inhalers using cortisone-like steroids and epinephrine are among the most effective ways to prevent and control asthma attacks. This fact should give us a major clue that asthma can be aggravated by adrenal glands that are tired and depleted because they are working overtime due to chronic stress and they are trying to produce stress hormones such as cortisol and adrenaline (which is related to epinephrine). If your body's best natural defense against an asthma attack is to pump out some adrenal hormones, and it is unable to do so because the adrenal glands are depleted, the inhaler is the next best thing as a temporary stopgap measure. But to the extent that this is a problem in a child or adult, there is a serious depletion that needs to be addressed. It is very important that parents find the cause behind their child's asthma attacks, and treat that.

If you are suffering from asthma that's serious enough to compromise everyday life, your best bet is to combine some type of counseling with avoiding environmental triggers and lifestyle changes such as managing stress and good nutrition. Tackling any one of those three causes (emotional, environmental, lifestyle) will help, but it usually takes working on all three to truly solve the problem.

Nutritional Prescription for Allergies and Asthma

1. Avoid processed foods such as chips, cakes, cookies, puddings, cheeses, canned foods and frozen foods that contain additives, preservatives, dyes or flavor enhancers such as MSG and hydrolyzed protein.
2. Avoid excessive sugar and refined white flour.
3. Avoid caffeine, which puts stress on the adrenal glands.
4. To treat asthma you can try taking some or all of the following supplements, in addition to what is recommended in the Six Core Principles for Optimal Health:
   - Vitamin C, 1000 to 4000 mg, three to four times a day (has antihistamine-like activity and supports the adrenal glands).
   - Vitamin A (preformed, not as beta-carotene), up to 50,000 IU a day in divided doses for up to two weeks to help heal mucous membranes and resist infection (do not take over

10,000 IU daily if you are pregnant or if you could become pregnant).

- Vitamin B6, 50 to 100 mg three times a day.
- Magnesium citrate, gluconate or glycinate, 200 to 300 mg three times a day.
- Cod liver oil daily for up to three weeks in the winter (make sure it has a natural preservative such as vitamin E).
- Evening primrose oil, borage oil or black currant oil for up to three weeks.
- N-acetyl cysteine (NAC), 500 mg two to three times a day.
- Ephedra tea (for adults), one to three cups daily (if it makes you jittery or irritable, or if you have high blood pressure, don't use it).
- Licorice root tincture to support the adrenal glands (follow directions on the container). Don't use for more than three weeks if you have high blood pressure.
- St. John's wort (Hypericum) to help control anxiety.
- Ginkgo biloba in a standardized extract, 60 mg one to three times daily.
- MSM (methylsulfonylmethane) is a form of organic sulfur. It binds to allergens, thus preventing allergic reactions, and it coats the intestinal lining to prevent dust mites and their droppings from playing havoc with allergies and worsening asthma. Take 1,000 mg, two to three times daily. You can take up to 6,000 mg daily.

Preventing and Treating Colds and Flus Naturally

We have been led to believe that we "catch" more colds in the winter because of the colder weather. But the common cold was unknown to the Eskimos before the white man went to the Arctic, bringing his refined white flour, sugar and alcohol with him. And why do some people regularly get colds and flus and others seem immune? Maybe it has something to do with lifestyle.

When the weather turns cold we tend to overheat our homes, creating dry, low-humidity air. Microorganisms (germs) multiply faster in your nasal passages when the humidity is low. When the heat goes on, a humidifier should go on with it.

When you feel cold or flu symptoms, act immediately. Even a few hours can make a big difference. Also get to bed early, stay warm, avoid junk food and drink plenty of clean water. Too much sugar will depress your immune system, making you more susceptible to opportunistic germs.

Colds and flus are passed on from one person to another more through shaking hands than any other cause. This is a good reason to keep your hands away from your face and to wash your hands before you eat, just like your mother told you! When the Japanese have a cold or flu they would never think of going out into a crowd without first donning a surgical mask over their nose and mouth.

Another major factor that contributes to cold/flu season is the holidays. Not only do family gatherings and travel stress us out, we tend to overeat more during the holidays and consume more alcohol and sweets that suppress the immune system.

The number-one, all-time most effective medicine for colds and flus is an ounce of prevention: a nutritious diet, plenty of clean water, exercise, enough sleep and relaxed time spent with loved ones. However, since we are by nature not perfect, here are some natural helpers for fending off and alleviating colds and flus. One of the most important keys to warding off a cold or flu is to start treating it early, at the first signs. If you wait until you have full-blown symptoms and feel miserable, the medicines only alleviate the symptoms somewhat.

ECHINACEA

Taken at the first sign of a cold or flu, echinacea will help boost the immune system. Many herbalists like to combine echinacea with goldenseal and astragalus.

CHINESE HERBS

The Chinese have dozens of tried and true herbal remedies called "patent medicines" that they have used for thousands of years. These are just starting to catch on in the United States. They are available at many health food stores and herb shops. There are two that work

SHOULD YOU GET A FLU SHOT?

Every fall Americans are put through the annual flu season vaccination ritual. The ritual goes like this: You go to your physician, he or she tells you that the flu can be deadly and that a flu shot will prevent it. You get the shot, feel terrible for a week, and a couple of months later, you get the flu along with everyone else. The next year rolls around and you ask yourself, should I or shouldn't I get a flu shot? That's a decision only you can make, but I'd like to give you a few facts about flu shots that you're not likely to hear from your physician.

Deaths from flu are increasing in spite of flu shots. The flu can be deadly. According to government statistics, P&I deaths (pneumonia and influenza) are among the top 10 causes of death in the elderly. And wouldn't it be wonderful if flu shots were the magic bullet they're made out to be? But, according to statistics released by the Centers for Disease Control, the P&I death rate has increased 59 percent since 1979. Even adjusting for the fact that there are increasing numbers of people over the age of 65, who are more susceptible to death from the flu, there is still a 44 percent increase in P&I deaths among people 65 and older. And this is in spite of the fact that an estimated 52 percent of the population aged 65 and older received flu shots in 1994, way up from an estimated rate of 20 percent in 1987, for example.

If flu vaccinations are working so well, why is this happening? One reason is that as you age, which is when you need the most protection from flu, your body's ability to create antibodies to the vaccine deteriorates. It is known that only about half of the elderly who receive flu shots can mount an antibody response strong enough to be protective. And because the strains of flu that sweep through North America are different every year, the antibody response will only be protective if the manufacturers of the vaccine are lucky enough to pick the right flu virus! A study from the Netherlands showed that among two groups of elderly people, one that received flu shots and one that received a placebo, the group receiving the flu shot only had a 1 percent lower incidence of flu than the placebo group!

Flu shots are not without side effects. Studies have shown that as many as one in 10 people who get a flu shot experience flu symptoms within a week. Meanwhile, a study in Newfoundland found that older people who take a multivitamin every day for a year have a much stronger immune system and fewer days of illness due to infections than those who don't take multivitamins.

If you feel it's important to follow your physician's orders and get a flu shot, by all means do it, but please don't fool yourself into thinking that a flu shot is highly protective and that you don't need to take care of yourself to prevent the flu.

well for warding off colds and flus. Ganmaoling tablets are a general cold/flu remedy. If you're starting to get a cough or other symptoms in your lungs, try Sangchu tablets. These herbs work very specifically to balance the body and work best if they are taken alone, without any other medication.

HOMEOPATHICS

Many people respond well to homeopathic medicines. Coldcalm by Boiron works well for colds and many people swear by Oscillococcinum for the flu. Boericke and Tafel makes an excellent cough syrup called B & T Homeopathic Cough and Bronchial Syrup.

HERBAL TEAS

There are quite a few tea mixtures that can help with cold/flu symptoms. Chamomile tea works well and Celestial Seasonings' Sleepytime tea contains chamomile and other soothing and relaxing herbs. The same company makes Mama Bear's Cold Care tea, which is mostly peppermint and licorice and works well for soothing a cough. There are many types of cold/flu herbal tea mixtures on the market. For respiratory ailments look for teas containing licorice, fennel and horehound. For sinus ailments and headaches look for chamomile, echinacea, goldenseal and bayberry.

GINSENG

Studies have shown that 100 mg a day of ginseng extract significantly cuts your chances of catching a cold or flu bug.

VITAMIN C

Take at least 2,000 mg a day of vitamin C. The esterfied C type works best for a sensitive stomach. Along with its antioxidant activity, the vitamin C will lower your histamine level, giving you relief from sinus congestion, watery eyes, sniffling and sneezing.

YOUR NATURAL REMEDY TRAVEL KIT

You can keep preventive medicine in your desk drawers at work so that if you feel a cold or flu coming on you don't have to wait until you get home to treat it. When you travel, always plan ahead by bringing natural remedies for colds and flus, indigestion, insomnia and tension or stress. It's especially important to plan ahead during the holiday season, when we often combine extra-stressful travel, cold weather, too many immune-depressing sugary foods and family tensions. Also remember to drink plenty of clean water and take your multivitamin every day. Here are suggestions for your travel kit:

- ✓ Melatonin, sublingual (under the tongue) tablets for insomnia and jet lag.
- ✓ Ginger capsules or ginger tea for nausea and gas.
- ✓ Chewable papaya tablets for indigestion after a big meal.
- ✓ Echinacea, astragalus, goldenseal capsules or tincture for cold and flu prevention.
- ✓ Zinc lozenges combined with vitamin C and propolis for cold prevention. Zinc has a direct effect in boosting the immune system and may have some antiviral properties as well.
- ✓ An herbal throat spray that includes echinacea and goldenseal to prevent a sore throat from taking hold.
- ✓ White willow bark capsules or tincture to treat a headache or other types of pain.
- ✓ Kava or St. John's wort capsules, tablets or tincture for stress and anxiety.
- ✓ Chromium picolinate tablets (200 mcg) to balance blood sugar.
- ✓ *Oscillococcinum*, a homeopathic remedy, to prevent the flu. Open one tube, pour it into your mouth and suck on the contents until gone (it's tiny sugar pellets). Since this is a homeopathic remedy, it is important not to consume caffeine, menthol or peppermint within 30 minutes of taking it. Take every six hours. If it doesn't work after three tubes it's probably not going to. Oscillococcinum's action is fast and dramatic when it works.
- ✓ Vitamin C in Emergen-C packets. Vitamin C supports the immune system on many levels. At the tissue level, it counteracts histamines, which cause inflammation and congestion, and is needed for tissue repair. At the cellular level, it acts as an antioxidant and is essential to the functioning of the white blood cells that fight disease. Take at least one packet every two hours when you feel a cold or flu coming on, for up to 12 hours.

COLD/FLU KIT FOR KIDS

Sick kids aren't about to swallow some yucky-tasting medicine and with their sensitive taste buds it's easy to get a yuck. Fortunately kids find most of the cold/flu essentials easy to tolerate. The Oscillococcinum tastes like sugar—no problem. Most kids like zinc lozenges, especially when they're coming down with a cold, and chewable vitamin Cs are easy to find. They'll probably hate the throat spray—it does pack a punch—but it's worth a try.

ZINC LOZENGES

Alternative health professionals have been telling you for at least a decade to suck on zinc and vitamin C lozenges to shorten the duration of a cold, and finally a scientific study has been published in the *Annals of Internal Medicine* confirming this. Of 100 cold sufferers, half were given lozenges with zinc and half without. The zinc group got better in an average of four days, while the nonzinc group got better in an average of seven days. (It generally takes conventional medicine at least a decade to catch up with the progress made and implemented in alternative medicine. Yet another reason to work with an alternative health care practitioner.)

In spite of the hype you'll hear about how only one special type of zinc works, that is hogwash. Any type of zinc chelate will work just fine. There are many excellent zinc lozenges available. Look for one with at least 5 mg of zinc and follow directions on the container.

PROTECTING YOUR SINUSES AND THROAT

Many colds begin with an infection in the sinuses, which then drips down the back of the throat and infects the throat and then moves on to the lungs. If you can do it, rinse your sinuses with a water, salt and baking soda mixture, 1 cup water, ¼ to ½ tsp. of salt and a pinch of baking soda. Do this over a sink. You can either use a rubber ear syringe, a shallow cup or the palm of your hand. Tip your head to one side, block the bottom nostril, insert the syringe into the other nostril and gently squeeze the water in, allowing it to go up the nose and drain out the top of the mouth. If you're doing it in your palm, you have to gently sniff the water up the nostril—this takes a bit more finesse. You can also find nasal irrigators at most health food stores. These look like little ceramic pitchers with a long spout that you can place in one nostril.

If you have a sore throat, go after the bacteria on the throat by gargling with salt water, a strong mouthwash such as Listerine or an herbal spray that contains goldenseal and propolis.

Special Treatments for Viruses

Although your best defense against a virus is a strong immune system, there are some natural supplements you can take that will greatly aid your body in fending them off.

SELENIUM

Selenium is a trace mineral that we only need in microgram amounts, but a deficiency can make us much more susceptible to the flu. There is new evidence that taking larger doses of selenium can make a major difference in helping the body fight off a virus. A normal daily dose of selenium is 50 to 200 mcg, but if you're fighting a cold or flu you can take up to 800 mcg daily for three days. Selenium also works well to help fight off the herpes virus, in the same dosages.

ELDERBERRY

European black elderberries (*Sambucus nigra L.*) have been used as a folk remedy for flu, colds and coughs for at least 2,500 years. Even Hippocrates mentioned it in his writings. If you're from the American Midwest, chances are your grandparents made elderberry wine and sipped it on winter evenings as a tonic.

More recently, an Israeli scientist named Madeleine Mumcuoglu was in Switzerland researching viruses and looking for a doctoral thesis. Her supervisor suggested that, since he had 22 pounds of elderberries in his freezer, she investigate their power to fight the flu. She took his advice and was able to isolate some proteins that deactivated a flu virus in the laboratory.

20 WAYS TO SUPERCHARGE YOUR IMMUNE SYSTEM AND PREVENT COLDS AND FLUS

1. Stretching helps your lymphatic system do its job of removing toxins from your body. Be sure to stretch your neck muscles, your torso, and to stretch your arms over your head.

2. Get an extra hour of sleep or go to bed early with a cup of chamomile tea and an uplifting book.

3. Zinc lozenges are powerful weapons in the fight against winter colds. Try the varieties with propolis and vitamin C added.

4. The homeopathic remedy Oscillococcinum will quickly knock out many kinds of flu. The only way to find out if it will work for what you've got is to try it.

5. Reduce the stress in your life through meditation and exercise. Chronic stress depletes your adrenals, which play a vital role in immunity.

6. Stock up on the vitamin C and bioflavonoids. If you feel something coming on, take 1,000 mg of vitamin C and a bioflavonoid such as grapeseed and/or green tea extract every hour.

7. Drink plenty of clean water which will help your body keep itself detoxified.

8. Eat plenty of fiber to keep things moving through the digestive system.

9. Eat yogurt once a day for the calcium and beneficial intestinal flora. The friendly bacteria in your intestines are your best weapon against unfriendly bacteria.

10. Skip the candy and soda pop. Try a piece of fruit or some nuts instead.

11. Keep alcohol consumption low. A glass of wine with dinner is fine. More than that and your liver has to work too hard.

12. Eat your vegetables—fresh and preferably organic.

13. Are you allergic to dairy products? Wheat? Corn? Chronic allergies can weaken your immune system.

14. Eat more complex carbohydrates and less refined white flour which causes blood sugar jumps and constipation.

15. Try shiitake or reishi mushrooms with your veggies—the Chinese use them to bolster the immune system.

16. Take two droppersful or two capsules of echinacea tincture three times a day at the first sign of a cold or flu. Some people like the echinacea and goldenseal combination. Don't take it for more than two weeks in a row or your body will become desensitized to it.

17. If you have a late night or stressful day, balance things out by getting extra rest.
18. If you're going to be traveling on a plane, take plenty of vitamin C and echinacea for a few days ahead of time.
19. Seek out the company of loved ones or volunteer for someone less fortunate than you.
20. Exercise keeps everything in the body ship-shape, but if you feel weak or tired, don't push it too hard.

Mumcuoglu theorized that the elderberry worked because viruses cannot replicate themselves on their own. They invade living cells and alter their DNA. If you can stop the virus from entering cells, it can't get to the DNA to replicate itself. The flu virus invades cells by puncturing cell walls with tiny spikes called hemagglutinin that cover its surface. After watching viruses and elderberry in the laboratory, Mumcuoglu found that the active ingredients in elderberry actually disarmed the spikes by binding to them and preventing them from piercing the cell membrane. The viral spikes are covered with an enzyme called neuraminidase. This enzyme acts to break down the cell wall. Mumcuoglu believes that bioflavonoids, also present in high concentration in elderberries, may inhibit the action of this enzyme.

Back in Israel nearly a decade later, Mumcuoglu and her colleagues found that their elderberry extract deactivated other flu viruses in the test tube. The next step was to do a double-blind study with a group of people suffering from the flu. Half the group was given an elderberry extract, and half was given a placebo. Within 24 hours, flu symptoms of fever, cough and muscle pain in the elderberry group had dramatically improved in 20 percent of the patients. By day two another 75 percent had clearly improved, and by day three more than 90 percent of the group was better. In contrast, among those taking the placebo, only 8 percent showed any improvement after 24 hours, and the remaining 92 percent took about six days to improve. Nobody in the elderberry group complained of any side effects.

The elderberry group also had a higher level of antibodies to the flu, indicating an enhanced immune system response. If a pharmaceutical drug or the flu shot had anywhere near this type of response, everyone would have some in their medicine cabinet!

Mumcuoglu has also done studies that show great promise in combating other viruses with elderberry extract, including HIV, herpes and Epstein-Barr virus.

If you take elderberry syrup or extract at the first sign of a cold or flu, chances are excellent it will work. And if you live in an area where elderberries grow, you may want to consider reviving the tradition of sipping elderberry wine on chilly winter evenings! You can find elderberry remedies at most health food stores. Follow the directions on the label.

CHAPTER 12

Drugs for Pain Relief and Their Natural Alternatives

AMERICANS LOVE TO take pills for pain. We gobble up *billions* of pain reliever pills each year to the tune of $30 billion a year. The large drug companies that sell over-the-counter pain-relieving drugs like acetaminophen (Tylenol), ibuprofen and aspirin are always fighting for a share of that huge market, and we buy right into their advertising and marketing, believing that the only way to deal with pain is to make it go away with a pill. And after all, who doesn't want their pain relieved, and the sooner the better.

The urge to simply suppress pain can be harmful in the long run. Pain is your body's way of telling you something is wrong. It is a warning signal that has been called the guardian of health, and the sooner you act to heal the source of your pain, the better off you'll be.

If you suffer from some type of chronic pain you are not alone. Just in the United States, over 100 million people suffer from chronic pain. About 37 million of those suffer from arthritis, 30 million from headaches, and 15 million from the pain caused by cancer. Another 32 million suffer from other types of chronic pain such as back pain, osteoporosis and nerve pain.

If you are suffering from severe pain that requires prescription medication, be aware that prescription drugs for pain have the potential to be abused and to cause you harm and even death. On the other hand, nobody should ever suffer unnecessarily from pain out of fear of becoming addicted to a pain drug. If you have acute or temporary severe pain caused by recovering from surgery or a broken bone, for example, it's wonderful to be able to take advantage of the relief that pain-killing drugs can give you. That's what they should be used for.

Managing and preventing pain effectively involves much more than just taking a pill to make it go away. It's important to treat the underlying cause of the pain as well. Acute or short-term pain, and chronic or long-term pain need to be treated differently. Short-term pain can often be helped by treating both cause and symptom at once, such as ice and some aspirin for a pulled muscle, but chronic pain requires a whole other set of solutions, which will be covered in more depth at the end of the chapter.

In the United States, the terminally ill tend to be *under* treated for pain. If you have severe, intractable, untreatable pain, you should never avoid pain relief medication out of a sense of guilt or shame, or concern that you will become dependent on it.

If you have chronic pain caused by a disease such as arthritis or fibromyalgia, the waters become a little bit muddier in terms of deciding when and how to take pain medication. Most pain-killing drugs don't work for very long or very well for these types of pain. The most important part of managing chronic pain is preventing and eliminating the source of the pain. You'll find solutions that generally work much better than pain-suppressing drugs at the end of this chapter. Please read the chapter on addictive drugs if you are dealing with severe pain or think you may be hooked on pain-killing drugs.

OVER-THE-COUNTER PAINKILLERS

Because the over-the-counter painkillers such as aspirin, ibuprofen and acetaminophen are so common and we can buy them without a prescription, we tend to think they're harmless and that we can take them every day, but they actually have side effects that can range from uncomfortable to deadly. The most commonly reported side effect is gastrointestinal bleeding caused by aspirin and ibuprofen-type drugs, also called NSAIDs (nonsteroidal anti-inflammatory drugs). It is estimated that 41,000 people a year are hospitalized from the side effects of taking too many NSAIDs and some 6,000 people a year die from complications directly related to NSAIDs. Some 30 percent of hospitalizations and deaths related to peptic ulcer disease are attrib-

NSAIDS AND MELATONIN DON'T MIX

Melatonin is a wonderful hormone for treating jet lag, occasional insomnia in younger people and chronic insomnia in older people. This amazing hormone is secreted in the human brain in response to darkness, and is truly important to a good night's sleep.

Some drugs, including NSAIDs, interfere with the brain's production of melatonin. In fact, just one dose of normal aspirin can cut your melatonin production as much as 75 percent. If you're taking these drugs, take the last dose after dinner. Other drugs that can interfere with melatonin production in the brain include the benzodiazepines such as Valium and Xanax, caffeine, alcohol, cold medicines, diuretics, beta-blockers, calcium channel blockers, stimulants such as diet pills, and corticosteroids such as prednisone.

If you're in the habit of having a midnight snack, some of the foods that can boost the production of melatonin include oatmeal, corn, barley, bananas and rice. A hot bath before bed can also raise melatonin levels.

uted to aspirin- and ibuprofen-type drugs. When you combine aspirin or ibuprofen-type painkillers with alcohol, you are four times as likely to develop gastrointestinal bleeding.

Acetaminophen, advertised as a safe alternative to the NSAIDs that cause stomach upset, is not a harmless panacea. Although it is an over-the-counter drug, it can have serious side effects, such as liver and kidney damage. Each year many thousands of people are unknowingly harmed by liver damage caused by acetaminophen. This is especially true of children whose parents carelessly give them liquid acetaminophen at the least sign of discomfort.

It's important that you understand very clearly that while aspirin, ibuprofen and acetaminophen can be very useful for the odd headache or sprain, they are potent drugs with serious side effects that should never be taken for more than a few days in a row or more than a few days a month.

WHAT CAUSES ARTHRITIS PAIN?

One of the most common types of pain is arthritis pain. Osteoarthritis is the most common form of arthritis and affects more than 40 million Americans. It affects 80 percent of people over the age of 50.

Although conventional medicine doesn't have much to offer in the way of relief from arthritis aside from pain-killing drugs, we do know a lot about what causes arthritis and alternative medicine has great success with treating it.

The major risk factors for arthritis are well-known. Smoking has been proven over and over again to increase the risk of arthritis. A recent study of twins done in Great Britain compared arthritis in those who smoked and those who didn't, and found that those who smoked had a much higher risk of arthritis.

Side Effects of NSAIDs

NSAID	Action	Side Effects
acetaminophen (Tylenol)	relieves pain, reduces fever	liver and kidney damage, rash, dizziness; do not combine with alcohol or take for a hangover
aspirin	reduces fever, relieves pain, reduces inflammation	allergic reactions, stomach upset, gastrointestinal bleeding, ulcers, ringing ears; should not be used by pregnant women or children
ibuprofen (Advil)	reduces fever, relieves pain, effective for menstrual pain, reduces inflammation	skin rashes, itching, stomach upset, digestive problems
ketoprofen (Orudis)	reduces fever, relieves pain, reduces inflammation	stomach upset, digestive problems, dizziness, itching, skin rashes
naproxen (Aleve)	relieves pain, reduces fever, reduces inflammation	skin rashes, itching, stomach upset, digestive problems, dizziness

Obesity may be the single biggest cause of arthritis. According to an article in the *American Journal of Clinical Nutrition,* the single biggest risk factor for osteoarthritis in the hips and hands of people older than 60 is being overweight. Reducing the symptoms of this painful disease should be a great inspiration to drop those pounds! Gentle movement and exercise are highly recommended for all types of arthritis.

Naturopathic doctors have discovered that food allergies are often a direct culprit in arthritis pain. Crippling arthritis can clear up simply by eliminating the nightshade family of plants from the diet (tomatoes, potatoes, eggplant). Other common food allergens are citrus fruits, dairy products, wheat, corn and soy.

Long term, the NSAIDs and acetaminophen can actually aggravate arthritis, because they inhibit collagen synthesis and accelerate the destruction of cartilage. Collagen is the glue that holds tissues together, and any chronic pain relief program should be building collagen, not destroying it.

TRACK DOWN THE CAUSE OF YOUR HEADACHE

As estimated 30 million Americans suffer from chronic headaches, and 90 percent of those are thought to be "tension headaches." This doesn't necessarily mean these headaches are caused by emotional tension (though that is often the case), it means they are caused by tension in the muscles of the shoulders, neck and head, and by constriction or congestion of the blood vessels in the head. Tension headaches have literally dozens of potential causes, and often a combination of causes.

Another 20 to 30 million people suffer from occasional headaches, sometimes called "too much" headaches. This includes "too much" sugar, alcohol, drugs, staying up late, stress, sun or whatever else it is that gives you a pain in the head. Eyestrain, sinus infection and allergies, ear infection and fever are also well-known culprits.

Prescription and over-the-counter drugs are probably the single most common cause of headaches in older people. In fact, so many drugs can cause headaches that if you're taking any type of medication, you can assume first that it's the culprit and go from there. If you're taking more than one medication, chances are even better they are the culprit.

Lesser-known causes of tension headaches are constipation, hypothyroidism (low thyroid), high blood pressure, hypoglycemia, caffeine withdrawal and adrenal exhaustion. Allergies or sensitivities to substances such as perfume, car exhaust, paint fumes and cigarette smoke can also cause headaches.

Migraine headaches afflict fewer people but make up for that in the intensity of the pain they inflict. The good news is that the causes of migraines are fairly easy to track down once you know how.

For women, hormone imbalance is a common cause of headaches: Some 6.1 percent of men compared to 14 percent of women have four or more headaches a month. Three times as many women than men suffer from migraines, and many women's migraines occur premenstrually. (Whenever women are suffering from an ailment twice as much as men, or vice versa, it's a good tip-off that the underlying cause is hormonal.) The culprit in these cases is usually a progesterone deficiency and a resulting excess of estrogen. Synthetic hormone replacement therapy (i.e., Premarin, Provera, Prempro) is probably the most common cause of headaches among menopausal women. Read the book, *What Your Doctor May Not Tell You About Hormone Balance* by John R. Lee, M.D. (Warner Books, 1996) for details on how to balance your hormones naturally.

After stress, food allergies are probably the most common cause of both tension and migraine headaches, especially in children. There have been controlled double-blind studies showing that elimination of allergenic foods cures migraines in a majority of patients. In one study, 83 percent of the patients who eliminated allergenic foods, drugs or inhalants cured their migraines. The foods that most often cause migraines are dairy products, wheat, citrus, chocolate, coffee, nuts, eggs, the artificial sweetener aspartame, the flavoring MSG (monosodium glutamate) and other artificial additives and preservatives.

Many people who get migraines are sensitive to foods containing large amounts of the amino acid tyramine. These include aged and fermented foods such as aged cheeses, vinegar, beer, wine and miso; pickled foods including sauerkraut; meats such as sausages and bologna and avocados.

If you take migraine drugs for pain relief, you should know that the side effects are significant and some of them are so toxic that they are only prescribed for five days at the maximum.

BACK PAIN

Acute back pain is among the easiest types of pain to prevent. You do it by lifting properly and keeping your back and stomach muscles strong. Chronic back pain is an extremely common type of pain, especially in older Americans who are simultaneously putting on weight and suffering from chronic stress. Although back-strengthening exercises have permanently eliminated back pain in many people, there is undeniably an emotional component to the majority of back pain.

If you or someone you love has back pain, read the book *Healing Back Pain* by John Sarno, M.D. (Warner Books, 1991). This book was written by an M.D. who had seen thousands of patients with back pain and had little success in treating them until he began addressing the emotional components of this type of pain. It's an illuminating and useful book, and his suggestions are easy to do.

CARPAL TUNNEL SYNDROME

Carpal tunnel syndrome is a repetitive motion disorder caused by repeating one movement over and over again with the wrist. Those who work intensively on computers, cashiers and waitresses are among those who most commonly suffer from carpal tunnel syndrome.

Once you have carpal tunnel syndrome it can be very difficult to heal, so pay attention to early symptoms and treat them right away by not doing the repetitive motion. It's easy to brush off early pain by telling yourself you don't have the time to solve the problem, but if you wait too long you may solve the problem by being out of a job. You'll get some nutritional pointers for treating carpal tunnel at the end of the chapter.

DRUGS FOR PAIN RELIEF

Acetaminophen

ACETAMINOPHEN (Tylenol, Children's Feverall, Acephen, Abenol, Apacet, Aceta, Myapap, Maranox, Genapap, Panadol, Neopap, Silapap, Anacin-3, Redutemp, Arthritis Foundation Pain Reliever, Dapa, Ridenol)

Acetaminophen is one of the most overused and abused drugs on the market today because clever advertising and marketing have told us that it is harmless. However, it is potent medicine with great potential to do harm, especially in children. Please use it only when necessary.

Acetaminophen is also used in dozens of prescription and over-the-counter cold, cough, flu, arthritis and headache remedies in combination with other drugs. Read labels.

WHAT DOES IT DO IN YOUR BODY?

Relieves pain and reduces fever by increasing the dissipation of body heat. It also relieves pain from inflammation, but does not reduce inflammation.

WHAT IS IT PRESCRIBED FOR?

Most commonly it is prescribed for headaches, pain from earaches, teething, toothaches, menstruation, for the common cold or flu, as well as arthritic and rheumatic conditions. It is also prescribed for people who are allergic to aspirin.

WHAT ARE THE POSSIBLE SIDE EFFECTS?

Acetaminophen is notoriously hard on the liver, and for that reason alone should be used with caution. If you have any type of liver disease or dysfunction, or if you are drinking alcohol, you should avoid this drug altogether. Other possible side effects include open sores, fever, jaundice, hypoglycemic coma, low white blood cell count, easy bruising and excessive bleeding.

CAUTION! THINK TWICE ABOUT TAKING THESE TYPES OF DRUGS IF . . .

- You have severe allergies.
- You are a chronic alcoholic, drink excessively or even have one drink a day. The combination of this drug and alcohol can produce significant liver dysfunction.
- You have liver disease or a liver dysfunction.

WHAT ARE THE INTERACTIONS WITH OTHER DRUGS?

Acetaminophen may raise levels or prolong the effects of these drugs:

↑ alcohol*   lithium*

The following drugs may be reduced in potency or decreased in the amount of time they are effective when combined with acetaminophens:

↓ ACE inhibitors*   Lamotrigine
  Anticholinergics   Loop diuretics*
  Beta-blockers*   Zidovudine (Retrovir)
  Charcoal, activated

These drugs may increase the effects or prolong the action of acetaminophen:

↑ Alcohol   Probenecid
  Beta-blockers

These drugs may reduce the effects of acetaminophen and/or increase its potential to cause liver damage:

↓ Barbiturates*   Oral contraceptives
  Carbamazepine*   Phenytoin
  Charcoal, activated   Rifampin*
  Hydantoins*   Sulfinpyrazone*
  Isoniazid*

---

* Potentially dangerous interaction.

WHAT ARE THE INTERACTIONS OF ACETAMINOPHEN WITH FOOD?

In general, eating foods while taking this drug decreases or delays the drug's absorption. Eating large amounts of cruciferous vegetables such as cabbage and Brussels sprouts, carbohydrates such as crackers, dates and jellies and foods high in pectin such as apples increases the effects of acetaminophen.

Aspirin and Similar Drugs (Salicylates)

ASPIRIN (Bayer, St. Joseph's, Bufferin, Alka-Seltzer)

CHOLINE SALICYLATE (Arthropan)

DIFLUNISAL (Dolobid)

MAGNESIUM SALICYLATE (Bayer Select Maximum Strength Backache)

SALICYLATE COMBINATIONS (Tricosal)

SALICYLSALICYLIC ACID (Amigesic)

SODIUM SALICYLATE

SODIUM THIOSALICYLATE (Rexolate)

Aspirin is a near miracle drug, especially if you have a "too much" headache or a minor ache or pain. But it can easily and quickly cause serious gastrointestinal bleeding, it can increase the risk of some eye diseases, and it interacts dangerously with a long list of other drugs, so please use it with caution and don't use it regularly. Aspirin has been loudly and widely touted as a cure-all for heart disease when taken daily in small doses, because of its ability to thin the blood, but it's not worth the risk of gastrointestinal bleeding. See page 89 for more about aspirin and heart disease.

WHAT DO THEY DO IN YOUR BODY?

Lower elevated body temperatures while also reducing inflammation and pain.

WHAT ARE THEY PRESCRIBED FOR?

Relief from mild to moderate fevers, inflammation, aches and pains. Aspirin is also prescribed for reducing the risk of heart attacks, although the risks of gastrointestinal bleeding outweigh the benefits for heart disease, especially considering how many other natural supplements can do the same thing without the side effects. Simply taking 300 to 500 mg of magnesium and 400 IU of vitamin E daily will likely do your heart a world more good than aspirin.

Aspirin is prescribed for a variety of inflammatory conditions such as rheumatic fever, rheumatoid arthritis and osteoarthritis.

WHAT ARE THE POSSIBLE SIDE EFFECTS?

Aspirin is particularly hard on the digestive tract and can cause nausea, upset stomach, massive intestinal bleeding and peptic ulcers. It can also cause temporary liver dysfunction and skin discomforts such as hives and rashes. Anemia, low white cell blood count, prolonged bleeding, easy bruising are also possible with this drug, as well as severe allergies, mental confusion, dizziness, headaches and depression. Ringing in the ears or tinnitus is a sign that you have taken too much aspirin.

CAUTION: THINK TWICE ABOUT TAKING THESE TYPES OF DRUGS IF . . .

- You are scheduled for surgery in a week or less (to avoid postoperative bleeding).
- You are allergic to any salicylates or nonsteroidal anti-inflammatory drugs (NSAIDs).
- Your child or teenager has chicken pox or flu. **A physician should check for Reye's syndrome, a rare but serious disease before giving a child or teenager salicylates.**
- You have asthma. Some asthmatics are intolerant of aspirin and can go into shock.
- You have liver damage, poor clot formation or vitamin K deficiency.
- You have kidney disease or dysfunction. Aspirin may aggravate your condition.

- You have gastric ulcers, mild diabetes, gout, gastritis or bleeding ulcers.
- You have hemophilia or hemorrhagic states.
- You have advanced kidney dysfunction due to magnesium retention. Do not take magnesium salicylate.

WHAT ARE THE INTERACTIONS WITH OTHER DRUGS?

Salicylates may raise levels or prolong the effects of these drugs:

↑ Alcohol (one aspirin an hour before drinking can raise alcohol blood levels 26 percent of normal)
Anticoagulants*
Daranide*
Diabetes drugs (oral)
Diamox*
Methotrexate*
Neptazane*
Nitroglycerin
Penicillin
Probenecid
Valproic acid

The following drugs may be reduced in potency or decreased in the amount of time they are effective when combined with salicylates:

↓ ACE inhibitors
Beta-blockers
Gout drugs
Ibuprofen and related drugs
Loop diuretics*
Probenecid
Spironolactone
Sulfinpyrazone

These drugs may increase the effects or prolong the action of salicylates:

↑ ACE inhibitors*
Alcohol (may increase stomach irritation)
Ammonium chloride
Anticoagulants*
Carbonic anhydrase inhibitors

These drugs may reduce the effects of salicylates:

↓ Antacids   Corticosteroids

*Potentially dangerous interaction.

WHAT ARE THE INTERACTIONS WITH FOOD?

In general, eating foods of any kind delays or decreases the absorption of these drugs.

WHAT NUTRIENTS DO THEY THROW OUT OF BALANCE OR INTERACT WITH?

Aspirin and similar drugs block vitamin C from getting into the cells and lower levels of iron, folic acid and potassium.

WHAT ELSE TO TAKE IF YOU TAKE THESE DRUGS

Increase your intake of foods high in vitamin C and potassium and be sure to follow the Six Core Principles for Optimal Health (Chapter 8) to insure an adequate intake of vitamins and minerals. Be sure you're getting 200 mcg daily of folic acid, especially if there's any possibility of becoming pregnant.

Ibuprofen and Similar Drugs

DICLOFENAC (Cataflam, Voltaren)

ETODOLAC (Lodine)

FENOPROFEN (Nalfon)

FLURBIPROFEN (Ansaid)

IBUPROFEN (Motrin, Advil, Midol IB, Bayer Select Pain Relief, Nuprin, IBU)

INDOMETHACIN (Indocin)

KETOPROFEN (Orudis, Oruvail, Actron, Ketoprofen)

KETOROLAC (Toradol)

MECLOFENAMATE SODIUM (Meclomen)

MEFENAMIC ACID (Ponstel)

NABUMETONE (Relafen)

NAPROXEN (Aleve, Naproxen, Naprosyn, Naprelan)

OXAPROZIN (Daypro)

PIROXICAM (Feldene)

SULINDAC (Clinoril)

TOLMETIN SODIUM (Tolectin)

The ibuprofen-like painkillers are another example of an over-the-counter medication that is a potent drug with serious side effects when taken by the wrong person for more than a few days. Ibuprofen is a potent anti-inflammatory drug so it is often used to treat arthritis pain. As many women are well aware, the ibuprofen-type drugs can bring welcome relief from menstrual cramps. (This is probably a result of reduced prostaglandin synthesis.) What many arthritis sufferers and women with menstrual cramps don't realize is that if you have a sensitive stomach, taking ibuprofen just a few days a month can cause chronic digestive problems all month long. Ibuprofen is closely related to aspirin, and can cause diarrhea, constipation, heartburn, gas, gastrointestinal bleeding and chronic stomach pain and irritation. Taking it with food will help, but doesn't eliminate the problem.

Hundreds of thousands of people get stuck on the drug treadmill when they take these types of drugs. Here's the scenario: They take ibuprofen or a similar drug for arthritis pain nearly every day and develop chronic stomach irritation, so their physician recommends Tagamet, which blocks the production of stomach acid. As a result of lower stomach acid, nutrients aren't being properly broken down or absorbed, and the process of low level malnutrition begins. The irritated digestive tract precipitates food allergies, which aggravates the arthritis, prompting ever-higher doses of pain medication and Tagamet. Pretty soon sleeping pills are prescribed to help get through the night, and the person is groggy during the day. Just a few months of this type of scenario is enough to land an independent elderly person in a nursing home. Please don't underestimate the potency of these drugs.

What Do They Do in the Body?

Relieve pain from inflammation and lower elevated body temperatures.

What Are They Prescribed For?

Rheumatoid arthritis, osteoarthritis, mild to moderate pain, tendonitis, bursitis, acute gout, fever, sunburn, migraine headaches, menstrual cramps and discomforts, and acne.

What Are the Possible Side Effects?

The most common and one of the most dangerous side effects of the ibuprofen-like drugs is damage to the digestive system. They can cause nausea, vomiting, diarrhea, constipation, cramps, gas, as well as serious bleeding and ulcers, particularly if you are elderly.

These drugs are hard on both the liver and kidneys. They can cause hepatitis, jaundice and elevated liver enzymes, as well as urinary tract infections, urinary frequency and a wide variety of kidney problems.

Other side effects include dizziness, headaches, drowsiness, fatigue and nervousness. They can aggravate a wide range of behavioral problems including depression and psychosis. They can also cause muscle weakness or cramps, numbness, changes in blood pressure, vision disturbances and damage, hearing disturbances, shortness of breath, rashes, blood sugar changes, weight gain or loss, mineral imbalances, menstrual problems, impotence and breast enlargement in men, and a wide range of blood disorders, including anemia. Like aspirin, these drugs can prolong bleeding time by as much as three or four minutes.

Caution: Think Twice About Taking These Types of Drugs if . . .

- You are elderly. Serious side effects are more likely to happen to you if you are over the age of 65.
- You have had an allergic reaction to these or to other similar drugs such as aspirin.
- You have kidney or liver disease or dysfunction.
- You have an ulcer, inflammation or a history of bleeding in your intestinal tract or rectum.

- You have a history of anemia, excessive bleeding or poor clotting.
- You are scheduled for surgery in a week or less.
- You have a heart condition or pancreatitis.
- You have eye problems.
- You have an existing controlled infection. These drugs can mask the symptoms of infection.
- You are sensitive to sunlight.

WHAT ARE THE INTERACTIONS WITH OTHER DRUGS?

Ibuprofen and similar drugs may raise the levels or prolong the effects of these drugs:

↑ Alcohol
Anticoagulants*
Cimetidine
Cyclosporine
Digoxin
Dipyridamole (may increase water retention)

Hydantoins
Lithium*
Methotrexate*
Penicillamine
Sympathomimetics

The following drugs may be reduced in potency or decreased in the amount of time they are effective when combined with ibuprofen and similar drugs:

↓ ACE inhibitors*
Beta-blockers*

Loop diuretics*
Thiazide diuretics*

These drugs may increase the effects or prolong the action of ibuprofen and similar drugs:

↑ Cimetidine
Cyclosporine

Probenecid

---

*Potentially dangerous interaction.

These drugs may reduce the effects of ibuprofen and similar drugs:

↓ Cimetidine   Salicylates
  DMSO/sulindac*   Sucralfate

WHAT ARE THE INTERACTIONS WITH FOOD?

Generally, any time you eat food and take these types of drugs, the food will delay or decrease the absorption of the drug. Always take these drugs with food.

WHAT NUTRIENTS DO THEY THROW OUT OF BALANCE?

Iron levels may be reduced because of blood loss due to gastrointestinal bleeding.

WHAT ELSE TO TAKE IF YOU TAKE THESE DRUGS

If you are a premenopausal woman and taking these drugs for more than a few days (which is not recommended), take a low-dose (2 to 5 mg) iron supplement, or make sure you're getting some iron in your multivitamin.

NONNARCOTIC PAINKILLER COMBINATIONS

NONNARCOTIC ANALGESIC COMBINATIONS (Vanquish, Pamprin, Extra Strength Excedrin, Midol, Cope, Anacin, Saleto, Gelpirin, Supac, Extra Strength Tylenol Headache Plus, Equagesic, Gensan)

NONNARCOTIC ANALGESICS WITH BARBITURATES (Fiorinal, Esgic, Fioricet, Repan, Amaphen, Butace, Endolor, Femcet, Two-Dyne, Bancap, Triaprin, Lanorinal)

These drugs generally combine acetaminophen or aspirin with a barbiturate, meprobamate or antihistamine for sedative effects, caffeine to help constrict blood vessels and relieve headaches, belladonna alkaloids to reduce muscle spasms, and pamabrom as a diuretic. They are sold both as prescription and over-the-counter drugs.

WHAT DO THEY DO IN YOUR BODY?

These drugs are used as painkillers with specific added effects such as sedation or muscle relaxation.

WHAT ARE THEY PRESCRIBED FOR?

They are prescribed for a wide variety of pain conditions including arthritis, headaches and muscle pain.

WHAT ARE THE POSSIBLE SIDE EFFECTS?

The side effects can be severe because they are drug *combinations* and thus, more dangerous. Many of these drugs are available without a prescription. If you are going to take them, read the directions!

Migraine Drugs

SUMATRIPTAN SUCCINATE (Imitrex)

Other migraine drugs not covered here because they are so rarely used include: methysergide maleate (Sansert), ergotamine tartrate (Ergomar), dihydroergotamine mesylate (D.H.E.45) and the combination drugs Cafatine-PB, Cafetrate, Catergot, Ercaf, Midrin and Wigraine.

WHAT DOES IT DO IN YOUR BODY?

Sumatriptan relieves pain from migraine headaches by constricting the blood vessels in the brain.

WHAT IS IT PRESCRIBED FOR?

Relieving pain from migraine headaches.

WHAT ARE THE POSSIBLE SIDE EFFECTS?

Sumatriptan has a powerful constricting effect on the heart and blood vessels and as a result has caused fatal heart spasms and possibly fatal strokes. Migraine headaches are unbearable, but they aren't worth dying over. If you have any type of heart disease or are at risk for heart disease, do not take this drug. Your physician should fully evaluate your heart disease risk before prescribing this drug, and the first dose should be given in the physician's office.

Taken regularly, sumatriptan can cause damage to the eyes.

It often causes a tingling sensation which is not harmful. It can also cause dizziness, a sensation of tightness or heaviness, numbness, coldness or warmth, drowsiness, weakness, a stiff neck and flushing.

Other possible side effects include: allergic reactions, kidney and liver impairment, impotence, jaw or chest tightness, seizures, joint pain, stiffness and swelling, mental confusion, sleep disturbance, depression, suicidal tendencies, skin rashes and flu symptoms. In addition, you could experience diarrhea, unusual thirst, asthma, blood sugar imbalances, weight gain or loss, intestinal bleeding, peptic ulcer, breast tenderness, abortion, speech or voice disturbance, deafness, allergy to sunlight, and shock.

CAUTION: THINK TWICE ABOUT TAKING THIS DRUG IF . . .

- You have heart disease or risk factors for heart disease.
- Your migraine headache is different than usual.
- You tend to have hypersensitivity or severe allergic reactions.
- You have kidney or liver disease.
- You have a history of seizures.
- You have eye problems, especially glaucoma.

WHAT ARE THE INTERACTIONS WITH OTHER DRUGS?

The following drugs may raise levels or prolong the effects of sumatriptan:

↑ Ergot-containing drugs   MAO inhibitors

WHAT ARE THE INTERACTIONS WITH FOOD?

Eating food delays absorption by 30 minutes.

Central Analgesics

TRAMADOL (Ultram)

These drugs aren't exactly classified as opiates or narcotics, but they have an abuse and addiction profile similar to the opiates. Use with great caution. The only central analgesic commonly used these days is tramadol (Ultram), which is the one that will be covered here.

WHAT DOES IT DO IN YOUR BODY?

It blocks the perception of pain and produces a state of euphoria.

WHAT IS IT PRESCRIBED FOR?

Pain management.

WHAT ARE THE POSSIBLE SIDE EFFECTS?

Addiction, seizures, liver and kidney damage, respiratory depression, increased intracranial pressure, dizziness and vertigo, nausea, constipation, headaches, sleepiness, vomiting, itching, nervousness and anxiety, weakness, sweating, heartburn, dry mouth, diarrhea, fainting, hypotension (low blood pressure), irregular heartbeats, loss of appetite, gas, stomach pain, rash, visual disturbances, urinary tract disturbances, menopausal symptoms.

CAUTION: THINK TWICE ABOUT TAKING THIS TYPE OF DRUG IF . . .

- You have a history of substance abuse, kidney or liver damage. Please try to avoid this drug if at all possible.

WHAT ARE THE INTERACTIONS WITH OTHER DRUGS?

These drugs may increase the effects or prolong the action of tramadol:

↑ MAO inhibitors*

---

*Potentially dangerous interaction.

These drugs may reduce the effects of tramadol:

↓ Carbamazepine   Quinidine

Narcotic Painkillers

ALFENTANIL (Alfenta)

CODEINE

COMBINATIONS (Propacet, Roxicet)

FENTANYL (Sublimaze, Duragesic-25)

HYDROCODONE (Lortab, Hydrogesic, Vicodin)

HYDROMORPHONE (Dilaudid)

LEVOMETHADYL (ORLAAM)

LEVORPHANOL TARTRATE (Levo-Dromoran)

MEPERIDINE (Demerol)

METHADONE (Dolophine)

MORPHINE SULPHATE (Astramorph, Duramorph, MSIR, MS Contin, Roxanol)

OPIUM (Pantopon, Opium Tincture, Paregoric)

OXYCODONE (Roxicodone)

OXYMORPHONE (Numorphan)

PROPOXYPHENE (Darvon, Dolene)

REMIFENTANIL (Ultiva)

SUFENTANIL (Sufenta)

These are addictive, mind-altering drugs that are among the top-selling drugs in the U.S. It's likely that tens of thousands of people are addicted to hydrocodone and its relatives. The fact that these drugs are such bestsellers tells us that this is an area where both the pharmaceutical industry and the conventional medical industry (physicians, hospitals, insurance companies, HMOs) are profiting from the addictive nature of these drugs. Hydrocodone and codeine are often found in combination painkillers, of which there are dozens, so if it's not on this list, that doesn't mean it's not dangerous and addictive. Don't let your physician become your drug pusher!

Please don't avoid these drugs if you really need them for pain. Nobody should suffer unnecessarily. If you do need to take them for more than a few days, be aware that you will go through a withdrawal reaction and work with a responsible health care professional to withdraw from the drug gradually.

Please don't take these drugs unless absolutely necessary, and if you have a history of drug or alcohol abuse, go off of them gradually and under the close supervision of a health-care professional.

WHAT DO THESE DRUGS DO IN YOUR BODY?

These drugs relieve pain and induce states of euphoria.

WHAT ARE THEY PRESCRIBED FOR?

The relief of moderate to severe pain, as medication prior to and/or during surgery and as cough suppressants.

WHAT ARE THE POSSIBLE SIDE EFFECTS?

The most important side effect of these drugs is that they are addictive. For that reason alone, don't take them unless you must! These drugs alter your perception of pain and reality. Some of their side effects are euphoria, drowsiness, apathy and mental confusion. They also reduce your respiratory rate and heart rate which can result in fainting, heart attack, shock and seizures.

Because they slow down your digestive system, constipation and urine retention can also happen with these drugs as well as nausea, vomiting and abdominal pain. These drugs also cause allergic reactions such as skin rashes, water retention and hypertension. Frequently these drugs cause lightheadedness, dizziness, sedation, face

THE SIGNS OF WITHDRAWAL FROM NARCOTIC DRUGS

The earliest signs include yawning, sweating, tearing eyes, runny nose. Later the symptoms can include dilated eyes, flushing, heart palpitations, twitching, shaking, restlessness, irritability, anxiety, loss of appetite. Signs of severe withdrawal can include muscle spasms, fever, nausea, diarrhea, vomiting, severe backache, abdominal and leg pains and cramping, hot and cold flashes, inability to sleep, repetitive sneezing, heart rate and breathing rate.

flushing and sweating. Other side effects include palpitations, allergic reactions and jaundice.

CAUTION: THINK TWICE ABOUT TAKING THESE DRUGS IF . . .

- You are suicidal or prone to addiction. Drug abuse can and does happen with prolonged use of these drugs. People who are prescribed narcotics for medical purposes over a period of one or two weeks do not develop dependence. But prolonged use of narcotics can lead to psychological and physical dependence and then uncomfortable and difficult withdrawal.
- You are an alcoholic; have bronchial asthma or if you have trouble breathing; if you have a head injury or brain tumor; if you have chronic obstructive heart disease, liver or kidney dysfunction.
- You are on MAO inhibitors or have been within 14 days. Do not take meperidine.
- You have an acute abdominal condition. These drugs can obscure an accurate diagnosis.
- You have lung or respiratory disease. Be careful—cough reflex is suppressed with these drugs.

WHAT ARE THE INTERACTIONS WITH OTHER DRUGS?

Narcotics may raise levels or prolong the effects of these drugs:

↑ Alcohol*   Diazepam*
Carbamazepine   Droperidol/fentanyl
Chlorpromazine   Warfarin
Cimetidine*

These drugs may increase the effects or prolong the action of narcotic agonist analgesics:

↑ Barbiturate anesthetics   Furazolidone
Chlorpromazine   Monoamine oxidase inhibitors
                                  (MAO inhibitors)*

These drugs may reduce the effects of narcotic agonist analgesics:

↓ Hydantoins   Rifampin

WHAT ARE THE INTERACTIONS WITH FOOD?

High-fat foods may increase the effects of morphine. Foods that acidify the urine cause a decrease of potency. Foods that alkalinize the urine decrease the ability of the body to excrete morphine.

Narcotic Agonist-Antagonist Painkillers

BUPRENORPHINE (Buprenex)

BUTORPHANOL (Stadol)

DEZOCINE (Dalgan)

NALBUPHINE (Nubain)

PENTAZOCINE (Talwin, Talacen)

---

*Potentially dangerous interaction.

What Do They Do in Your Body?

Relieve pain and induce euphoric mood changes.

What Are They Prescribed For?

Relieving pain, particularly for postoperative patients.

What Are the Possible Side Effects?

These drugs are potent pain-relieving substances which have a lower abuse potential than pure narcotics, but they can still be addictive, and usually are!

These drugs can cause sweating, chills, flushing, water retention, heart or pulse irregularity, nausea, vomiting, abdominal pain, muscular pain, slowed breathing, rashes, slurred speech, blurred vision, hallucinations, dizziness, urinary frequency, heart attacks, seizures, and skin and muscle damage.

Caution: Think Twice About Taking These Types of Drugs if . . .

- You have an allergic reaction to these drugs.
- You have a drug dependence problem.
- You have liver or kidney dysfunction or disease.
- You have a head injury.
- You have heart disease.
- You must drive or operate machinery (that includes cars).
- You have severe allergic reactions (particularly to sulfur).
- You have acute asthma or other significant respiratory problems.

What Are the Interactions with Other Drugs?

These drugs may increase the effects or prolong the action of narcotic agonist-antagonist analgesics:

↑ Alcohol*
Barbiturate anesthetics

Central nervous system depressants such as tranquilizers and sedatives

NATURAL REMEDIES FOR PAIN

Most of the pain we suffer we can do something about. We have a pretty good grasp of what causes the pain of headaches, and in alternative medicine we have many effective ways to treat arthritis. Most back pain can be prevented and healed using a combination of physical and emotional healing, and with lifestyle changes alone the pain of osteoporosis can be often prevented. This means that millions of people can avoid the use of pain-killing drugs and their side effects.

If you have an acute pain such as a muscle sprain, you may need to warm up before you exercise in the future. If you have chronic pain such as back pain, you may need to do exercises to strengthen your back muscles. Exercise is the single best cure for chronic back pain. If you have chronic pain such as from arthritis, try an elimination diet to find out whether a food sensitivity is causing inflammation in your joints. Or it could be a side effect of a prescription drug. The anticholinergic drugs can cause muscle stiffness and neck pain, for example. Headache pain is often caused by stress, allergies or sensitivities to food or chemicals.

The Best Natural Remedies for Occasional Pain Relief

There are many ways to alleviate chronic pain before reaching for the NSAIDs. Here are a few favorite natural pain relievers. All of the supplements can be found at your health food store.

HOT AND COLD PACKS

Ice is one of the best and simplest remedies for pain caused by inflammation. The cold very effectively reduces the inflammation. Use a cold pack for 20 minutes every few hours for sprains and strains. For a muscle sprain or strain that's been around for a few days, or swelling caused by a bruise, first use a 20-minute cold pack then a 20-minute hot pack. The cold will reduce the inflammation, and the heat will encourage blood flow into the area and help break up damaged tissue so that healing can take place.

One of the simplest, cheapest and most effective ways to relieve chronic pain (with the exception of headaches) is with what is known as moist heat. You can apply moist heat by taking a long, hot shower and aiming the shower head at the area that hurts. You can take a long, hot bath with relaxing herbal oils, or you can use a hot pack or a hot water bottle. If you have access to a Jacuzzi, you can aim the jets of water at the places that are painful. Sometimes we resist the simple remedies. But this one is important to use daily if you're suffering

DIGESTIVE ENZYMES

If you have pain from a muscle injury or arthritis, try digestive enzymes. There are new clinical studies showing that enzymes help reduce inflammation caused by arthritis, injuries to joints and other connective tissues such as muscle sprains, and can even relieve back pain. Enzymes tend to speed up the rate at which many bodily processes work, and injuries are no exception. Enzymes work at the site of an injury to remove damaged tissue, which reduces swelling, and to help the body repair itself. Bromelain, which comes from pineapples, is an enzyme that has anti-inflammatory properties. One of the best combinations is quercetin, an antioxidant, and bromelain.

DL-PHENYLALANINE (DLPA)

This is a combination of L-phenylalanine, an essential amino acid, and D-phenylalanine, a nonnutrient amino acid that helps promote the production of endorphins, natural painkillers made in the brain. DLPA is very effective in the relief of chronic pain such as arthritis and back pain. While in most studies there have been no side effects at all from DLPA, it has raised blood pressure in a few people. Although this is unlikely to happen, if you have high blood pressure, please monitor it if you take DLPA. Don't use DLPA in combination with antidepressant drugs or if you have phenylketonuria (PKU).

VITAMINS AND MINERALS

There are vitamins and minerals that can play a part in reducing inflammation. These include vitamin C, vitamin E and the B-complex vitamins. Taking a magnesium/calcium supplement can relieve the pain of muscle spasms and often relieves chronic headaches. A copper deficiency can cause inflammation in the joints, as well as fragile skin and connective tissue. The bioflavonoids such as grapeseed extract and quercetin can help reduce inflammation reactions.

HERBS FOR PAIN

White Willow Bark *(Salix spp.)*: White willow bark was used as a pain reliever long before a chemist at the Bayer company in Germany synthesized acetylsalicylic acid, or aspirin, from one of its active ingredients in 1897. Aspirin is a synthetic drug (not found in nature), but various teas, decoctions, tinctures and poultices of trees of the salix species, most commonly known as willow and poplar, have been used to relieve pain for many centuries. White willow bark doesn't cause gastric bleeding or ringing in the ears as aspirin does, and is a very effective pain reliever, especially for headaches and arthritis pain. Traditionally a tea of the inner bark was used (a small handful of bark to a cup of tea) to treat headaches. A bath, wash or poultice was used to treat aches and pains in the joints. You can find white willow bark in capsule or tincture form at your health food store.

Feverfew *(Chrysanthemum parthenium)*: Nearly 2,000 years ago, the Roman doctor Dioscorides, one of the first to write a medical textbook, recommended the herb feverfew for headaches. Feverfew is still the most effective treatment known for migraines. It is the only medicine that will help migraine headaches without side effects. This member of the daisy family is also called bachelor's buttons. Feverfew has undergone much testing and research as a migraine remedy as pharmaceutical companies try to find the active ingredient so they can isolate it and synthesize it. However, the lowly feverfew is not revealing its healing secrets, and the freeze-dried herb in capsules, or a tincture of the fresh leaves, is still the best way to take the plant. Feverfew has also been used successfully to treat arthritis.

Treating Chronic Pain

As scientists research pain, they're finding that a wide variety of techniques which induce relaxation and increase body awareness can be used very effectively to beat the demon of chronic pain. In fact, an expert panel concluded at the National Institutes of Health that there is enough positive research data to now integrate behavioral and relaxation therapies into standard treatment of chronic pain and insomnia. This does not mean it's "all in your head," which implies that somehow it's your fault you're in pain. It means there are techniques you can use to induce deep relaxation and become more aware of stress points in your body, and how to relax them.

People in chronic pain tend to tense specific areas of muscle, such as the neck and shoulder area, creating other areas of pain and skeletal imbalances. This creates a vicious cycle, with a new area of pain leading to increased tension, which creates yet more pain. Pretty soon, pain seems to exist everywhere in the body and the person in pain doesn't want to move at all—the worst thing you can do for most pain!

Emotional factors such as tension, anxiety, depression, loneliness, anger, an inability to communicate, a sense of being a victim, and a sense of being estranged from the world can all contribute to more severe pain by blocking the body's production of natural painkillers called endorphins. People who strive to become more aware of their pain—exactly where it is located, what causes it, what makes it worse and what makes it better, for example, rather than blocking it with analgesics and narcotics—tend to have a great sense of empowerment and less severe pain. Our first tendency for most of us when we're in pain is to try and block it, usually with medication. It's ironic that the reverse approach of becoming more aware and paying more attention can be the key to coping effectively with chronic pain.

Two of the most powerful techniques for both increasing body awareness and inducing relaxation are meditation and the Asian movement disciplines such as yoga, qi gong or tai chi.

MEDITATE YOUR PAIN AWAY

Meditation can bring a greater awareness of what we're doing with our consciousness in any given moment. It may begin simply by paying attention to breathing, and progress to a "detached observing" of what is happening with the mind and emotions. As people learn to separate their physical sensations from their thoughts, pain will often begin to dissipate some. A favorite basic meditation that can be used anytime by anyone for relieving stress or tension is this: Breathe deeply and slowly in through the nose to the slow count of five, hold the breath for the slow count of five, and breathe out to the slow count of five. Repeat at least three times. A few rounds of this elegantly simple technique and you'll be amazed at how relaxed you can feel.

Another simple meditation technique is to repeat one word silently over and over. Many meditation disciplines use the word *om*. You can use any word or phrase you want as long at it has a positive association.

A form of meditation especially designed to induce relaxation is called visualization or guided imagery. In these techniques you sit or lie down, close your eyes and take three long, deep breaths. Then you visualize the most relaxing place or situation you can think of, and make it your "vacation spot" that you visit whenever you feel tense. Many people like to envision themselves on a tropical beach. As you visualize, engage all of your senses: The sky is deep blue and the water turquoise; you sift the warm, white sand between your fingers and feel the hot sun; you hear the waves breaking and the palm trees rustling; you smell the salt water and sweet aromas of tropical flowers.

A technique you can use to help you become more aware of your body is to lie on your back in a comfortable place with your eyes closed, perhaps with some soothing music on. Starting at your toes, slowly and in turn, become aware of every part of your body, and as you become aware of it, gently tense the muscles around it for 5 to 15 seconds (keep breathing), and then relax them. For example, feel each toe on your right foot by wiggling it, and then curl all five of them forward. Do the same with your foot and ankle, move to your other foot, then move up to your calves, your knees and your thighs, tensing and relaxing each area. By the time you finish with your face, you'll be deeply relaxed.

Exercise Your Pain Away

It is extremely important to exercise in whatever way you can when you're suffering from chronic pain. If you do exercises such as yoga or chi gong, sometimes called "enlightened exercise," you will stretch, tone and strengthen your muscles, limber up your joints, improve your circulation, coordination and balance, get your lymph system flowing, bring greater alignment to your musculo-skeletal system, improve your posture, increase relaxation, and become more aware of your body. People who do these practices regularly claim that they also speed healing, boost the immune system, improve digestion, increase energy and improve mood. Studies show they can also reduce blood pressure.

Much pain, particularly back pain, results from poor posture and improper use of the spine (i.e., lifting something without bending your knees). Greater body awareness will alert you when you're doing something that creates pain. These types of exercise also teach you to move away from habitual patterns of movement and into new, more healing patterns. With any exercise, especially yoga, remember to stop whatever you're doing if you experience any pain. Contrary to the "no pain, no gain" philosophy, adopt a new philosophy of "there's no gain in pain." Stretching is an essential part of all the forms of enlightened exercise. You can stretch gently anytime you're starting to feel pain or tension.

Although much pain is caused by the improper use of the muscles and spine, it is also caused by muscles that aren't used and aren't toned. For almost all lower back pain caused by strained muscles, there are specific exercises you can do that will, in effect, cure the problem. You can get these exercises from almost any physician or physical therapist. Yoga instructors usually have their own set of back exercises, which are equally effective.

TREATING CHRONIC PAIN WITH HERBS

One of the biggest problems in chronic pain is stress and tension: physical, emotional and mental. When you hurt all the time, you tend to tense muscles all over your body, creating additional areas of pain. People who suffer from chronic pain often become anxious and fearful, and feel helpless, which is understandable. Waking up and going to bed with pain as a constant companion is a traumatic experience.

For that reason you can try the herb kava with the goal of relieving anxiety and tension, and secondarily to relieve pain. Sometimes a little herbal help in relaxation can help start you on the path to healing.

Kava *(Piper methysticum)*: If you're suffering from depression and anxiety caused by chronic pain, an herb called kava might do the job for you. This member of the pepper family grows as a bush in the South Pacific. Kava is a sedative and muscle relaxant. The South Pacific Islanders, who use it in much the same way many people in North America use alcohol, describe kava as a calming drink that brings on a feeling of contentment, well-being and encourages socializing.

Kava is also a pain reliever, and can often be used in place of the NSAIDs. In a European study, people with anxiety symptoms given a 70 percent kavalactone extract in the amount of 100 mg three times a day, were found after four weeks to have a significant reduction in anxiety symptoms such as feelings of nervousness, heart palpitations, chest pains, headaches, dizziness and indigestion. All with no side effects noted.

For over 100 years, scientists have been trying to figure out exactly what it is in kava that gives it sedative and antidepressant properties. Although they have isolated chemical compounds named *kavalactones*, which do act as sedatives and antidepressants when given alone, an extract of the whole root has always worked better. Kava also has a different action on the brain than any of our other antidepressants or sedatives, possibly working in the limbic brain, the seat of our emotions. In medicinal doses, Kava has no known side effects. In very high doses it can cause sleepiness, and high doses over a long period of time can cause skin irritation.

The best way to take kava is powdered, in a capsule or as an extract.

St. John's wort *(Hypericum perforatum)* is a medicinal plant with a beautiful yellow flower that's been used by the Chinese, the Greeks, the Europeans and the American Indians for centuries to treat heart disease, anxiety, insomnia and depression. In a study of 105 patients who had symptoms of mild to moderate depression, half the patients took 300 mg of St. John's wort extract three times a day for four weeks, and the other half took a placebo. Some 67 percent of the group taking the St. John's wort had positive results, compared to only 28 percent of the placebo group. Another study comparing St. John's wort to two standard antidepressants, amitriptyline (Elavil) and imiprimine (Tofranil) showed that the St. John's wort had a better positive result. This amazing herb has also been used in studies alongside the antidepressant SSRIs such as Prozac, and found to be as effective. And, you guessed it, those taking the prescription antidepressants suffered from drowsiness, constipation and dry mouth, while those taking St. John's wort reported no side effects.

Healing Headache Pain Naturally

Headaches are a source of pain that bothers all of us at some time or another, but they can almost always be avoided with a bit of alertness to what might bring them on. Of course nobody outside of yourself can help you solve the problem of "too much" headaches, as in too much alcohol, sugar, staying up late, TV watching or internet surfing.

How you cure your chronic headaches is going to be a matter of uncovering the cause and that will take some sleuthing. Once you have a few leads, you can track down the perpetrator and say good-bye to pain. It will be up to you to put together your own personal headache profile, but once you do, avoiding headaches will be a matter of common sense solutions.

Headaches are an extremely personal matter, in the sense that the cause tends to be a little bit different for everyone. Harry cured his headaches by eliminating certain foods from his diet. Sarah started using natural progesterone cream and taking magnesium, and her migraines disappeared. Francine banished her tension headaches by swimming at her local YMCA three or four times a week, and taking a yoga class where she learned some breathing exercises for muscle relaxation.

For most people headaches are caused by a sequence or combination of triggers. It might be a combination of emotional stress and chocolate; or too much time in front of the computer combined with low blood sugar; or a glass of red wine with Chinese food containing MSG. Ultimately, you will be your own best headache detective.

YOUR BRAIN HAS A MIND OF ITS OWN

The human brain may be the most miraculous creation on earth, aside from life itself. Its inner workings are so complex and instantaneous that it puts even the most sophisticated computer to shame. And com-

ALTERNATIVE MEDICINE TREATMENTS THAT WORK FOR CHRONIC PAIN

There are literally dozens of safe, effective alternative medicine techniques for healing pain that don't involve surgery or medication. Here are some that have been proven over time to work for some people:

Acupressure
Acupuncture
Alexander Technique
Biofeedback
Chiropractic
Feldenkrais
Hydrotherapy

Hypnosis
Massage
NLP (Neuro Linguistic Programming)
Rolfing
TENS (Transcutaneous Electrical Stimulation)

puters don't even have our rich interplay of thoughts, emotions, creativity, intuitions and instincts.

An entire new field of scientific study, known as psychoneuroimmunology, is devoted just to studying the connection between our emotions, our brains and our bodies. For example, did you know that serotonin, one of the brain's neurotransmitters that affects mood, is also found abundantly in the small intestine? Have you ever gotten bad news, or been about to perform in front of an audience, and clutched your stomach because it was suddenly and violently queasy? That's right, your brain lives in your stomach, as well as in your head. In fact it lives all over the body. The gray matter in your head is just the main terminal.

In his book *Healing Back Pain* (Warner Books, 1991), John Sarno, M.D., an expert who has spent more than 20 years in his field, explains how feelings such as anger, fear and anxiety that we don't want to be aware of can be the cause of pain almost anywhere in the body. He says we create pain in the body to distract us from these unwelcome feelings. Try reading Sarno's book if your headaches don't respond to the other treatments mentioned here. Everything he says about back pain can also apply to headaches.

Stress factors such as overwork, lack of sleep, anxiety and depression can all cause or contribute to headaches. Stress causes us to tense muscles we don't even know we have, which deprives them of oxygen and causes pain. Any type of tension that centers in the shoulders, neck, face or head can affect muscles and blood vessels, causing pain. It is estimated that 50 percent of tension headaches are caused by stress.

PREVENTING AND TREATING HEADACHES

There are some very simple, basic steps you can take both to prevent and treat headaches. Following the Six Core Principles for Optimal Health is your best bet for a headache-free lifestyle.

Exercise. This is such a simple solution to headaches that it's often overlooked. Moving your body improves circulation and increases oxygen in the blood, improves hormone balance, reduces stress and is relaxing, reduces anxiety and depression, and stimulates our brain's natural mood enhancers and painkillers called endorphins.

Magnesium. If there had to be one magic bullet for both migraine and tension headaches it would be the mineral magnesium. It's not clear whether magnesium banishes migraines by relieving muscle spasms or changing brain chemistry, but there have been many, many successes curing migraines with this simple solution. If you get migraine headaches, include magnesium in your daily vitamin regimen. You can take 400 mg twice daily (one with breakfast and one before bed) and if you feel a migraine coming on, take 400 mg immediately.

In one study done in Germany, 81 migraine sufferers were given 600 mg of magnesium daily or a placebo. After two to three months, those taking the magnesium had 42 percent fewer migraines, while those in the placebo group had only 16 percent fewer migraines.

Feverfew. The herb feverfew is another safe, natural and effective remedy for both tension and migraine headaches. If you tend to get migraines, it's best to take feverfew daily as a preventive until you've found the underlying cause. You can use it in capsule or tincture form, but since it tastes absolutely terrible you might want to stick with the capsules! Follow the instructions on the container.

Coffee. If you feel a headache coming on, a cup or two of coffee can constrict your blood vessels enough to prevent it. On the other hand, too much coffee can cause a headache, as can coffee withdrawal. Coffee is a stimulating drug and should be treated as such.

Relaxation. Almost anything that helps you relax will help prevent and treat headaches. That includes massage, breathing exercises, visualization techniques and meditation. Soothing herbal teas such as chamomile, skullcap and passionflower can be helpful, and when necessary you can use the more powerful antianxiety and antidepressant herbs St. John's wort or kava.

Treating Arthritis Pain Naturally

Sometimes you can take care of arthritis naturally, covering all your bases with nutrition and exercise, and still get a painful flare-up that leaves permanent damage to joints. Mary is a good example. A couple of years ago Mary's pain and stiffness had been increasing in her hands and her hips, and the aspirin she had been taking to keep it under control was causing stomach pain. She started taking glucosamine and EFAs (essential fatty acids) and started easing off the aspirin gradually, over a period of two weeks. She also tried an elimination diet. Within a few months her arthritis was virtually gone.

But a few months after that, Mary experienced a painful flare-up of her arthritis that left her with a permanent knob on the knuckle of one of her hands. After closely examining her lifestyle changes during the flare-up, Mary realized that during the summer months she had been eating fresh tomatoes at least once a day, sometimes twice. Tomatoes belong to the nightshade family (along with potatoes, eggplant, bell peppers, hot peppers, tobacco), and are renowned for aggravating arthritis in some people. As soon as Mary stopped eating the tomatoes, her arthritis symptoms eased up entirely.

To avoid permanent damage caused by a severe flare-up of arthritis, it's important to treat the symptoms *immediately*, as well as look for the underlying cause and eliminate it as soon as possible. For immediate treatment of symptoms, you can keep a cortisone cream on hand, and rub it on the affected area every few hours until the pain begins to subside. (Cortisone creams are easily available in your pharmacy. They are not ever to be used long-term, but are very effective in reducing inflammation short-term.) For minor flare-ups you can use a cream containing capsaicin (cayenne).

In addition to the cortisone cream, you can take the supplements listed at the end of this section. Most important is to play detective, and make a list of everything you've done differently in the week preceding the flare-up, to track down the culprit.

Other factors besides dietary allergens that may cause an arthritis flare-up are primarily related to inflammation. These can include exposure to environmental toxins such as pesticides; excessive estrogen caused by HRT (hormone replacement therapy); a leaky gut caused by taking NSAIDs (nonsteroidal anti-inflammatory drugs such as aspirin and ibuprofen); overdoing it with exercise or some other type of physical exertion; or a sudden onset of stress such as can happen when traveling and visiting family.

If the culprit is stress, resist the temptation to blame the stress on the outer cause (travel, family, illness of a loved one, for example), and work on your inner response to the stress. You can't control your outer environment much of the time, but you can always control your inner environment, and that is one of the great secrets to serenity.

Delayed Food Allergies Are the Biggest Culprits

Alternative health care professionals are finding that nearly all of their patients with arthritis can be helped at least some by eliminating food allergens from the diet, and some patients can be cured this way. You can find out how to accomplish elimination of food allergies in detail in the chapter on digestion. According to a Scandinavian study, delayed food allergy tests (such as the ELISA) do not seem to be good predictors of foods that cause arthritis. This means that the very best course of action at this time is an elimination diet. This is one step that everyone with arthritis should take.

Glucosamine

There's a natural treatment for arthritis that in clinical studies relieved the symptoms of osteoarthritis and in some cases reversed the disease. This substance is glucosamine, a naturally occurring compound in the body that may help keep cartilage strong and flexible, and can also play a role in repairing damaged cartilage.

Like bones, the cartilage found in tendons, ligaments and other connective tissue is very much alive. When it becomes damaged in a healthy person it is slowly but surely replaced by new cartilage. As we grow older, it appears that our bodies become less efficient at repairing cartilage.

Glucosamine is a key substance in the cartilage rebuilding process. It provides basic cartilage building blocks and stimulates the growth of cartilage. Animal studies have also shown that through a presently unknown mechanism, glucosamine reduces inflammation.

There have been at least five excellent studies done comparing the effects of glucosamine versus NSAID drugs such as acetaminophen, ibuprofen and aspirin. In each study the NSAIDs group improved faster during the first two weeks, but after a month the effectiveness began to wear off and side effects such as stomach and digestive problems began to appear. In contrast, after four to eight weeks the glucosamine groups showed a high degree of relief from pain, joint tenderness and swelling. A study that did before-and-after electron micrographs of cartilage taken from both a placebo and a glucosamine group showed continuing arthritis in the placebo group and nearly healthy cartilage in the glucosamine group. None of the glucosamine groups reported any significant side effects.

If you are suffering from osteoarthritis, bursitis, joint pain, swelling or tenderness, you might want to try glucosamine. Take one 500-mg capsule three times a day for eight weeks, and then taper it down to one 500-mg capsule daily for maintenance.

FISH OIL CONTINUES TO BE A WINNER

Research continues to indicate that omega-3 fatty acids found in fish oil can reduce arthritis pain considerably. A study from the Fred Hutchinson Cancer Research Center in Seattle that looked at diet and arthritis found that people who ate baked or broiled fish more than twice a week had less risk of rheumatoid arthritis. Other kinds of fish, such as fried fish, didn't have an effect. You can take fish oil capsules, but watch for rancid oil, which will do you more harm than good. Your best bet is to eat cold water fish two or three times a week.

You can also get omega-3 fatty acids from flax oil, but it's not recommended in high doses long term, as it can suppress both "good" and "bad" prostaglandins, the hormone-like substances that create or subdue inflammation. If you use flax oil, be sure it comes in a dated, refrigerated, light-proof container, and use it up within two weeks.

DHEA Is Good for Arthritis, Too

A researcher from the National Institutes of Health was the author of an article in the *Journal of Rheumatology* stating that men and women with rheumatoid arthritis tend to have lower than normal levels of DHEA (dehydroepiandrosterone), and men have low testosterone levels. For many of the chronic problems of aging, including arthritis, you can try taking a DHEA supplement of 5-25 mg daily or every other day for women and 25 mg daily for men.

Vitamin C Saves Joint Tissues

A study from a researcher at Boston Medical Center in the journal *Arthritis and Rheumatism* reported that people with rheumatoid arthritis who had higher levels of vitamin C had significantly less progression of the disease and less knee pain, due to a reduction in the loss of cartilage. Cartilage is made from collagen, and vitamin C is a key component of collagen. You can take up to 3,000 mg daily in divided doses to prevent and treat arthritis.

Other Supplements to Reduce Inflammation

One of the first steps in cooling down an arthritis flare-up is reducing inflammation, which should be done as quickly as possible. Here are some herbs, vitamins and other nutrients that reduce inflammation. As a preventive measure you can take them in one of the many arthritis formulas that contain combinations of these supplements. For flare-ups, increase the dose of the formulas or take them separately.

To prevent both chronic arthritis and flare-ups, it's extremely important to follow the Six Core Principles for Optimal Health, taking the vitamins and drinking plenty of water, and getting some exercise. Keeping muscles strong will support joints better, and movement helps move toxins out of the joints.

Pregnenolone, a steroid hormone, can be very helpful in treating arthritis. Most of the studies were done decades ago, but interest in it as an arthritis treatment was dropped because it can't be patented. It has no known side effects, and often improves memory as well. You can take 100 mg two to three times daily.

Bromelain (from pineapple) is an enzyme that helps heal tissues and speed up the removal of inflammatory waste products from the joint. Other digestive enzymes such as papain (from papaya) can also be helpful.

Turmeric or **curcumin** (curcumin is the active ingredient of turmeric), which you mainly know as a spice, is a powerful anti-inflammatory that works as well as cortisone for some people during arthritis flare-ups. For a flare-up you need to take 300 to 600 mg of curcumin, three times a day in capsules. (If you take turmeric, you may need as much as 50 grams a day, which is overdoing it!)

Cat's Claw or **Una de Gato** (*Uncaria tomentosa*) is a South American tree. Its inner bark is used to treat arthritis. You can take it as a tea (the way the natives take it), in capsules or tincture form. Take 1 to 6 grams for a flare-up, or drink a cup or two of the tea a week as a preventive measure.

Ginger is one of the best healing herbs that is effective in reducing inflammation of all kinds.

The extract of a new ginger subspecies called EVEX-33 (Zihaxin) has been shown in clinical studies to reduce the symptoms of osteoarthritis, rheumatoid arthritis, bursitis and fibromyalgia.

EVEX-33 inhibits prostaglandin production (which causes short-term joint problems) and leukotrienes (which can produce long-term joint problems). A major U.S. study is currently underway to research these effects in more detail.

It's interesting to note that there were no side effects in any double blind animal study done with this extract. In one study of older dogs with joint problems (dogs up to 100 pounds received one capsule daily and dogs over 100 pounds received two capsules daily), all showed great improvement within 30 days.

You can take one capsule twice daily.

Vitamin D is important to healthy joints. Recent research has shown that low levels of vitamin D can contribute to the progression of osteoarthritis. Be sure you're getting out in the sunlight for at least 15 minutes a week, summer and winter, and if you live in a cloudy climate you may want to include 200 to 400 IU of vitamin D in your daily vitamin intake during the winter months.

Treating Carpal Tunnel Syndrome Naturally

Although the general wisdom is that carpal tunnel syndrome (CTS) is caused by repetitive movement, our great-great grandparents did plenty of repetitive movement—just think of plowing, spinning, sewing and churning butter, to name a few! And yet carpal tunnel syndrome was unknown until the past few decades. Repetitive motion may just be final insult to already aggravated wrist nerves.

It's very likely that there are nutritional and hormonal factors associated with CTS that are important to pay attention to. It's clear that a vitamin B6 deficiency is involved in carpal tunnel syndrome, and a B6 deficiency may have even more to do with carpal tunnel syndrome than repetitive motion. Pyridoxal-5'-phosphate, the active form of vitamin B6, is a co-catalyst for a large number of enzymes. It reduces inflammatory reactions in connective tissue and promotes collagen repair. Vitamin B6 is also essential to the production of progesterone, a hormone that balances excessive estrogen.

Women get carpal tunnel syndrome more than men do, some women get it when they're pregnant, and both sexes get it around middle age, leading us to suspect that hormonal imbalance may aggravate or precipitate CTS. We also know that low thyroid and birth control pills are associated with CTS.

When estrogen is present in excess it can cause salt and fluid retention, it interferes with thyroid hormone, reduces the level of oxygen in all cells, and reduces vascular tone. All of these conditions aggravate carpal tunnel syndrome. We're living in a sea of xenoestrogens (environmental estrogens) from pesticides, plastics, and even soaps, not to mention exposure through hormone-treated meat, so that even men are exposed to excessive amounts of estrogen.

A woman named Beth who uses the computer for a living began to have wrist pain and stopped using her computer immediately. The pain persisted, so she tried taking vitamin B6 and that helped some, but she had to take large doses to get relief. Then Beth realized she was eating a snack food every day that contained yellow dye No. 5 (tartrazine), which depletes vitamin B6. Within days of avoiding yellow dye her wrist pain began to go away.

According to Alan Gaby, M.D., author of the book *The Doctor's*

Guide to Vitamin B6 (Rodale Press, 1984), other causes of vitamin B6 depletion include: the chemical hydrazine, found in rocket and jet fuel and cigarette smoke; isoniazid, a drug used to treat tuberculosis; hydralazine, a prescription drug used to treat high blood pressure; the antidepressant phenelzine; the herbicide maleic hydrazide; the deadly chemical pollutants PCBs, and possibly rancid unsaturated vegetable oils.

Once carpal tunnel gets established in the nerves of the wrist it is very difficult to treat. It's important to pay attention to any type of pain in the wrist that doesn't go away after a few days and to stop doing the aggravating motion immediately.

To aid in healing carpal tunnel, in addition to 50 to 100 mg of vitamin B6 daily you can take ginkgo biloba to improve blood supply to the affected area. Since ginkgo improves circulation to the extremities, it seems a logical choice for CTS. You can also try taking glucosamine or EVEX-33, since they aid the body in repairing cartilage and tendons.

CHAPTER 13

Antibiotics, Antifungals and Their Natural Alternatives

ANTI-INFECTIVES IS THE general term describing the drugs we take to fight all kinds of infections such as bacteria, fungus, parasites and viruses. In this chapter, antibiotics and antifungals are the types of anti-infectives that will be covered.

WHEN SHOULD YOU TAKE ANTIBIOTICS?

Your life may depend on avoiding antibiotics until you really need them.

Kill the germ with an antibiotic, and your infection problem—sinus congestion, ear ache, urinary tract infection, cough—is solved. Right? Well, for the past 50 years, this is how conventional medicine has been treating patients. But 98 percent of those infections would have gotten better with some very basic care, like rest and fluids. And antibiotics do nothing to get rid of a virus when you have the flu.

The notion that the neat solution to every infection is to find the right antibiotic is not only incorrect, it has led us into big trouble. We are addicted to antibiotics. We think they'll cure everything from cholera to a hangnail. If you think this is an exaggeration, check out these numbers: among American physicians, ob/gyns and internists alone write out 40,610,000 prescriptions for antibiotics every *week*. But pediatricians and family practitioners write out even more prescriptions than that for ear infections alone! And if you think antibiotic abuse isn't about money, think about the *billions* of dollars those millions of prescriptions represent.

Alexander Fleming, who discovered penicillin, warned us nearly a century ago that the overuse of antibiotics would create resistant bacteria. Even Louis Pasteur, the father of germ warfare using antibiotics, is said to have admitted on his deathbed, "The terrain is everything, the bacteria is nothing." This was his way of saying that a healthy body and a healthy immune system will fight off most infections, and an unhealthy body and immune system will be susceptible to infection.

In fact, antibiotics are a major cause of recurrent infections, and our overuse of them is breeding highly resistant strains of "superbugs" that are immune to all known types of antibiotics. To add insult to injury, we have lost the war on infectious diseases, even with all these antibiotics and better hygiene. According to a recent press conference held by the American Medical Association, infectious diseases have reemerged as a serious health threat. Just in the past decade, death from infectious diseases has risen a stunning 58 percent worldwide. Even after subtracting the deaths caused by the HIV virus, it's still up by 22 percent. Most of these deaths are caused by infections in the lungs and the blood that are resistant to antibiotics.

By using antibiotics as a cure-all, the magic bullet has come back to bite us. Every time we take antibiotics, we are giving harmful bacteria a new opportunity to become resistant. The consequence of this is that many antibiotics are useless. An increasingly common scenario in American hospitals is hospitalized patients who get a hospital-based staph infection or pneumonia that is totally resistant to antibiotics. People with antibiotic resistant diseases often die. The cost to treat these people is $1.2 *billion* each year in the U.S. Tuberculosis is making a comeback because it is now resistant to most antibiotics, along with highly resistant strains of pneumonia. Think twice and question your physician very closely before using an antibiotic.

Superbugs are just one of the downsides of these drugs. Antibiotics kill our beneficial gut bacteria, which provide a frontline defense system against harmful bacteria, viruses and other environmental irritants such as allergens and toxins such as pesticides. Antibiotics also weaken the immune system, promote the growth of harmful candida, create a friendly environment for parasites, and cause excessive loss of vitamins and minerals through digestive problems. They cause diarrhea and create a susceptibility to food allergies by destroying the protective bacteria that line the gut, a setup for chronic fatigue.

Clearly we need to find other ways to fight infections and to support our immune systems when we get sick. Antibiotics should only be used as a final resort in fighting a potentially life-threatening infection. Before he or she prescribes an antibiotic, your physician should do a culture to find out, (1) if bacteria are present, and if so, (2) what strain of bacteria is present and thus what type of antibiotic to give you. Avoid wide spectrum antibiotics whenever possible.

If You're Taking Antibiotics, Don't Reach for an Antacid

Antibiotics can play havoc on your digestive system, bringing on unpleasant symptoms such as gas, diarrhea, abdominal cramping and indigestion. It would be natural to rifle through your medicine cabinet for Tums, Pepto-Bismol or another brand of antacid to relieve yourself of these discomforts. But don't. If you take an antacid with most antibiotics (particularly tetracycline or quinolone antibiotics), you'll be reducing their effectiveness by 50 to 90 percent. When taking an antibiotic, hold yourself back from taking an antacid or you'll undermine the antibiotic's ability to fight your infection.

AN OVERVIEW OF ANTIBIOTICS

Antibiotics are anti-infective drugs which destroy specific types of bacteria. Penicillin, cephalosporins, tetracycline, macrolides, and aminoglycosides are some of the more common types of antibiotics. There are many different types of penicillin drugs, but by far the most prescribed penicillins are amoxicillin and the combination amoxicillin and potassium clavulanate (another antibiotic). Some of the brand names of amoxicillin are Amoxil, Amoxicillan, Trimox or Augmentin, which you will probably recognize if you have been a parent in the past few decades.

Penicillins stress the kidneys significantly and are particularly hard on children's kidneys. If your child has been prescribed a penicillin, make sure your physician monitors his or her kidney and liver function.

Cephalosporins are broad spectrum antibiotics. The most prescribed of these drugs are Cefaclor, Cephalexin, Duricef, Lorabid, Cefzil, Ceftin, and Suprax.

Fluoroquinolones are synthetic broad-spectrum bacterial agents. The most common brand name of this drug is Cipro. Side effects can be very serious with this drug, including allergic reactions to sunlight. It also interacts badly with any food that contains caffeine and can produce insomnia, the jitters and heart palpitations. It can also cause ruptured tendons.

Tetracycline used to be prescribed much more often than it is today. The most common tetracycline prescribed today is doxycycline. It is prescribed for acne as well as some dangerous infections such as Rocky Mountain spotted fever. This drug is so hard on your liver and kidney that your physician should monitor the function of these organs periodically to avoid kidney and liver damage.

Macrolide antibiotics are also tough on your body. They are effective for limiting the growth of a variety of infections but their serious side effects could stay with you permanently. Some patients who had severe reactions to this drug like hearing loss, hallucinations and abdominal pain had a recurrence of these allergic reactions even after they stopped taking the drug. So don't take macrolides unless you absolutely have to!

Neomycin sulfate is the most frequently prescribed aminoglycoside antibiotic. This drug suppresses intestinal bacteria and also has potentially dangerous side effects which necessitate monitoring of both kidney and nerve function during the course of therapy. In fact, the side effects are so common that 8 to 28 percent of patients who take this drug develop impairment of their kidney function. This is another anti-infective to stay away from unless you really need it.

Antifungal agents, of course, fight fungal infections and fluconayole is the most popular drug in this class. A single dose of this drug can bring on unpleasant side effects such as nausea and vomiting. Several doses can cause severe reactions including liver dysfunction and seizures.

Because antibiotics are limited in the types of infections they can effectively fight, physicians are supposed to—but rarely do—determine exactly what kind of infection a patient has *before* prescribing an antibiotic. Not only does testing tell the physician if the infection is bacterial or viral in nature, but also exactly what kind of virus or bacteria it is. Again, antibiotics only destroy specific kinds of bacteria. If you have an infection that is caused by a bacteria or virus other than the type your prescribed drug kills, then taking that drug will prolong your illness, waste your money and subject you to unnecessary side effects.

Antibiotics can be very effective in combating bacterial infections. However, many people are allergic to antibiotics and experience severe allergic reactions—even fatal ones. There are many varied reactions that you can experience, but they usually begin with skin rashes, followed by one or more of the following: itching, hives, severe diarrhea, shortness of breath, wheezing, sore throat, nausea, vomiting, fever, swollen joints, and unusual bleeding or bruising. If any of these symptoms occur after taking an antibiotic, contact your physician immediately.

ANTACIDS THAT INTERFERE WITH ANTIBIOTICS

Aluminum hydroxide gel	Mylanta II
Amitone	Phillips' Milk of Magnesia
Calcium carbonate	Riopan
Chooz	Riopan Plus Di-Gel
Dicarbosil	Rolaids
Di-Gel Advanced Formula	Rolaids Calcium Rich/Sodium Free
Gas-X	Rulox
Gaviscon	Rulox Plus
Gaviscon Cool Mint Flavor	Simaal 2 Gel
Gaviscon ESR	Titralac
Gaviscon-2	Titralac Plus
Gelusil	Tums
Kudrox	Tums Anti-Gas
Maalox HRF	Tums E-X Extra Strength
Milk of magnesia	WinGel
Mylanta Double Strength	

ANTIBIOTICS MAY REDUCE THE EFFECTIVENESS OF BIRTH CONTROL PILLS

Antibiotics kill bacteria in the digestive tract that are key players in maintaining blood levels of contraceptive hormones. Studies have shown that unintended pregnancies have occurred from a birth control pill and antibiotic interaction. (The same reaction may be true for antifungal medications too.) Even the most vocal critics of this theory recommend that women receiving broad spectrum antibiotics with oral contraceptives should use alternative means to protect themselves from unplanned pregnancies.

Antibiotics That May Affect Oral Contraceptives

Achromycin V	Dynapen	Robitet
Ala-Tet	Geocillin	Spectrobid
Amcill	Geopen	Staphcillin
Amoxil	Ledercillin	Sumycin
Augmentin	Minocin	Tegopen
Azlin	Monodox	Terramycin
Bactocill	Nallpen	Tetracap
Beepen-VK	Omnipen	Tetracyn
Betapen-VK	Panmycin	Tetralan
Bikomox	Pathocil	Totacillin
Biomox	Pentids	Trimox
Cloxapen	Pen-V	Unipen
Coactin	Pen-Vee K	Uri-Tet
Declomycin	Polycillin	V-Cillin K
Doryx	Polymox	Veetids
Doxy-Caps	Principen	Vibramycin
Doxychel	Prostaphlin	Vibra-Tabs
Dycill	Robicillin VK	Wymox
Dynacin		

ANTIBIOTICS

Penicillins

AMOXICILLIN (Amoxil, Trimox, Augmentin, Biomox, Polymox, Wymox)

AMPICILLIN (Polycillin-N, Amicillin, Omnipen, Totacillin, Principen, D-Amp)

AMPICILLIN WITH PROBENECID (Probampacin)

AMPICILLIN AND SULBACTAM (Unasyn)

BACAMPICILLIN HCl (Spectrobid)

CARBENICILLIN INDANYL (Geocillin)

CLOXACILLIN (Tegopen, Cloxapen)

DICLOXACILLIN (Pathocil, Dynapen, Dycill)

METHICILLIN (Staphcillin)

MEZLOCILLIN (Mezlin)

NAFCILLIN (Unipen, Nafcil, Nallpen)

OXACILLIN (Bactocill, Prostaphlin)

PENICILLIN G (Pfizerpen, Pentids, Wycillin, Permapen, Bicillin)

PENICILLIN V (Veetids, V-Cillin, Beepen, Betapen, Robicillin)

PIPERACILLIN (Pipracil)

PIPERACILLIN AND TAZOBACTAM (Zosyn)

TICARCILLIN (Ticar)

TICARCILLIN AND CLAVULANATE (Timentin)

WHAT DO THEY DO IN YOUR BODY?

Halt bacterial infections.

WHAT ARE THEY PRESCRIBED FOR?

Treating mild to moderately severe penicillin-sensitive bacterial infections including pneumonia, some respiratory tract infections, ear infections, some sexually transmitted diseases and meningitis.

WHAT ARE THE POSSIBLE SIDE EFFECTS?

Mild to serious and occasionally fatal immediate allergic reactions. These reactions can include skin rashes, fever, problems with breathing, wheezing, abnormality of the tongue, sore throat, swollen joints, chills, water retention, breathing problems and death.

Penicillins also can create distress in the digestive and eliminative systems such as cramping, abdominal pain, gas, vomiting, bloody diarrhea, rectal bleeding, upset stomach, taste abnormalities, and kidney inflammation.

Possible side effects also include imbalance of blood chemistry including suppression of the immune system and anemia. These drugs can also produce lethargy, dizziness, convulsions, anxiety, depression, combativeness, insomnia, seizures and hyperactivity.

These drugs are particularly hard on young kidneys. Your child's physician should be monitoring your child's organ system function closely when your child is taking this type of drug.

If you are receiving this drug through an IV drip, you should know that potassium or sodium is added to the solution and can cause an imbalance of those minerals in your body.

CAUTION: THINK TWICE ABOUT TAKING THESE TYPES OF DRUGS IF . . .

- You have an allergic reaction to any type of penicillin.
- You have asthma, hay fever, and/or other allergies. If you take penicillin or any other antibiotic, your allergic reactions to it could be immediate and severe.
- You bleed or bruise easily or have any kind of kidney dysfunction.

WHAT ARE THE INTERACTIONS WITH OTHER DRUGS?

Penicillins may raise levels or prolong the effects of these drugs:

↑ Anticoagulants   Erythromycin*

The following drugs may be reduced in potency or decreased in the amount of time they are effective when combined with penicillins:

↓ Atenolol   Erythromycin*
  Beta-blockers   Oral contraceptives (use additional
  Chloramphenicol*   birth control when taking penicillin)

These drugs may increase the effects or prolong the action of penicillins:

↑ Allopurinol   Erythromycin*
  Beta-blockers   Probenecid

These drugs may reduce the effects of penicillins:

↓ Chloramphenicol*   Tetracyclines
  Erythromycin*

WHAT ARE THE INTERACTIONS WITH FOOD?

Taking food with most penicillins reduces their effectiveness. (Amoxil, Augmentin and Trimox are exceptions. They can be taken without regard to food.)

Having an alcoholic drink while taking these drugs can produce uncomfortable symptoms such as headaches, stomach cramping and vomiting.

Acidic fruit juices, sodas, wines, carbonated drinks, syrups and other acidic beverages decrease the effectiveness of penicillins. Don't take penicillins with acidic food or drink.

---

*Potentially dangerous interaction.

WHAT NUTRIENTS DO THEY THROW OUT OF BALANCE OR INTERACT WITH?

Vitamin K, amino acids, calcium, folic acid, magnesium, potassium, vitamin B6 and B12 are all depleted.

WHAT ELSE TO TAKE IF YOU TAKE THESE DRUGS

Supplements of the above. Take them two hours after a meal. Also be sure to take probiotics during and after a course of antibiotics (see natural alternatives at the end of this chapter).

Cephalosporins

CEFACLOR (Cefaclor, Ceclor)

CEFADROXIL (Duricef)

CEFAMANDOLE (Mandol)

CEFAZOLIN (Ancef, Kefzol, Zolicef)

CEFEPIME (Maxipime, Kefurox, Zinacef)

CEFIXIME (Suprax)

CEFMETAZOLE (Zefazone)

CEFONICID (Monocid)

CEFOPERAZONE (Cefobid)

CEFOTAXIME (Claforan)

CEFOTETAN (Cefotan)

CEFOXITIN (Mefoxin)

CEFPODOXIME PROXETIL (Vantin)

CEFPROZIL (Cefzil)

CEFTAZIDIME (Fortaz, Tazidime, Ceptaz, Tazicef)

CEFTIBUTEN (Cedax)

CEFTIZOXIME (Cefizox)

CEFTRIAXONE (Rocephin)

CEFUROXIME (Ceftin)

CEPHALEXIN (Keflex, Keftab, Biocef)

CEPHALOTHIN (Keflin, Neutral)

CEPHAPIRIN (Cefadyl)

CEPHRADINE (Velosef)

LORACARBEF (Lorabid)

WHAT DO THEY DO IN YOUR BODY?

They are related to penicillins and destroy specific bacterial infections.

WHAT ARE THEY PRESCRIBED FOR?

Halting bacterial infections.

WHAT ARE THE POSSIBLE SIDE EFFECTS?

Allergic reactions, particularly for people who have a history of allergy, asthma or hay fever. These reactions include rashes, open sores, breathing difficulties, vaginal infections, dizziness, drowsiness, nervousness, insomnia, confusion, anemia.

Intestinal problems are common when using these drugs. They can cause nausea, vomiting, diarrhea, stomach and abdominal cramping, gas and heartburn. A more serious side effect is colitis or inflammation of the colon. This problem results in colicky-like cramps, either diarrhea or constipation and is caused by a depletion of vitamin K as well as an imbalance of the friendly and unfriendly bacteria in the intestinal tract.

These drugs are also particularly hard on kidney and liver function and have caused liver dysfunction, jaundice and kidney failure. Because of this, your physician should monitor you closely if you are elderly or debilitated. Children should also be watched closely for any indications of kidney or liver system dysfunction. These drugs can cause seizures in people with kidney problems.

Like penicillin, these drugs also create changes in blood chemistry which suppress the immune system and can cause abnormal and heavy bleeding and mineral imbalances such as anemia.

CAUTION: THINK TWICE ABOUT TAKING THESE TYPES OF DRUGS IF . . .

- You have or have had asthma, hay fever, or an allergic reaction to this type of antibiotics.
- You have kidney dysfunction or kidney disease.
- You have a problem with excessive bleeding.
- You have liver dysfunction or liver disease.
- You have colitis or any other problem with your digestive tract.

WHAT ARE THE INTERACTIONS WITH OTHER DRUGS?

Cephalosporins may raise levels or prolong the effects of these drugs:

↑ Alcohol (can produce alcohol   Anticoagulants
   intolerance)*   Polypeptide antibiotics
   Aminoglycosides

This drug may increase the effects or prolong the action of cephalosporins:

↑ Probenecid

WHAT ARE THE INTERACTIONS WITH FOOD?

Do not take these drugs with food. Food delays or reduces the absorption of these drugs into your system. (Cephalexin, Duricef, Ceftin are exceptions.)

---

*Potentially dangerous interaction.

What Nutrients Do They Throw Out of Balance or Interact With?

Vitamin K, copper, sodium, vitamin B6, B12, zinc, amino acids, calcium, folic acid, magnesium, potassium may all be depleted by antibiotics.

What Else to Take If You Take These Drugs

Take supplements of the above nutrients and be sure to use probiotics (see natural alternatives at the end of this chapter).

Fluoroquinolones

Ciprofloxacin (Cipro)

Enoxacin (Penetrex)

Lomefloxacin (Maxaquin)

Norfloxacin (Noroxin)

Ofloxacin (Floxin)

Sparfloxacin (Zagam)

What Do They Do in The Body?

These drugs are synthetic antibacterial agents with specific components not present in antibiotics which enhance their ability to efficiently destroy some infections.

What Are They Prescribed For?

Patients over 14 who have cystic fibrosis and who experience exacerbated lung problems from infection, with malignant external ear infections or with tuberculosis.

Patients over 18 who have lower respiratory infections, skin infections, bone and joint infections, urinary tract infections, infectious diarrhea, typhoid and gonorrhea.

WHAT ARE THE POSSIBLE SIDE EFFECTS?

Allergic reactions—particularly to light of any kind. The reactions include skin burning sensation, redness, swelling, blisters, rash or itching. Other allergic reactions can range from serious to fatal. They include loss of consciousness, tingling, water retention in the face, dizziness, drowsiness and itching. There have also been reports of cataract development.

Convulsions, tremors, confusion and hallucinations have occurred with these drugs.

Colon inflammation that can occur from these drugs ranges from mild to life-threatening in severity and can result in chronic diarrhea or constipation.

These drugs can also cause respiratory problems, heart attacks, vaginal infections, intestinal bleeding and stomach disturbances.

These drugs are hard on the eliminative systems and can cause kidney damage and kidney failure as well as jaundice and hepatitis.

These drugs also caused lameness in immature dogs from permanent cartilage lesions and joint destruction. More recent reports on these drugs are that they can cause ruptured tendons, even for some time after the drugs have been discontinued. If you must take these drugs you should be extremely cautious about exercise, and inform your physician if you experience any type of pain or swelling after taking the drugs.

CAUTION: THINK TWICE ABOUT TAKING THESE TYPES OF DRUGS IF . . .

- You are allergic to these drugs or other antibacterial agents such as cinoxacin and nalidixic acid.
- You have eye problems such as cataracts or are sensitive to sunlight or to light from sunlamps.
- You have pressure from fluids or growths under the skull.
- You have or suspect any brain disorder such as severe cerebral arteriosclerosis, epilepsy or other factors which make you susceptible to seizures.
- You have diarrhea or colitis.
- You have kidney disease or kidney problems of any kind.

WHAT ARE THE INTERACTIONS WITH OTHER DRUGS?

Fluoroquinolones may raise levels or prolong the effects of these drugs:

↑ Anticoagulants   Digoxin
Caffeine   Theophylline*
Cyclosporine

The following drug may be reduced in potency or decreased in the amount of time it is effective when combined with fluoroquinolones:

↓ Hydantoins

These drugs may increase the effects or prolong the action of fluoroquinolones:

↑ Azlocillin   Probenecid
Cimetidine

These drugs may reduce the effects of fluoroquinolones:

↓ Antacids   Nitrofurantoin
Antineoplastic agents   Sucralfate
Bismuth subsalicylate   Zinc salts

WHAT ARE THE INTERACTIONS WITH FOOD?

Food in general delays the absorption of these drugs. Take them two hours after a meal. (Cipro is an exception. It is absorbed better without food but may be taken with food to avoid stomach upset.)

These drugs interact poorly with mineral supplements of any kind. Take them two hours after taking a mineral supplement.

Avoid coffee or tea while taking these drugs. Fluoroquinolones intensify the caffeine effect and can give you jitters, insomnia and heart

---

*Potentially dangerous interaction.

palpitations. Check labels for products which contain caffeine that you may not be aware of.

WHAT NUTRIENTS DO THEY THROW OUT OF BALANCE OR INTERACT WITH?

Acid/alkaline balance is often upset. Vitamin K, amino acids, calcium, folic acid, magnesium, potassium, vitamins B6, B12 can all be depleted.

WHAT ELSE TO TAKE IF YOU TAKE THESE DRUGS

Plenty of water! Supplements of the above. Take two hours after ingesting these drugs. Also, be sure to use probiotics during and after taking them (see natural alternatives at the end of this chapter).

OTHER TIPS ON THESE DRUGS

If you are taking these drugs for a prolonged amount of time, your physician should periodically assess your kidney, liver function as well as your blood chemistry.

Do not take antacids within four hours before or two hours after taking these drugs.

These drugs require sufficient fluids to ensure that you maintain the correct amount of water in your system and enough urine to eliminate required amounts of these drugs from your system.

MEDICINES THAT CONTAIN CAFFEINE

Anacin	Excedrin Extra-Strength
Aqua-Ban Plus	NoDoz
Bayer Select Maximum Headache Capsules	Quick Pep
	Tirend
BC Headache Powders	Vanquish Caplets
Caffedrine	Vivarin

Since these drugs can cause dizziness or lightheadedness, do not drive or perform tasks that require alertness or coordination.

Tetracyclines

DEMECLOCYCLINE (Declomycin)

DOXYCYCLINE (Doxychel, Vibramycin, Monodox, Doxy Caps, Doryx)

METHACYCLINE (Rondomycin)

MINOCYCLINE (Dynacin, Minocin)

OXYTETRACYCLINE (Uri-Tet, Terramycin)

TETRACYCLINE (Achromycin, Sumycin, Tetralan, Panmycin, Robitet, Teline, Tetracyn)

WHAT DO THEY DO IN YOUR BODY?

Tetracyclines inhibit the multiplication and the growth of bacteria but do not kill the bacteria.

WHAT ARE THEY PRESCRIBED FOR?

Severe acne, infections in the excretory and reproductive systems, a type of conjunctivitis, different kinds of infections related to gonorrhea and Rocky Mountain spotted fever. Sometimes tetracyclines are used to prevent diarrhea from occurring while one is traveling in foreign countries. They are also prescribed for early stages of Lyme disease. However, their efficacy has been questioned.

WHAT ARE THE POSSIBLE SIDE EFFECTS?

Allergic reactions—particularly to sunlight and sun lamps, weakness, shortness of breath, heart abnormalities, headaches, dizziness, open sores and rashes.

These drugs are very hard on both the kidney and liver and can impair the function of both of these vital organs. Because of this you may experience kidney impairment or liver poisoning, hepatitis or an increase in liver enzymes. In fact, it is so hard on these organs that your physician should monitor your liver and kidney functions periodically. In addition, physicians are warned that prescribing an additional drug that is also hard on your liver could be dangerous to you.

Headaches and blurred vision are possible with these drugs.

These drugs can also cause nausea, vomiting, diarrhea, indigestion, sore throat, abnormalities of the tongue, colitis, hernias, discoloration of teeth and nails and ulcers in the esophagus.

It has also been reported that they can discolor the thyroid gland to a brown-black color.

There are increasing reports that minocycline, commonly prescribed for acne in young people, can cause a lupus-like reaction that can last for more than a year after going off the drug. It's not worth it.

CAUTION: THINK TWICE ABOUT TAKING THESE TYPES OF DRUGS IF . . .

- You are allergic to sulfites. Allergic reactions can be life-threatening and can create severe asthmatic episodes.

WHAT ARE THE INTERACTIONS WITH OTHER DRUGS?

Tetracyclines may raise levels or prolong the effects of these drugs:

↑ Anticoagulants   Lithium
  Digoxin*   Methoxyflurane*
  Insulin

The following drugs may be reduced in potency or decreased in the amount of time they are effective when combined with tetracyclines:

↓ Lithium   Penicillins
  Oral contraceptives

---

*Potentially dangerous interaction.

These drugs may increase the effects or prolong the action of tetracyclines:

↑ Alcohol   Methoxyflurane*
  Digoxin

These drugs may reduce the effects of tetracyclines:

↓ Alcohol   Carbamazepine
  Antacids containing aluminum,   Cimetidine
    calcium, zinc or magnesium   Hydantoins
    (upto 90 percent do!)   Iron supplements
  Anticonvulsants   Phenytoin
  Barbiturates   Sodium bicarbonate
  Bismuth salts

WHAT ARE THEIR INTERACTIONS WITH FOOD?

Eating food with these drugs decreases their absorption. (Doxycycline is an exception. Take with food.) Take these drugs with a full glass of water. Avoid eating dairy products within two hours of taking them.

Iron, calcium, magnesium, riboflavin, vitamin C, zinc or any mineral supplements taken at the same time as tetracyclines can reduce their absorption and reduce absorption of these nutrients. Take these supplements two hours before or after taking tetracycline.

Also avoid antacids, laxatives or iron or magnesium-containing products. If you must take an antacid, take it at least two hours before or after tetracycline.

Caffeine enhances the effects of tetracycline.

WHAT NUTRIENTS DO THEY THROW OUT OF BALANCE OR INTERACT WITH?

Vitamin K, riboflavin, vitamin C, amino acids, copper, folic acid, vitamin B2, B6, B12, potassium, zinc, and calcium can all be depleted by antibiotics. These drugs can cause severe headaches when taken with high doses of vitamin A. Be sure to use a probiotic during and after a course of antibiotics. See the natural alternatives at the end of this chapter.

WHAT ELSE TO TAKE IF YOU TAKE THESE DRUGS

Supplements of the above nutrients and probiotics.

OTHER TIPS ON THESE DRUGS

Children under the age of eight should not be given these drugs.

During long-term therapy, your physician should periodically monitor your organ systems including kidney and liver functions and blood chemistry.

Macrolide Antibiotics

AZITHROMYCIN (Zithromax)

CLARITHROMYCIN (Biaxin)

DIRITHROMYCIN (Dynabac)

ERYTHROMYCIN (Ery-Tab, E-Mycin, Robimycin, E-Base, Eryc, Ilosone, Eramycin, EryPed)

TROLEANDOMYCIN (Tao)

WHAT DO THEY DO IN YOUR BODY?

These drugs either kill or stop multiplication and growth of specific bacteria.

WHAT ARE THEY PRESCRIBED FOR?

Tonsillitis, sinus infections, chronic bronchitis, pneumonia, skin infections, ear infections and acne; or for the prevention or destruction of bacteria/fungal infections in advanced HIV patients.

Azithromycin: This drug is prescribed for all of the above as well as bacterial infections of patients with chronic obstructive pulmonary disease or community acquired pneumonia.

Erythromycin: This drug is prescribed for moderately severe upper and lower respiratory infections, whooping cough, diphtheria, conjunctivitis of newborn, pneumonia of the infant, genital infections during pregnancy, syphilis, Legionnaire's disease, rheumatic fever, prolonged diarrhea, and early Lyme disease.

WHAT ARE THE POSSIBLE SIDE EFFECTS?

The most frequently reported side effects are related to the digestive system. They include diarrhea, nausea, abnormal taste, upset stomach, abdominal cramping, headache and vaginal infections. In children: diarrhea, vomiting, abdominal pain, rash, and headache.

Allergic reactions can range from life-threatening to mild. These can include loss of hearing, rashes, behavioral disorders, disorientation, dizziness, hallucinations, insomnia, nightmares, vertigo, palpitations, chest pain, liver dysfunction, abnormal heartbeats and death. Allergic reactions have reoccurred in patients using azithromycin and erythromycin even after they stopped taking the drugs.

Erythromycin (e.g., E-Mycin) interacts dangerously with many common drugs such as some calcium channel blockers and the cholesterol-lowering drug lovastatin (e.g., Mevacor), as well as some not-so-common drugs such as vinblastine (e.g., Velban), a chemotherapy drug. Clearly, erythromycin is a drug to be used with extreme caution or not at all. It raises levels of many other drugs due to its blocking action on certain enzymes in the liver responsible for metabolizing the drugs. This means it could affect hundreds of other drugs that simply haven't been studied yet, and even substances such as coffee and alcohol. Your best bet is to stay away from a drug like that unless you are in a life-threatening situation.

CAUTION: THINK TWICE ABOUT TAKING THESE TYPES OF DRUGS IF . . .

- You are taking terfenadine or astemizole and have a preexisting heart problem like irregular heartbeat, have a slow heartbeat, have ischemic heart disease, have had congestive heart failure or electrolyte disturbances or have heart problems of any kind.

- You have colitis or inflammation of the intestinal tract or severe diarrhea or constipation.
- You have liver or kidney disease or dysfunction—particularly if you are elderly.

WHAT ARE THE INTERACTIONS WITH OTHER DRUGS?

Macrolides may raise levels or prolong the effects of these drugs:

↑ Alfentanil	Hismanal*
Anticoagulants*	Lovastatin
Antihistamines*	Methacholine
Astemiyole	Methylprednisolone
Bromocriptine	Midazolan
Carbamazepine*	Penicillins
Cisapride*	Simvastatin
Cyclosporine	Terfenadine
Digoxin*	Theophyllines*
Disopyramide	Triazolam
Ergot alkaloids	Warfarin*
Felodipine	Zidovudine

The following drugs may be reduced in potency or decreased in the amount of time they are effective when combined with macrolides:

↓ Lincosamides	Zidovudine
Penicillins	

This drug may increase the effects or prolong the action of macrolides:

↑ Fluconazole

These drugs may reduce the effects of macrolides:

↓ Antacids	Theophyllines

---

*Potentially dangerous interaction.

What Are the Interactions with Food?

Food delays the absorption of these drugs. Take one hour before or two hours after a meal. Acidic fruits or juices, carbonated drinks, sodas, wines and syrups decrease the effectiveness of these drugs. Alkaline foods such as milk, dairy products and vegetables also decrease the effectiveness of these drugs.

What Nutrients Do They Throw Out of Balance or Interact With?

Amino acids, calcium, vitamin B6, B12, folic acid, potassium and vitamin K may be depleted.

What Else to Take If You Take These Drugs

Supplements of the above. Take two hours after taking macrolides. Be sure to take probiotics during and after a course of antibiotics. See the natural alternatives at the end of the chapter.

Aminoglycosides

Amikacin (Amikin)

Gentamicin (Garamycin, Jenamicin)

Kanamycin (Kantrex)

Neomycin (Neo-Tabs, Mycifradin, Neo-fradin)

Netilmicin

Paromomycin (Humatin)

Streptomycin

Tobramycin (Nebcin)

What Do They Do in Your Body?

They block the proliferation of intestinal bacteria.

WHAT ARE THEY PRESCRIBED FOR?

Suppression of intestinal bacteria. Because of the high potential for toxicity from these drugs, they are only prescribed for periods shorter than two weeks.

WHAT ARE THE POSSIBLE SIDE EFFECTS?

The side effects of these drugs are serious. Therefore, monitoring of kidney and nerve function are critical. Eight to 28 percent of patients who took these drugs for several days or more developed renal (kidney) impairment. Toxicity is so prevalent that physicians are warned against prescribing additional drugs that are at all difficult on kidney and/or liver.

Hearing loss, fainting, ringing in the ears, skin tingling, muscle twitching and convulsions. Hearing loss that occurs with these drugs may be irreversible.

These drugs also cause problems in the digestive tract and inhibit absorption of nutrients. This can produce nausea, vomiting, diarrhea and colitis, not to mention malnutrition.

CAUTION: THINK TWICE ABOUT TAKING THESE TYPES OF DRUGS IF . . .

- You have muscular disorders such as Parkinson's disease. These drugs can worsen muscle weakness.
- You have open sores in your intestinal tract or have digestive problems.
- You have kidney or liver problems of any kind.
- You have hearing problems.
- You have an electrolyte imbalance.

WHAT ARE THE INTERACTIONS WITH OTHER DRUGS?

Aminoglycosides may raise levels or prolong the effects of these drugs:

↑ Anticoagulants   Polypeptide antibiotics*
Neuromuscular blockers*

---

*Potentially dangerous interaction.

The following drugs may be reduced in potency or decreased in the amount of time they are effective when combined with aminoglycosides:

↓ Digoxin   Methotrexate

These drugs may increase the effects or prolong the action of aminoglycosides:

↑ Cephalosporin antibiotics   Loop diuretics
  Indomethacin   Penicillins

This drug may reduce the effects of aminoglycosides:

↓ Penicillins

WHAT ARE THE INTERACTIONS WITH FOOD?

Acidic foods taken with these drugs can increase the effects and length of effectiveness of the drug. Alkaline foods can decrease the effectiveness of these drugs.

WHAT NUTRIENTS DO THEY THROW OUT OF BALANCE OR INTERACT WITH?

Magnesium, calcium, potassium, vitamin A, carbohydrates, vitamin K.

WHAT ELSE TO TAKE IF YOU TAKE THESE DRUGS

Take supplements of the above several hours apart from taking an aminoglycoside, and be sure to use a probiotic during and after a course of antibiotics. See natural alternatives at the end of the chapter for details.

Antifungal Agents

AMPHOTERICIN B (Abelcet, Amphotec, Fungizone)

FLUCONAZOLE (Diflucan)

FLUCYTOSINE (Ancobon)

GRISEOFULVIN (Fulvicin, Grifulvin, Grisactin)

ITRACONAZOLE (Sporanox)

KETOCONAZOLE (Nizoral)

MICONAZOLE (Monistat)

NYSTATIN (Mycostatin, Nilstat)

TERBINAFINE (Lamisil)

Most of the antifungal drugs have very nasty side effects and dangerous interactions with a long list of other drugs. Be extremely cautious with their use. It has become something of a fad in alternative medicine to prescribe antifungal drugs for intestinal candida infections that are diagnosed by symptoms. The long-term effect of this treatment is that the candida returns, worse than ever, within a year. You are better off treating candida infections, both vaginal and intestinal, with one of the suggested alternatives at the end of this chapter that support your good bacteria.

Antifungals are also notoriously ineffective for treating toenail fungus. Again, chances are it will come back worse than ever, even after a long course of the drugs.

WHAT DO THEY DO IN YOUR BODY?

They inhibit fungal growth.

WHAT ARE THEY PRESCRIBED FOR?

Fungal infections. Most commonly, vaginal infections from candida, the prevention of fungal infections during surgery and for meningitis.

What Are the Possible Side Effects?

These drugs can be prescribed for women with yeast infections, but they have 10 percent more side effects than intravaginal agents which accomplish the same thing. See the section on natural alternatives.

Side effects can include headache, nausea, abdominal pain, diarrhea, dizziness, drowsiness. Patients receiving multiple doses may experience all of the above side effects plus seizures, skin disorders and serious liver reactions.

Injury to your liver is possible. Toxicity is rare but has ranged from mild to fatal.

Allergic reactions can occur such as rashes, shortness of breath, and dizziness. Some people have had serious skin disorders from these drugs which have produced open sores.

Caution: Think Twice About Taking These Types of Drugs If . . .

- You have malignant cancer or AIDS.
- You have any dysfunction of the liver or liver disease.
- You have kidney dysfunction or kidney disease.
- You have a serious skin disorder.

What Are the Interactions with Other Drugs?

Antifungal agents may raise levels or prolong the effects of these drugs:

↑ Anticoagulants
Anticonvulsants (Dilantin, Mesantoin, Peganone)*
Antihistamines, nonsedating*
Calcium channel blockers
Cisapride
Corticosteroids
Cyclosporine
Digoxin
Phenytoin
Quinidine
Sulfonylureas (could result in hypoglycemia)
Terfenadine/Itraconazole*
Theophyllines
Thiazide diuretics
Triazolam and midazolam
Warfarin*
Zidovudine

*Potentially dangerous interaction.

The following drugs may be reduced in potency or decreased in the amount of time they are effective when combined with antifungal agents:

↓ Anticoagulants/griseofulvin   Oral contraceptives
Cyclosporine/griseofulvin   Salicylates (aspirin)/griseofulvin

These drugs may increase the effects or prolong the action of antifungal agents:

↑ Amphotericin/flucytosine   Hydrochlorothiazide
Cytosine/flucytosine

These drugs may reduce the effects of antifungal agents:

↓ Antacids   Isoniazid
Barbiturates   Oral contraceptives
Carbamazepine   Rifampin
Cimetidine and other H2 blockers

NATURAL ALTERNATIVES TO ANTIBIOTICS

When penicillin was discovered, we thought we had discovered a magic bullet that would kill any and all infections. Physicians tend to prescribe it for anything from a cut to a cold, knowing all the while that it doesn't kill the viruses that cause colds, it only kills bacteria. We Americans have become hooked on antibiotics. If our physician didn't write us out a prescription for them, we go to another physician.

The bacteria in our bodies that antibiotics are supposed to kill have an intelligence all their own when it comes to building resistance to these drugs. Every time we take antibiotics, or get them in dairy products or meat, we are giving bacteria a new opportunity to become resistant. The consequence of this is that many antibiotics have become useless—a wide variety of bacteria that are the cause of many serious illnesses are resistant to them. Clearly we need to find other ways to fight infections and to support our immune systems when we get sick.

Use Probiotics When You Take Antibiotics

One of the most serious side effects of taking antibiotics is the killing off of the bacteria that live in your intestines. The colon, in contrast to the germ-free stomach and small intestine, is lavishly populated with bacteria, which are normal intestinal flora that keep the "bad" bacteria under control. These bacteria, also called probiotics, are also found in the mouth, the urinary tract and the vagina. There are about 100 trillion of these bacteria living in our bodies and over 400 species. The three most common friendly bacteria are called *Lactobacillus acidophilus*, *Lactobacillus bulgaricus* and *Bifidobacterium bifidum*.

Probiotics are also intimately tied into how our immune system works. They manufacture the B vitamins. They help us digest our food, reduce cholesterol and help keep hormones in balance. If you take an antibiotic and kill them off, it will seriously compromise your health. Steroids such as prednisone, poor digestion, nutritional deficiencies and stress can also kill off these good bacteria, leaving an overgrowth of the bad guys, most of whom are a fungal yeast called *Candida albicans*. An overgrowth of yeast in the intestines can cause fatigue, bloating, gas, diarrhea, constipation, skin problems, and a long list of secondary symptoms such as headaches, mental fogginess, achy joints and pollen allergies.

If you must take antibiotics for some reason, be sure to take probiotics both during and after the course of antibiotics. Take them at least two hours away from when you take the antibiotic and keep taking them for at least two weeks after you finish the antibiotics.

Probiotic supplements are "alive" and have a relatively short shelf life of a few months. If you use probiotic supplements, please stick to the refrigerated brands. A good probiotic supplement will contain fructooligosaccharides (FOS), which promote the growth of good bacteria.

There is much disagreement among health professionals and probiotic manufacturers about which types of probiotic supplements are best. Most people do just fine with a mixture of lactobacillus, bifidus and acidophilus. The loose powder is the ideal way to get a concentrated dose of probiotics, but if this is going to be too much trouble, take it in capsules. When we're talking about billions of bacteria, the loss of a few million won't hurt too much! You need to keep them refrigerated when you get them home. Since stomach acid rises when you eat, you'll get more of them into your digestive system by taking them in-between meals.

You can get probiotics in your diet by eating yogurt with live cultures (this is listed on the label). Many supermarkets and health food stores also sell *acidophilus,* a milk product containing live cultures.

Natural Remedies for Resisting Infections

The best way you can create hostile terrain for bacteria is to follow the Six Core Principles for Optimal Health and make it a way of life. That will give your body a solid foundation from which to fend off bacteria and viruses. It's important to be aware that we are always being exposed to billions of potentially infectious germs, and our bodies naturally fend them off. When your immune system is weakened through poor nutrition, high stress levels, not enough sleep and the rigors of travel, the germs have the opportunity to get a foothold in your body.

One of the keys to resisting an infection is to begin helping your body fight it as soon as you are aware it's there. We all know the symptoms: fatigue, achiness, sore throat, swollen glands, runny nose, cough and fever. If you have a sore throat and ignore it, stay up late and eat a bowl of ice cream, it's bound to get worse. If you gargle with salt water, go to bed early with a cup of chamomile tea and avoid sugary foods, chances are it will be gone by morning.

Here are some simple, specific steps you can take to stay free of infections:

Cleanliness is next to godliness when it comes to fighting infections. Clean terrain is hostile terrain for bacteria. Keep your hands away from your face and mouth, and wash your hands before eating. Keep kitchen surfaces clean and be extremely careful in public restrooms about what you touch.

If you're coming down with a sore throat, one of the simplest and most effective solutions is to gargle with a germ-killing mouthwash (make sure the gargle reaches your throat) or a simple salt water solution (1 tsp salt to 1 cup of water). A sore throat is often caused by mucus from the sinuses dripping down the back of the throat, so giving that area an antibacterial bath can work wonders. There are some herbal throat sprays on the market that are excellent for banishing throat infections.

A great remedy for an encroaching sinus infection is to rinse the sinuses with a salt water solution (1 tsp. of salt and a pinch of baking soda per 1 cup of water). This remedy takes some discipline and focus, and it's not recommended for most children. You need to put the salt water solution in the palm of your hand or a clean, wide container such as a wide, short water glass. Hold one nostril closed, then put your other nostril in the water and inhale the water slowly and gently into your sinuses until you can feel it draining down the back of your throat. If you can, spit out the water rather than swallow it. If you "snort" the water it will be very uncomfortable and only further irritate your sinuses, but if you can manage this technique it works wonders. Many health food stores sell little sinus irrigation pots with a spout that can be put into the nostril.

As your body fights infection it needs extra nutrition. It uses extra vitamins and minerals in its battle against bacteria, and it's up to you to supply the extras needed. You can double your intake of your multivitamin for up to a week to help fight an infection.

On the other hand, sugar and alcohol will make it much harder for your body to do its job. Both suppress the immune system, leaving you wide open to whatever germs are around.

There's nothing like vitamin C for fighting infections *and* viruses. If you take 1,000 to 2,000 mg every three to four hours as soon as you feel a cold coming on, drink plenty of water and avoid sugar, you can often knock it out before it ever gets started. Vitamin C will work even better if you combine it with bioflavonoids.

The other important infection-fighting supplement is vitamin A. It is an immune stimulant that boosts thymus gland function and helps maintain healthy cells in your mucus membranes. You can take 10,000 to 30,000 IU daily for a week to help fight off an infection. (If you're pregnant don't take more than 10,000 IU daily.)

Your two most important infection-fighting minerals are zinc and selenium. There are a wide variety of lozenges available at your health food store that contain zinc, selenium and vitamin C. Pass on those with a lot of sugar.

Bacteria are also adverse to high temperatures, which is why we sometimes get a fever when we get infections. This is why it's important not to bring down a fever unless it's dangerously high. The fever is the very thing that will kill the bacteria or virus that's making you sick. It is especially important to allow children to have a fever, up to 103 or 104 degrees F. (talk to your physician). This is part of the body's mechanism for training the immune system to recognize hostile bacteria and viruses and forming antibodies that will recognize them in the future. If you suppress the fever with acetaminophen (Tylenol), your child is more likely to get sick again the next time the bug comes to visit.

A product you can use if you feel an infection coming on is grapefruit seed extract, sold under a variety of brand names. It is a grapefruit bioflavonoid concentrate that works well to help knock out a cold. You can take one 100-mg tablet every four to five hours or a few drops of the liquid. There are anecdotal reports from women that grapefruit seed extract will effectively cure urinary tract infections.

The herb echinacea, sometimes combined with goldenseal in formulas, is an effective immune stimulant, but works best when used early on in an infection.

Natural Prescription for Preventing Colds and Flus

Here's a suggested course of action when you feel a cold or flu coming on:

- Reduce stress and get plenty of sleep.
- Stop eating all sugars.
- Take echinacea and goldenseal.
- Take high levels of vitamin A, 15,000 to 30,000 IU two times a day for three to five days only. Use proportionately less for children. (Use under 10,000 IU daily if pregnant.)
- Take vitamin C as much as you can without getting loose stools. If you get loose stools, cut back proportions until your elimina-

tions are normal. Most people who are getting sick or are sick can tolerate up to 10,000 mg daily in divided doses.

- You can also take colloidal silver, 1 tsp. at first. Then 1 tsp. four times a day for adults—proportionately less for children.
- For colds, take zinc lozenges 10 to 20 mg two to four times a day—for up to five days.

Viral Infections

- Take elderberry extract (follow directions on the container).
- Take 1 to 2 mg of selenium daily for up to five days.
- Take olive leaf extract: 500 mg three to four times a day.

Bladder Infections

For bladder infections, drink 4 oz. of unsweetened cranberry juice or take 1 capsule of cranberry concentrate three times a day along with grapefruit seed extract.

Chronic Infections

For recurrent, chronic infections:

- Avoid sugars.
- Take as much vitamin C as you can tolerate.
- Take 10 to 15 mg of zinc daily for up to two weeks.
- Take a high-potency multiple vitamin/mineral formula.
- Take 25,000 IU of vitamin A one to two times a day for up to two weeks.

Ear Infections

For recurring ear infections:

- Eliminate sugar.
- Identify and eliminate food allergies.
- Take vitamin C to tolerance.
- Take vitamin A, 10 to 15,000 IU a day for up to two weeks.

Internal Fungal Infections

Candida is a common fungus that grows out of control in many people, thanks to too many antibiotics and too much sugar. Your best strategy for fighting a fungal infection is to boost your body's natural resources as much as possible, so that your own "good" bacteria can fight off the candida.

It's extremely important to eliminate sugar from your diet if you're fighting a candida infection, and it helps to eliminate or cut back on fermented foods such as beer, wine, vinegar, aged cheeses and anything made with yeast.

If you suspect you have a serious candida overgrowth in your intestines, read the book *Optimal Wellness* by Ralph Golan, M.D. (Ballantine Books, 1995). He covers the subject in detail, and gives an excellent protocol to follow for bringing candida under control.

Grapefruit seed extract, garlic oil and oregano oil are all very effective antifungals. It's certainly worth giving them a try before taking a potent antifungal drug. Be sure to take probiotics to enhance your body's production of its own "good" bacteria.

Vaginal Yeast Infections

Vaginal yeast infections are an overgrowth of candida, usually caused by taking antibiotics. They cause itching and redness and a white discharge from the vagina. Yeast infections can also be caused when the pH of the vagina is altered, creating a favorable environment for candida growth. The pH of the vagina can be altered by frequent sex, because semen creates a more alkaline environment in the vagina. It can also be altered by the use of commercial douches, which in general cause a lot more unpleasant odors than they cover up.

Fortunately vaginal yeast infections are usually easy to treat, especially when caught early. The first thing you can try is douching at least twice a day with a vinegar and water solution, ¼ cup white or apple cider vinegar to 1 quart of water. You can also use a yogurt douche for the probiotics in it, although it's probably easier and less messy just to insert a probiotic gelatin capsule into the vagina.

To avoid future yeast infections, use a vinegar douche once a day if you are having frequent sex and avoid using commercial douches. If you are taking antibiotics, and you have a tendency to get yeast infections, take your probiotics orally and vaginally!

Toenail Fungus

Toenail fungus is an unsightly and uncomfortable and can cause the loss of toenails. It's extremely difficult to get rid of, and conventional drugs used to treat it are ineffective or dangerous. The imidazole antifungal drugs can cause headaches, dizziness, rashes, digestive problems and photosensitivity, and they interact dangerously with a long list of other drugs including antihistamines, any drug that puts extra stress on the liver, and alcohol. Drugs that suppress stomach acid can reduce the effectiveness of antifungals. Birth control pills can be made ineffective by antifungal drugs. Many of the antifungal drugs, but especially ketoconazole (Nizoral) can cause acute liver toxicity.

The worst part is that toenail fungus often comes back after the drugs are discontinued. There must be another way, right? Well, you can beat toenail fungus naturally, but you need to be rigorous about it for months and sometimes more than a year. Going barefoot in clean areas can help, because your feet stay dry and aired out, but avoid going barefoot in gyms and other public areas. You must keep your feet clean and dry as much as possible, and not wear shoes that cause your feet to sweat.

To avoid reinfecting yourself you'll need to douse your shoes with an over-the-counter antifungal powder to kill any lingering fungus there, and be sure to wash your socks in hot water and detergent. Also wipe down the bathroom, shower and any other place you go barefoot with a mixture of soap and tea tree oil to kill fungus there.

Tea tree oil, garlic and vinegar are effective antifungals. Here's a natural strategy for banishing toenail fungus: Every night before bed soak your feet in a vinegar and water solution (1 cup per ½ gallon of water) for 10 minutes. Then soak them in a mixture of tea tree oil and if you can stand the smell, garlic oil (six to eight drops of each) and warm water for half an hour. After that, thoroughly dry your feet and apply tea tree oil directly to the nails and wear white cotton socks to bed. You will have to do this for at least three months to get rid of the fungus.

Just as with an internal fungus infection, it's important to support your body by avoiding sugar and taking probiotics.

CHAPTER 14

Drugs for Insomnia, Anxiety and Depression and Their Natural Alternatives

LACK OF SLEEP is one of the most common causes of fatigue and, conversely, one of the most important keys to maintaining a high energy lifestyle. Whether it's not being able to get to sleep, or waking several times each night, or never feeling as though you've gotten a good night's sleep, insomnia can take a huge toll on your quality of life. Fortunately for most people, it's relatively easy to remedy restless nights. The most obvious sleep robbers are the most common ones: stress, lack of exercise, caffeine and prescription drugs. Having to get up at night repeatedly to urinate can disturb sleeping patterns enough to cause problems, as any man coping with an enlarged prostate gland can tell you. For women, menopause may bring on hot flashes and night sweats which disturb sleep.

Often when people are under stress and feel helpless to do anything about it, they lie awake at night tossing and turning with repetitive "tapes" going through their heads, or they wake up very early in the morning and can't get back to sleep. Big decisions, the illness or troubles of a loved one, major life changes, financial difficulties, and any number of the other lumps and bumps life hands out, can all cause sleeplessness. Depression and anxiety will often cause sleeplessness, which creates a vicious circle of more depression and more sleeplessness.

DEPRESSION: PART OF BEING HUMAN

With very few exceptions, we all have cycles in our lives when we're down, cycles when we're up, and cycles when we're somewhere in-between. It's quite normal to feel some level of depression before, during or after a major life change such as the death of someone close, illness or injury, birth, marriage, divorce, job change, or a move, for example. Ten to 20 percent of people who go to see a physician are depressed.

When we're very "high" or excited about something, we'll normally have a corresponding dip in our emotions afterward. These emotional ups and downs are all part of being human, and most of us learn to cope with them pretty well by the time we're middle-aged. Some people suffer from depression with the coming of winter. Eighty percent of those who suffer from seasonal affective disorder, or SAD, are women. Winter's shortened daylight hours and cloudy skies change circadian rhythms. The carbohydrate cravings, increased appetite, more time spent sleeping and fatigue characteristic of SAD have been treated successfully with natural therapies such as bright artificial light, herbal remedies and nutritional changes.

Depression can also be a symptom of a deficiency of thyroid hormone (hypothyroidism). If you are gaining weight, feel cold much of the time and lack energy in addition to feeling down, see a health professional to rule out thyroid problems.

Debilitating depression that makes a person nonfunctional for weeks or months at a time is another story, and should be treated by a competent health care professional.

Minor depression can be a form of "time out" for adults. Sometimes it's nature's way of giving us a rest, or perhaps we need to go within ourselves and be reflective. Maybe it's a message from the psyche telling us we need to re-evaluate our lives. This re-evaluation is most often an inner call to align ourselves with a sense of purpose or mission in life—to go for what we *really* want, to reach for our dreams, even if they seem completely out of reach.

THERE ARE ALTERNATIVES TO SEDATIVES AND ANTIDEPRESSANTS

We've all heard countless horror stories about people who take sedatives and antidepressants. Let's face it, most of the time prescription drugs don't work very well for anxiety and depression, and the only category of "safe" they fall into is the FDA's. Would you consider a medicine that has unacceptable side effects at normal doses and is addictive to be "safe and effective"? And, believe it or not, one of the most common side effects of sedatives and antidepressants is depression!

Thanks to a massive, multimillion-dollar public relations campaign on the part of the giant pharmaceutical companies which sell drugs such as Prozac, millions of people are suffering under the illusion that if they aren't feeling wonderful all the time, something must be wrong with them and they need to fix it by taking a pill. Physicians are handing out prescriptions for antidepressants and anti-anxiety drugs like candy. Never mind that the pills are expensive, addictive and have serious side effects.

The following information covers the most-prescribed sleeping pills, antidepressants and anti-anxiety drugs, but if you take them, please remember they are not lightweight drugs. They all have the potential for abuse and/or addiction, and none should be used long term. According to an organization called CANDID (Citizens Against Drug-Impaired Drivers), prescription and over-the-counter medications that cause drowsiness contribute to more than 100,000 car crashes a year. If your drug insert warns against driving while under the influence of the drug, please take that warning seriously!

PRESCRIPTION DRUGS FOR SLEEP

ZOLPIDEM TARTRATE (Ambien)

WHAT DOES IT DO IN THE BODY?

This drug has a hypnotic, sedative, muscle relaxant effect, which it achieves by altering neurotransmitter channels in the brain.

SOME DRUG-INDUCED SIDE EFFECTS MIMIC PARKINSON'S

Harvard researchers have discovered that thousands of elderly patients prescribed tranquilizers may be suffering from drug-induced Parkinson's disease. Instead of checking whether the medication is causing the symptoms, most physicians then prescribe anti-Parkinson's drugs (i.e., L-dopa or Sinemet), which have many undesirable side effects and don't work for drug-induced Parkinson's anyway. Real Parkinson's tends to come on gradually. A sudden onset of this disease should be cause to go off any tranquilizers, sedatives or sleeping pills to see if symptoms improve. Some of the drugs that most commonly cause side effects that mimic Parkinson's include tricyclic antidepressants, antipsychotics, carbamazepine, methyldopa, metoclopramide (Reglan), trimethobenzamide and reserpine.

What Is It Used For?

A sleep aid.

What Are the Potential Side Effects/Adverse Effects?

In clinical trials of this drug, 4 to 6 percent of subjects stopped taking Ambien because they were so bothered by side effects. The most common is headache. Others include: drowsiness, dizziness, lethargy, a "drugged" feeling, lightheadedness, depression, abnormal dreams, amnesia, anxiety, nervousness, sleep disorder, allergy, back pain, flu-like symptoms, chest pain, fatigue, nausea, stomach upset, diarrhea, abdominal pain, constipation, loss of appetite, vomiting, muscle pain, upper respiratory infection, sinus and throat inflammation, runny nose, rash, urinary tract infection, palpitations and dry mouth. Dozens of other side effects may occur, but they are more rare.

Caution!

Ambien should only be used for seven to 10 days at a time. Insomnia may at its root be caused by an underlying physical or psychiatric disorder, and if you need to use drugs to get to sleep for more than a week to 10 days, you should look deeper and try to solve the problem. Other important tips:

- Be sure to use the smallest effective dose of this drug.
- If you have breathing problems such as asthma or emphysema use sedatives with caution, as they can depress the body's instinctual drive to breathe.
- If you have been addicted to any drug, you should know that zolpidem tartrate can be addictive.
- Any sedative or hypnotic drug can cause abnormal thinking and behavioral changes much like those caused by alcohol. Decreased inhibition and increased aggression, bizarre behavior, hallucinations, feelings of unreality and amnesia could be attributed to taking this drug.
- If you are suffering from depression, this drug may make it worse and even precipitate suicidal thinking.
- Abrupt discontinuation of Ambien can lead to withdrawal symptoms ranging from a mild downshift in mood and insomnia to abdominal or muscle cramps, vomiting, sweating, tremors and convulsions.
- This drug has a very rapid onset of action, so only take it right before going to bed. It may affect your ability to drive or operate machinery even the following day, so use caution.
- Those with impaired liver function should use this drug with caution if at all.
- If you are elderly or debilitated, you may have heightened sensitivity to this drug and you should be monitored carefully.

WHAT ARE THE INTERACTIONS WITH FOOD AND OTHER DRUGS?

Don't combine with alcohol or narcotics.

NONPRESCRIPTION ANTIHISTAMINE SLEEP AIDS

DIPHENHYDRAMINE (Dormin Caplets, Miles Nervine Caplets, Nytol, Sleep-Eze 3, Sleepwell 2-nite, Sominex 2, Extra Strength Tylenol PM, Aspirin Free Anacin P.M. Caplets, Bayer Select Maximum Strength Night Time Pain Relief Caplets, Sominex Pain Relief, Bufferin AF Nite Time Caplets, Excedrin P.M., Unisom with Pain Relief, Compoz Nighttime Sleep Aid, Sominex Caplets, Twilite, Compoz Gel Caps, Dormin, Maximum Strength Sleepinal Capsules and Soft Gels, Maximum Strength Unisom SleepGels, Nighttime Pamprin)

DOXYLAMINE (Unisom Nighttime)

WHAT DO THEY DO IN THE BODY?

These drugs contain antihistamines, which cause sleepiness. Some contain pain relievers to help those in pain sleep.

WHAT ARE THEY USED FOR?

Relief of insomnia and/or pain. More than 30 percent of adults use nonprescription drugs to help them sleep.

WHAT ARE THE POTENTIAL SIDE EFFECTS/ADVERSE EFFECTS?

Dry mouth and throat, constipation, ringing in the ears and blurred vision may occur. In older men, prostate enlargement and difficult urination can be a side effect of these drugs. Elderly people are prone to other side effects such as delirium, excitement, nervousness and agitation.

CAUTION! DON'T TAKE THESE DRUGS IF . . .

- You have asthma, chronic lung disease, glaucoma or prostate gland enlargement.
- You still need them after two weeks. See a health professional.

Never use over-the-counter sleep aids for more than two weeks at a time.

Avoid driving or other hazardous tasks requiring coordination or dexterity while using these medications.

WHAT ARE THE INTERACTIONS WITH OTHER DRUGS?

Any sedating drug will add to the depressant effects of sleeping pills. Avoid using prescription sedatives and alcohol with doxylamine or diphenhydramine.

ANTI-ANXIETY DRUGS

Benzodiazepines

ALPRAZOLAM (Xanax)

CHLORAZEPATE (Tranxene, Gen-Xene)

CHLORDIAZEPOXIDE (Librium, Mitran)

CLONAZEPAM (Klonopin)

DIAZEPAM (Valium, Zetran, Valrelease)

HALAZEPAM (Paxipam)

LORAZEPAM (Ativan)

OXAZEPAM (Serax)

PRAZEPAM (Centrax)

TEMAZEPAM (Restoril)

WHAT DO THEY DO IN THE BODY?

This class of drugs affects the action of neurotransmitter substances in the brain, bringing about relaxation and decreased anxiety.

WHAT ARE THEY PRESCRIBED FOR?

Very small doses quell anxiety. These drugs are prescribed in higher doses as sleep aids. Benzodiazepines are also used as antiseizure and anti-epileptic drugs and as muscle relaxants. They are prescribed for irritable bowel syndrome, nausea and vomiting caused by chemotherapy, panic attacks, depression and premenstrual syndrome (Xanax), acute withdrawal from alcohol addiction, and chronic insomnia (Ativan). They do not heal any of these health problems, they only temporarily relieve symptoms.

WHAT ARE THE POTENTIAL SIDE EFFECTS/ADVERSE EFFECTS?

Transient mild drowsiness in the first few days of use is common. This side effect may be more pronounced in the elderly or debilitated, who are more likely to experience loss of muscular coordination and confusion when starting out on a course of benzodiazepines.

Other possible side effects include: sedation, depression, lethargy, apathy, fatigue, decreased activity, lightheadedness, memory impairment, disorientation, amnesia, restlessness, confusion, crying, delirium, headache, slurred speech, loss of voice, stupor, seizures, coma, fainting, rigidity, tremor, abnormal muscle tone, vertigo, dizziness, euphoria, nervousness, irritability, difficulty concentrating, agitation, inability to perform complex mental functions, paralysis of half the body, unsteadiness, loss of coordination, strange dreams, glassy-eyed appearance, paradoxical reactions (increased anxiety or hyperactivity), behavior problems, hysteria, psychosis, suicidal tendencies, constipation, diarrhea, dry mouth, coated tongue, sore gums, nausea, changes in appetite, vomiting, difficulty swallowing, increased salivation, stomach inflammation, incontinence, changes in libido, urinary and menstrual problems, heart rhythm and blood pressure changes, cardiovascular collapse, retention of fluid in the face and ankles, palpitations, visual disturbances, twitching of the eyeballs, decreased hearing, nasal congestion, auditory disturbances, rashes, itching, hair loss or growth, hiccups, fever, sweating, tingling of the extremities, muscular disturbances, growth of breasts in males, milk production in the breasts of females, respiratory disturbances, increased levels of enzymes in the bloodstream indicating tissue damage, hepatitis or jaundice (both very rarely), changes in blood cell counts, decrease in body weight, swelling of lymph nodes and joint pain.

CAUTION!

Don't take this drug if you have a psychological disorder that doesn't have anxiety as a prominent feature and is mainly manifested as depression.

The long-term effectiveness (four months or more of treatment) of these drugs has not been assessed. Please don't use these drugs long term.

These drugs may cause drowsiness, so avoid driving or other tasks that require alertness.

Dependency can occur in as little as four to six weeks. Withdrawal symptoms may include anxiety, sensory disturbances, sleeping too much, flu-like symptoms, difficulty concentrating, fatigue, restlessness, loss of appetite, dizziness, sweating, vomiting, insomnia, irritability, nausea, headache, muscle tension or cramping, tremor, vocal changes, confusion, abnormal perception, depersonalization, muscle twitches, psychosis, paranoid delusions, hallucinations, memory impairment and grand mal seizures. If you have been using benzodiazepines for a while, decrease the dosage gradually.

Use caution if you have liver problems or if you are elderly or debilitated; you may need a lower dose.

WHAT ARE THE INTERACTIONS WITH OTHER DRUGS?

The following drugs may prolong the effects or raise levels of benzodiazepines:

↑ Cimetidine
Clarithromycin
Disulfiram
Fluoxetine
Isoniazid
Ketoconazole

Macrolide antibiotics
Metoprolol
Omeprazole
Propranolol
Propoxyphene
Valproic acid

The following drugs may decrease levels or reduce the effects of benzodiazepines:

↓ Antacids
  Oral contraceptives
  Ranitidine

Rifampin
Theophylline

Benzodiazepines may increase levels or prolong the effects of the following drugs:

↑ Alcohol
  Barbiturates
  Digoxin*
  Narcotics

Phenytoin
Probenecid
Sedating antihistamines

OTHER INTERACTIONS

Benzodiazepines may reduce levels or decrease the effects of levodopa.

When the antipsychotic drugs Clozaril or Loxitane are used with Ativan or Valium, difficulty breathing and very low blood pressure may result. Blue fingernails and lips and delirium or stupor are warning signs that you should get immediate medical attention.

WHAT ARE THE INTERACTIONS WITH FOOD?

Don't drink alcohol while using these drugs. Avoid charcoal-broiled foods, as they increase the rate at which this drug is emptied from your system. You can take benzodiazepines with water or food if stomach upset occurs, but this may slow down the absorption of the drug.

---

*Potentially dangerous interaction.

BUSPIRONE (BuSpar)

WHAT DOES IT DO IN YOUR BODY?

It is not known exactly how buspirone works.

WHAT IS IT PRESCRIBED FOR?

Treatment of anxiety.

WHAT ARE THE POSSIBLE SIDE EFFECTS?

Buspirone may cause temporary or permanent damage to the nervous system. It can also cause drug dependence, sedation and withdrawal reactions. Adverse reactions have included dizziness, drowsiness, restlessness, nervousness, insomnia, lightheadedness, nausea, numbness, headaches, fatigue, dream disturbances, tinnitus, sore throat, nasal congestion. There are dozens and dozens of individualized side effects possible with this drug, most having to do with interference with or damage to the nervous system.

CAUTION: THINK TWICE ABOUT TAKING THIS DRUG . . .

Please think twice about taking this drug, *period*. There are too many other safer alternatives.

WHAT ARE THE INTERACTIONS WITH OTHER DRUGS?

Buspirone may raise levels or prolong the effects of these drugs:

↑ Haloperidol   MAO inhibitors

ANTIDEPRESSANT DRUGS

BUPROPION (Wellbutrin, Zyban)

WHAT DOES IT DO IN THE BODY?

It weakly inhibits the reuptake of serotonin and dopamine, neuro-transmitters that play important roles in determining your mood. This drug doesn't fit into any of the categories most antidepressants do, and no one knows just exactly how it works.

WHAT IS IT USED FOR?

Treatment of depression, nicotine withdrawal.

WHAT ARE THE POTENTIAL SIDE EFFECTS/ADVERSE EFFECTS?

Ten percent of the people who took this drug in clinical trials stopped because of problems with side effects. The most common were rashes, psychological disturbances such as agitation and mental status changes, neurological disturbances such as seizures, headache and sleep disturbances, and gastrointestinal disturbances such as nausea and vomiting.

Other side effects may include: constipation, weight loss (may be up to five pounds), increased appetite, stomach discomfort, menstrual problems, dry mouth, excessive sweating, tremor, insomnia, auditory disturbances, blurred vision, taste disturbances, dizziness, cardiac arrhythmias, high blood pressure, palpitations, fainting, agitation, confusion, hostility, decreased libido, anxiety, euphoria, fever and chills.

CAUTION! DON'T USE THIS DRUG IF . . .

- You have a seizure disorder; it increases your risk of seizures.
- You have or have had bulimia or anorexia.
- You are switching from monoamine oxidase inhibitors (MAO inhibitors) to Wellbutrin. At least 14 days should elapse between your last dose of MAO inhibitors to the first of Wellbutrin. Don't take this drug with MAO inhibitors.
- You have recently had a heart attack or any other kind of unstable heart disease. Bupropion should be used with care.
- You are taking other antidepressants or antipsychotic drugs. If you have had head trauma, or have any history of seizures, you

are much more likely to experience seizures as a side effect of this drug. High doses or sudden changes in dosage of this drug can cause seizures.

- You have manic-depressive (bipolar) disorder. This drug may trigger manic episodes. Use with caution.

Your ability to drive or to perform other tasks requiring judgment or motor skills may be impaired. Wait a few days before operating a car or machinery to be sure the dose you're taking isn't too sedating.

Bupropion has been shown in animal studies to be toxic to the liver in large doses. If you already have liver or kidney impairment, you should avoid this drug altogether or start at a low dose.

If you start to feel extremely restless, agitated, anxious, or can't sleep when you start taking Wellbutrin, you may need to discontinue it. You may be sensitive to it and prone to delusions, hallucinations, psychosis, confusion or paranoia with continued use.

Take Wellbutrin in equally divided doses, three to four times a day, to minimize seizure risk.

WHAT ARE THE INTERACTIONS WITH OTHER DRUGS?

Bupropion may increase levels or prolong the effects of the drug levo-dopa, making adverse effects more likely.

MAO inhibitors* such as phenelzine increase levels of bupropion in the body, possibly resulting in deadly toxicity.

Don't take this drug with alcohol, as this combination can cause seizures.

VENLAFAXINE (Effexor)

WHAT DOES IT DO IN THE BODY?

Alters neurotransmitter activity in the brain. It is a weak inhibitor of the reuptake of the neurotransmitters serotonin, norepinephrine and dopamine.

---

*Potentially dangerous interaction.

WHAT IS IT USED FOR?

Treatment of depression.

WHAT ARE THE POTENTIAL SIDE EFFECTS/ADVERSE EFFECTS?

In clinical studies of Effexor, 19 percent of patients stopped taking it because of side effects. Nausea, sleepiness, insomnia, dizziness, abnormal ejaculation, headache, nervousness, dry mouth, anxiety, weakness, and excessive sweating were the adverse effects most often experienced with this drug.

While venlafaxine may help alleviate depression, it can increase feelings of anxiety or cause insomnia. If you are often anxious, this may not be the right drug for you. Loss of appetite and body weight, mania, seizures and elevated heart rate are other side effects to look out for.

CAUTION!

- Don't combine this drug with monoamine oxidase inhibitors (MAO inhibitors). High body temperature, sudden rapid muscular twitches, extreme agitation, delirium, and even coma and death have resulted from this deadly mix of drugs. Allow a minimum of 14 days between stopping MAO inhibitors and starting venlafaxine, and a minimum of seven days between stopping venlafaxine and starting MAO inhibitors.
- If you have hypertension, you should know that venlafaxine may cause a sustained increase in blood pressure. The higher the dose, the greater the increase.
- If you have kidney or liver impairment, use this drug with caution.
- Use of this drug for longer than four to six weeks has not been evaluated with clinical trials. Work with your physician to be sure that the drug is continuing to have benefit for you.
- If you have another illness that affects your blood pressure or metabolism, use caution when taking Effexor.

What Are the Interactions with Other Drugs?

The following drugs may raise levels or prolong the effects of venlafaxine:

↑ Cimetidine   MAO inhibitors*

Selective Serotonin Reuptake Inhibitors (SSRIs)

Fluoxetine (Prozac)

Paroxetine (Paxil)

Sertraline (Zoloft)

What Do They Do in the Body?

Neurons use a neurotransmitter substance called serotonin to relay messages through the nervous system. Researchers have found that some people who suffer from depression have low levels of serotonin in their synapses. SSRIs inhibit the reuptake of serotonin and so allow more of it to remain in the synapses for a longer period.

SSRIs also weakly inhibit the neuronal uptake of norepinephrine and dopamine, which also play a role in mood.

What Are They Used For?

These drugs are being prescribed for just about any ailment you can think of, for children and adults alike. In the not-too-distant future, widespread use and abuse of these drugs will be seen as one of the dark ages in medical history. Taking Prozac-like drugs for mild depression or personality quirks is the ultimate symptom of thinking we all should behave alike and should be happy all the time. It's a destructive mindset. SSRIs create a false sense of emotional detachment, and too many relationships and families have been pulled apart under their influence.

---

*Potentially dangerous interaction.

WHAT ARE THE POTENTIAL SIDE EFFECTS/ADVERSE EFFECTS?

Nervousness, insomnia, drowsiness, fatigue, weakness, tremor, increased sweating, dizziness, anxiety (especially with Prozac), headache (especially with Paxil), dry mouth (with Zoloft and Paxil), male sexual dysfunction (especially with Zoloft), loss of appetite, nausea, diarrhea, stomach discomfort (Prozac and Zoloft), altered appetite and weight, and constipation (Paxil).

In clinical trials of serotonin reuptake inhibitors, between 15 and 21 percent of those taking these drugs stopped due to unpleasant side effects.

Rash, fever, joint pain, abnormal changes in blood cell counts, swelling, excessive excretion of protein in the urine indicating liver or kidney damage, and elevated enzymes in the bloodstream (also indicating tissue damage) have occurred in some people who use Prozac. If you experience any of these symptoms, you probably are sensitive to it and should stop taking it. People who continue to use it after developing these symptoms may end up having a life-threatening anaphylactic reaction.

Doctors are recognizing a new disorder caused by SSRIs called "serotonin syndrome." It is usually caused by an overdose or an interaction with other drugs and it can be fatal. Symptoms include hallucinations, agitation, confusion, fluctuating blood pressure, seizures, fever, stiffness, irregular heartbeats.

We now also know there can be a withdrawal syndrome experienced when you stop taking SSRIs, especially with the short-acting SSRIs such as Paxil, Zoloft and Luvox. The effects of withdrawal can include dizziness, nausea, headaches, fatigue, poor concentration, mental fogginess and moodiness. If you're withdrawing from SSRIs, do it gradually, over a period of one to two weeks, and if you need to, use the natural alternatives given at the end of this chapter under the supervision of a health care professional who is familiar with their use.

CAUTION!

Clinical trials of most of these drugs have only lasted for 5 to 16 weeks. Studies of Prozac have lasted for up to a year. In other words, the long-term effects of these drugs have not been systematically studied.

- Don't take SSRIs with monoamine oxidase inhibitors (MAO inhibitors) or within 14 days of stopping MAO inhibitors.
- Please avoid these drugs if you have impaired liver function.
- If you tend to be manic, SSRIs may make you more so.
- Use caution when taking this drug if you have a history of seizures.
- If you are using diuretics to lower blood pressure, Prozac and Paxil can make it more likely that you will have electrolyte imbalances. These imbalances can cause heart rhythm disturbances.
- If you are diabetic, you should know that Prozac can make low blood sugar more likely, and high blood sugar can hit when the drug is stopped. Dosages of insulin and sulfonylurea drugs may require adjustment when taken with this drug.

SSRIs can cause drowsiness or dizziness. Use caution while driving, performing tasks requiring alertness, or operating machinery.

Don't take these drugs if you are already using tryptophan or 5 hydroxy tryptophan (5-HTP), which are natural precursors to serotonin, or St. John's wort, an herb with similar effects.

WHAT ARE THE INTERACTIONS WITH OTHER DRUGS?

FLUOXETINE (Prozac)

The following drugs may increase levels or prolong the effects of fluoxetine (Prozac):

↑ Benzodiazepines
Demerol
Dexfenfluramine*
Dextromethorphan (hallucinations have occurred)

Fenfluramine*
Imipramine
Meperidine
MAO inhibitors*
Tricyclic antidepressants

---

*Potentially dangerous interaction.

Prozac may increase levels or prolong the effects of the following drugs:

↑ Carbamazepine   Hydantoins
  Clozapine   Lithium*
  Dexfenfluramine*   Nonsedating antihistamines*
  Diltiazem   Pimozide
  Fenfluramine*   Propranolol
  Haloperidol   Warfarin

OTHER INTERACTIONS

The effectiveness of Prozac is decreased by the drug cyproheptadine.

The drug buspirone, when used with Prozac, may cause worsening of obsessive-compulsive disorder.

The drugs fenfluramine and dexfenfluramine can cause a dangerous condition in the body when used with Prozac or other SSRIs. Known as "serotonin storm," this interaction raises serotonin levels to toxic highs. Deaths have occurred, so avoid these combinations. Both fenfluramine and dexfenfluramine have been taken off the market in the U.S. at this time because they can cause heart valve problems.

The drug selegiline (Eldepryl), when combined with Prozac or the other SSRIs, has caused mania and hypertension.

PAROXETINE (Paxil)

The following drugs may increase levels or prolong the effects of Paxil:

↑ Cimetidine   MAO inhibitors*
  Imipramine   Meperidine

Paxil may increase levels or prolong the effects of the following drugs:

↑ Imipramine   Theophyllines
  Procyclidine   Warfarin

The following drugs may increase levels or prolong the effects of Paxil:

↑ Phenobarbitol   Phenytoin

---

*Potentially dangerous interaction.

Paxil may decrease levels of the following drugs:

↓ Digoxin   Phenytoin

SERTRALINE (Zoloft)

Zoloft may increase levels or prolong the effects of the following drugs:

↑ Benzodiazepines   Tolbutamide
  Lithium   Warfarin

WHAT ARE THE INTERACTIONS WITH FOOD?

You can take SSRIs with or without food. Avoid alcohol while taking SSRIs.

TRICYCLIC ANTIDEPRESSANTS

Amitryptyline (Elavil)

WHAT DOES IT DO IN THE BODY?

This drug belongs to a class of antidepressants known as tricyclics. They inhibit the uptake of norepinephrine and serotonin, two neurotransmitters that play a role in determining mood. They work through other mechanisms as well, generally decreasing the activity of certain biochemical pathways that affect mood.

WHAT IS IT USED FOR?

Treatment of depression or anxiety, usually in people at risk for abuse of the other medications for these problems. Chronic headaches, eating disorders, diabetic neuropathy, cancer pain, and arthritic pain are also treated with Elavil.

WHAT ARE THE POTENTIAL SIDE EFFECTS/ADVERSE REACTIONS?

Sedation, dry mouth, blurred vision, problems focusing, increased intraocular pressure which can lead to glaucoma, dilation of the pupils, constipation, dysfunction of parts of the small intestine, urinary problems, drastic dips in blood pressure when going from lying to sitting or from sitting to standing, high blood pressure, heart rhythm abnormalities, congestive heart failure, stroke, electrocardiogram changes (indicating damage to heart tissue), confusion (especially in the elderly), disturbed concentration, hallucinations, disorientation, impaired memory, feelings of unreality, delusions, anxiety, nervousness, restlessness, agitation, panic, insomnia, nightmares, mania, worsening of psychotic symptoms, drowsiness, dizziness, weakness, fatigue, headache, depression, excessive tension in the muscles or artery walls, sleep disorders, psychosomatic disorders, yawning, abnormal dreaming, migraines, depersonalization, irritability and mood swings, numbness, tingling, hyperactivity, lack of coordination, tremors, peripheral neuropathy, seizures, twitching, partial paralysis, allergic reactions including rash, itching and swelling, changes in blood cell counts, nausea, vomiting, loss of appetite, diarrhea, flatulence, trouble swallowing, strange taste in the mouth, increased salivation, abdominal cramps, inflammation of the stomach, throat or esophagus, black tongue, indigestion, breast development in males, testicular swelling, breast enlargement, spontaneous flow of milk, vaginitis and menstrual difficulties in women, changes in libido, painful ejaculation, voiding of urine during the night, cystitis, urinary tract infection, changes in blood glucose levels, increased secretion of the hormones prolactin and vasopressin (antidiuretic hormone), pharyngitis, laryngitis, sinusitis, coughing, spasm of the airways, nosebleed, shortness of breath, problems speaking, ringing of the ears, excessive tearing of the eyes, conjunctivitis, difference in the size of the pupils, inner ear inflammation, eye allergy symptoms, nasal congestion, excessive appetite, body weight changes, increased sweating, high body temperature, flushing, chills, hair loss, dental problems, abnormal skin odor, chest pain, fever, bad breath, thirst, back pain and joint aches. In some people, tricyclic antidepressants cause increased sensitivity to the sun.

Caution! Don't Use This drug If . . .

- You have recently had a heart attack. If you have any other heart problems, use extreme caution.
- You are taking MAO inhibitors.
- You have any of the following health problems: seizure disorders, difficulty urinating, spasm of the urethra or ureter, angle-closure glaucoma (even the average dose can cause an attack of glaucoma and permanent loss of vision), high intraocular pressure, high levels of thyroid hormone (hyperthyroidism) or if you are taking any kind of drug to regulate thyroid hormone levels, or kidney or liver disease. You should be closely monitored while taking Elavil.
- You are taking anticholinergic drugs such as those prescribed for Parkinson's disease. You may not react well to Elavil so use caution.

Your ability to drive and perform other hazardous tasks may be impaired while you are using this drug.

The symptoms of manic depression or schizophrenia may be worsened by tricyclic antidepressants.

You should stop taking Elavil for as long as possible before having elective surgery. Work with your doctor on this, though; don't stop cold on your own.

If you develop a fever or sore throat while taking this medication, it may be an indication of a serious drug-related side effect.

What Are the Interactions with Other Drugs?

The following drugs may raise levels or prolong the effects of Elavil:

↑ Cimetidine   Haloperidol
Disulfiram   Oral contraceptives
Estrogens (depending on dose) Phenothiazines
Fluoxetine

The following drugs may decrease levels or shorten the effects of Elavil:

↓ Barbiturates   Estrogens
   Charcoal   Smoking

Elavil may increase levels or prolong the effects of the following drugs:

↑ Anticholinergics   Dicumarol, an anticoagulant
   Clonidine

Elavil may decrease levels or shorten the effects of the following drugs:

↓ Bethanidine   Guanethidine
   Clonidine   Guanfacine
   Guanadrel   Levodopa

Stay away from monoamine oxidase inhibitors while using tricyclic antidepressants!*

NATURAL ALTERNATIVES FOR INSOMNIA, ANXIETY, DEPRESSION AND STRESS

We have become accustomed to running for the medicine cabinet for a drug when we're suffering from insomnia, anxiety or depression, but 90 percent of the time the cause of these problems is something that can be remedied without taking medication.

Sugar, alcohol and coffee are our legal American drugs and it's a good bet that these drugs plus food allergies contribute to the vast majority of insomnia, anxiety and minor depression. Both sugar and alcohol (which is high in sugar) can cause depression. Sometimes fatigue caused by sugar or alcohol is mistaken for depression. If you

---

*Potentially dangerous interaction.

have a sugar habit (and if you have one you know it), it's likely that fatigue is always dogging your tracks. Sugar stimulates your adrenal glands and taken in excess will wear them out. When your adrenals are tired, the rest of the body follows, and then, when you're stressed, you'll get irritable and depressed. If you think your depression might be fatigue, try cutting out all sugar for three weeks and see what happens. And yes, alcohol counts as sugar. Artificial sweeteners such as NutraSweet (aspartame) found in diet sodas are also not allowed, as they are brain stimulants, and may even give the adrenals the same signals that sugar does.

The balance of essential fatty acids in the bodies of depressed people tends to be imbalanced. Supplementation with borage oil and evening primrose oil, as well as eating plenty of fish, can help return the body to balance and give some relief. If you're taking drugs to lower your cholesterol levels and are feeling a bit down in the dumps, you should know that drug-induced low cholesterol has been linked with symptoms of depression. Quitting a smoking habit can also bring on a major depression. Both cholesterol-lowering drugs and smoking cessation affect serotonin levels.

Do you need to be told that coffee can cause anxiety? Coffee is a

IS YOUR MEDICATION MAKING YOU DEPRESSED?

One of the most common causes of depression is prescription drugs. Here is a list of some of the most common prescription drugs that can cause depression.

Amphetamines (including antihistamines)
Antibiotics
Anticonvulsants
Antidepressants
Barbiturates
High blood pressure drugs (beta-blockers, diuretics)

Hormones (estrogen, including Premarin, and synthetic progestins such as Provera)
Narcotics
Painkillers
Sleeping pills
Systemic corticosteroids (prednisone, cortisone, etc.)
Tagamet and Zantac
Tranquilizers (Halcion, Librium, Restoril, Xanax, etc.)

drug and should be treated as such. Among other things, it stimulates the production of adrenaline, one of the hormones secreted by the adrenal glands to help us in extreme emergency situations. Our adrenals evolved to give our early ancestors the extra strength and alertness needed to escape a saber tooth tiger attack, but we don't often need that much adrenaline these days. Like sugar, coffee constantly stimulates the production of adrenaline, putting excessive wear and tear on the adrenal glands. And let's not forget that green tea and black tea contain caffeine, and even decaf still contains some caffeine. If you're sensitive to caffeine it can keep you awake at night even if you haven't had any since noon. If you're suffering from insomnia, your best bet is to drink nonstimulating herbal teas such as chamomile or mint in the evening. If you need a boost in the afternoon, try a cup of ginseng tea.

More than a couple of alcohol drinks a day can cause enough ongoing stress to all systems of the body to bring on depression. Then you have a couple more drinks to banish the depression and you're in a vicious cycle. Like most things, alcohol in small amounts can be beneficial and in large amounts detrimental. You may escape temporarily from your problems, but excess alcohol is more likely to keep you up at night than put you to sleep, and robs your body of many nutrients.

Researchers are discovering that what you eat has a lot to do with how you feel. In a study of 275 people suffering from many different conditions including fatigue, insomnia and depression, elimination of allergenic foods resulted in significant improvement, with relief of nearly all symptoms. This is another reason to be moderate about your consumption of refined sugars, white flour, caffeine and chocolate.

Exercise Is Your Cure-All

Exercise is one of the best sleep aids around. Does this mean you need to get up in the middle of the night and run around the block? Not at all. The point is that if you've taken a brisk walk or gotten some other kind of exercise during the day, you'll sleep better and wake up more refreshed.

When we are depressed we tend to want to stop moving. When we are anxious we tend to move unproductively, such as not being able to sit still or pacing. If you've slowed down to a crawl and can't seem to get your engines started, or if you can't sit still or can't sleep, try some exercise. This sounds awfully simple, but sometimes it's the perfect antidote. Sometimes we need to get moving to get moving!

Track Down Your Sleep Robber

Many over-the-counter painkillers, cold and allergy remedies and appetite suppressants contain caffeine and other substances that can cause insomnia. Some examples of drugs that contain caffeine are Anacin, Extra Strength Excedrin, Bayer Select Maximum, Midol and Vanquish. Herbal products with zippy names and energy-boosting claims may be nothing more than concentrated ephedra, caffeine or guarana, a South American herb that contains high levels of caffeine.

Allergy and cold medicines may contain synthetic variations of ephedrine, such as pseudoephedrine (Sudafed), which can keep you awake. The asthma drug theophylline (Bronkaid and Primatene tablets, Tedral and others) is a stimulant that can make sleeping difficult.

The cortisones, such as prednisone, can also cause sleeplessness. The heart drugs propranolol, furosemide and lovastatin may cause insomnia, as can too high a dose of thyroid medication such as synthroid. Ironically, many of the antidepressants cause insomnia, which can cause depression due to lack of sleep!

Unfortunately, if one of these medications is keeping you awake at night your physician is most likely to write you out a prescription for a sleeping pill. In nearly all cases, that is the worst possible thing you can do for insomnia. Sleeping pills cause either dependence or outright addiction very quickly, they tend to lose their effectiveness over time, and have a rebound effect if you stop, causing worse insomnia than ever. They also tend to suppress your dream or REM sleep, sometimes resulting in severe mental disturbances and psychoses if used over a long period of time. If someone hands you a prescription for a sleeping pill, think twice.

If you're having trouble sleeping and you are taking any type of medication, including over-the-counter drugs, read the label or package insert to find out if it can cause insomnia, restlessness or irritability.

Don't drink a lot of fluids before bed, and if you're having prostate problems, use the herb saw palmetto. For details on treating prostate problems naturally, read the book *Dr. Earl Mindell's What You Should Know About Natural Health for Men* (Keats Publishing, 1996). For women, menopause may bring on hot flashes and night sweats that disturb sleep. For details on treating menopause symptoms naturally, read the book *Dr. Earl Mindell's What You Should Know About Natural Health for Women* (Keats Publishing, 1996).

If you like to watch TV at night before you go to sleep, choose nonviolent, upbeat shows. When you're sleepy your unconscious is particularly susceptible to suggestion. Violence and mayhem can show up in disturbing dreams that leave you feeling less rested in the morning. If you need a non-TV bedtime ritual, try reading (again, nothing too upsetting or violent) or a warm bath (not hot, that can be stimulating).

When you know that the next day is going to be busy or you have something coming up that you are tense about, make sure you are prepared. Sit down and make a list of things you need to remember, look at your schedule, and organize the day on paper.

If you are going to an important meeting you can visualize it coming out well (you don't need to visualize the whole thing, just the happy ending). That way you won't be worrying about it as you're trying to sleep. Another stress-beating strategy is to always do the hardest task or do the most difficult thing first in the morning. After that, everything is easy.

Should you eat right before you go to sleep? Some people say it gives them nightmares, and others say it helps them sleep better. This is very individual, and depends on your blood sugar, your digestion and your metabolism. However, if you do eat before bed, stick to simple foods like a piece of toast, a bowl of cereal (no sugar please), fruit (bananas work well) or crackers (low salt). Avoid white sugar, spicy foods and fat—they can keep you awake and fat is harder to digest.

Things That Go Bump in the Night

For those of us who travel a lot, live in a noisy neighborhood, have neighbors with a barking dog or a spouse who snores, noise can be a real sleep inhibitor. Some primitive part of us is on guard at night, ready to wake us up if something is wrong. Unfortunately this "guard" isn't always discriminating about what noises it deems important enough to wake up for.

Here's a sleeping tip that can work wonders: If there's a sound that's been waking you up at night, like a barking dog, sirens or garbage trucks, have a little conversation with the "part" of you that's waking up. Thank it for being attentive enough to wake you up, and explain that this particular sound is not a sign of danger. Tell it that it doesn't need to wake you up for those specific sounds, that it's perfectly safe to keep on sleeping. It may seem strange, but try it, it works!

When all else fails, ear plugs can be a real gift. Get the soft foam type at your local drugstore. Sleep masks are also available to remove sleep disturbances caused by light.

Melatonin

The hormone melatonin is secreted in tiny amounts from the pineal gland at the base of the brain. As each day draws to an end and darkness falls, melatonin gives us the hormonal signal that it's time to rest for the night. Because we live in a culture that stays up long into the night, with lights blazing, our pineal glands can get a little confused. Night shift work, newborn babies and crazy schedules also disrupt our natural circadian rhythms and quality of sleep suffers.

Melatonin production in the brain is important to a good night's sleep. As we age, our pineal gland secretes less melatonin and we tend to have more trouble going to sleep and sleeping through the night. Fortunately, thanks to the miracles of modern science, you can buy supplemental melatonin to help you get back into a pattern of deep, rejuvenating sleep.

It's best to take melatonin at least eight hours before you want to wake up, or you may experience some mild grogginess in the morning. Other than that, melatonin has repeatedly been shown to be completely free of side effects when used as directed, and is nonaddictive.

Since it regulates sleep-wake cycles, melatonin can also be very useful for banishing jet lag by adjusting circadian rhythms to match your geographic location. You do this simply by taking melatonin about an hour before you want to sleep in your new location. It will give your brain the message that it's time to sleep, regardless of what time zone you're in. One or two nights of melatonin should put you back on the right track.

As for the claims that melatonin is an anti-aging drug, we need to be cautious in making the leap from extending lifespan in a particular strain of mice, to extending lifespan in humans. In some studies mice that were given melatonin lived 20 percent longer, but other strains of mice in other studies died sooner. Some younger mice given melatonin developed cancer, and melatonin in high doses suppresses sex hormones. And besides, since mice are nocturnal, how much do those melatonin studies apply to humans?

You can use melatonin when you travel to erase jet lag. It can also work very well for older people who are having trouble sleeping, but be aware that we simply don't know the long-term effects of using melatonin every night. Any time we take a hormone in higher doses than the body would naturally produce, we're asking for an imbalance.

If you are over the age of 65 and your melatonin levels have dropped so far that you can't sleep at night, *and* you have eliminated other possible causes of your insomnia, then by all means, take 0.5 to 3 mg at night to help you sleep. In that case you are correcting a deficiency. It is also perfectly safe to take melatonin for an occasional bout of insomnia. Melatonin is a natural hormone, so when it is used occasionally your body should have no trouble excreting any excess.

If you need melatonin, it only takes a very small dose to help you sleep better. If low melatonin levels aren't your problem, even a big dose won't make any difference.

The melatonin sold in health food stores is manufactured, but is the exact same molecular structure as the melatonin made by the body. Sublingual forms of melatonin are more expensive but act more quickly. Look for a reputable brand that states on the label that it is pharmaceutical grade melatonin. Take melatonin tablets about one hour before you want to go to sleep, and the sublingual tablets half an hour before you want to go to sleep.

Some drugs, including NSAIDs (nonsteroidal anti-inflammatory drugs such as aspirin, ibuprofen and acetaminophen), interfere with the brain's production of melatonin. In fact, just one dose of normal aspirin can cut your melatonin production as much as 75 percent. If you're taking these drugs, take the last dose after dinner.

Other drugs that can interfere with melatonin production in the brain include the benzodiazepines such as Valium and Xanax, caffeine, alcohol, cold medicines, diuretics, beta-blockers, calcium channel blockers, stimulants such as diet pills, and corticosteroids such as prednisone.

Valerian

Sometimes at the end of a long day we're "wired but tired." The body is telling us it's time to sleep, but our mind is keeping us awake. When that happens you can try taking a dropperful of valerian tincture in water, and within 30 minutes you'll be fast asleep. Valerian (*Valeriana officinalis L.*) is a plant that has been used for thousands of years as a folk remedy for "nervous stomach" and as a sedative. Valerian has few, if any, side effects and is not habit-forming. Valerian can be taken as a tincture (a fluid extract of the herb, suspended in alcohol or glycerine) or in capsule form. If you can, get the fresh root tincture.

NATURAL REMEDIES FOR STRESS

There are many, many positive ways to cope with stress. One of them is to try a form of meditation that focuses on becoming aware of the mind and of your "self-talk" as well as on breathing and chanting techniques which can help focus the mind. If you are unconsciously saying negative things to yourself all day long, it can be more than enough to keep you up at night! Many forms of meditation will assist you in replacing that destructive self-talk with something more positive.

Another way to cope with stress is to talk to a trained therapist. Just talking out loud about a problem to another human who is willing to listen attentively can be enough to begin the emotional healing process. Often, when we talk about our problems out loud, resolutions begin to appear.

One technique that can be helpful when stress levels are high is to ask yourself, "What is one action step I can take to reduce my stress levels?" That might simply mean taking a walk in a beautiful place. Sometimes it's just a matter of getting to bed earlier or spending relaxing time with loved ones. For some it may be a hot bath or a meal at a favorite restaurant.

Stress causes a variety of biochemical imbalances in the body. The following herbs and supplements may be helpful to you in managing stress.

Panax Ginseng and Ashwagandha

Ginseng is used to remedy all sorts of ailments in Chinese medicine. Try 150 milligrams of standardized extract three times a day to relieve anxiety. Ashwagandha is an Ayurvedic herbal medicine; try 500 milligrams three times a day.

Calcium and Magnesium

Sometimes insomnia or anxiety can be caused by "universal" muscle tension, where it feels as if every muscle in your body is tense. People with this type of tension tend to get muscle cramps at night. When your grandmother gave you a glass of milk before bedtime she was wisely giving you a dose of calcium to relax your muscles and ease you into sleep. Magnesium regulates calcium uptake by cells, so take a magnesium/calcium combination for the greatest effect. You can try a combination of 600 mg calcium and 300 mg magnesium before bed.

TREATING DEPRESSION NATURALLY

Before getting into specific methods for treating depression naturally, let's first ask whether being down in the dumps or anxious for a few days now and then is cause for medication. We human beings are emotional creatures, and we naturally have our up times and our down times. Down times can also be the universe's way of pointing out to us that something needs fixing. If we push ourselves back up with a pill, without treating the cause, pretty soon we'll be depressed or anxious regardless of what we're taking.

If you're going through a down cycle, be sure to take time for yourself to be reflective about your life. Is there something in your relationship with yourself or someone else that needs healing? Do you have activities in your life that are important and meaningful to you? Have you been getting enough sleep? Are you taking a prescription drug that can cause anxiety or depression? How's your diet? Have you tried an elimination diet to find out if you're allergic to anything? All of these can be factors in anxiety and depression, as are major life changes such as children leaving home, divorce, major illness and the death of a loved one.

Being anxious or depressed isn't fun—we've all been there—but coming back into emotional balance can be a valuable exercise in learning how to take care of yourself better, and keeping your life on track. Most of the time these negative states of mind are caused by some combination of physical, emotional, mental or spiritual troubles, so it pays to check in with yourself at every level.

In North America and Europe we tend to believe all the TV ads that tell us we're not okay unless we're always vivaciously energetic, laughing, happy and ready to party at all times. In truth, what most of us need in our lives is more balance. Not wildly happy, not terribly sad, but balance. Being in balance could be experienced as a state of calm, well-being or peacefulness. Depression and anxiety are two extremes of being out of balance, but oddly enough, they tend to have similar root causes, and many people bounce back and forth between the two.

It's also natural to be depressed if you are in the midst of grieving over the death or serious illness of a loved one, a divorce, job loss or other significant life event. In these cases we sometimes can use some help, and when those times roll around you're way ahead if you start with natural remedies.

Kava

Kava, derived from a plant used by South Pacific islanders, can be a good, safe natural remedy for depression, anxiety or insomnia. If you're working on exercising and letting go of alcohol, sugar or coffee, but want some gentle, natural help along the way overcoming anxiety or depression, kava (*Piper methysticum*) might do the job for you. This member of the pepper family grows as a bush in the South Pacific. Kava root, ground up and mixed with coconut milk, is used by the South Pacific islanders in celebrations and ceremonies. If you've visited the South Pacific, you've probably been treated to a kava drink. Kava is described in medical terms as being a sedative and muscle relaxant, and in lay terms as a calming drink that brings on a feeling of contentment and well-being and encourages socializing. No wonder we know the South Pacific Islanders as being very easy to get along with! Kava is also a pain reliever, and can often be used in place of the NSAIDs (nonsteroidal anti-inflammatory drugs such as aspirin, acetaminophen and ibuprofen).

In Europe, numerous double-blind and placebo studies have consistently shown kava to be as effective in treating anxiety and depression as the so-called anti-anxiety agents such as the benzodiazepines (oxazepams such as Serax, diazepams such as Valium), without the side effects. Quite the opposite in fact. The benzodiazepines tend to cause lethargy, drowsiness and mental impairment. But in one double-blind placebo study done with 84 people with anxiety symptoms, taking 400 mg daily of kavain, a purified kavalactone (an active ingredient of kava), was shown to improve concentration, memory and reaction time. Other studies have shown no mental depression or interference with the ability to do tasks such as driving a car. In another study, people with anxiety symptoms given a 70 percent kavalactone extract in the amount of 100 mg three times a day, were found after four weeks to have a significant reduction in anxiety symptoms such as feelings of nervousness, heart palpitations, chest pains, headaches, dizziness and indigestion. And all with no side effects noted.

For over 100 years, scientists have been trying to figure out exactly what it is in kava that gives it sedative and antidepressant properties. Although they have isolated chemical compounds named "kavalactones," which do act as sedatives and antidepressants when given alone, an extract of the whole root has always worked better. Kava also has a different action on the brain than any of our other antidepressants or sedatives, possibly working in the limbic brain, the seat of our emotions.

In medicinal doses, kava has no known side effects. In very high doses it can cause sleepiness, and high doses over a long period of time can cause skin irritation and inflammation in the eyes.

The best way to take kava is powdered, in a capsule, or as an extract. For dosage, follow the directions on the label.

St. John's Wort

St. John's wort, which has been used medicinally for many centuries by the Chinese, the Greeks, the Europeans and the American Indians, is well-known for its positive effect on anxiety, insomnia, depression and a physical illness which has long been associated with stress: heart disease. It also seems to be effective as a treatment for seasonal affective disorder (SAD). This herb has been extremely well-studied in Europe, and found over and over again to be as effective as the SSRIs in treating depression, and as the benzodiazepines in treating anxiety. You may need to take it for a couple of weeks before it starts taking effect.

Take it in the dose recommended on the container. If you are coming off of an SSRI such as Prozac and want to try St. John's wort, allow a three-week period in between so that you don't end up with serotonin syndrome (a dangerous condition where too much serotonin remains in the synapses).

The B Vitamins

The B vitamins together and separately play important roles in nerve and brain function and in relaxing muscles. If you are older and not absorbing nutrients as well as you might be, your body may not be able to utilize the B vitamins in your food. It's important to include the B vitamins in a multivitamin. If you're having trouble with leg cramps at night, an extra 50 mg of vitamin B6 an hour before bed may help. Some people are cured of restless leg syndrome by taking an extra 400 mcg of folic acid before bed.

The B vitamins play an essential role in our neurological health, and yet most adult Americans are deficient in these vitamins. Although each of the B vitamins plays some role in brain function, vitamin B12 is best known for its ability to combat depression. For years alternative health professionals have given vitamin B12 shots as part of an overall treatment program for people who are extremely stressed out or depressed. Until recently this practice has been pooh-poohed, but now more and more M.D.s are jumping on the B12 bandwagon.

If you want to try B12 as an antidote for stress and/or depression, it's important to know that it's not well-absorbed when you take it orally (by mouth), which is why it is given in the form of injections. However, there are B12 supplements you can buy at your local health food store that are sublingual (dissolved under the tongue) and intranasal (in the nose). You'll want to take about 1,000 mcg (1 mg) at least every other day for treating depression.

The amino acid tryptophan, a precursor to melatonin, is a very safe and effective sleep remedy, and can also be a wonderful remedy for anxiety and depression. Unfortunately it was pulled off the market in the U.S. by the FDA when a contaminated batch from Japan caused death and illness in dozens of people. The illness it caused had nothing to do with the effects of uncontaminated tryptophan. In truth, tryptophan is very safe—far safer than sleeping pills and antidepressants, which it was competing with in a big way when it was pulled off the market. It's a good bet that tryptophan was pulled from the market to protect the profits of the big drug companies, not to protect your health. Ironically, tryptophan is still included in baby formulas and nutritional powders for senior citizens because it is an essential amino acid, but you can't get it by itself as a supplement in the U.S.

Tryptophan's effect on the brain is similar to that of drugs such as Prozac, except that it doesn't have the side effects and dangers and withdrawal problems those drugs have, it's much less expensive, and it's probably more effective. Tryptophan is trickling back onto the market in the U.S., and it can be purchased almost anywhere outside the United States. You can also try 5-hydroxy tryptophan (5HTP), a form of tryptophan which is available in health food stores.

One of tryptophan's primary effects on the brain is to reduce anxiety, which is often the culprit in insomnia. For the same reason it is often quite effective for treating depression, especially if there is an anxiety component to it. Some people purchase pharmaceutical grade tryptophan from veterinarians.

If you are taking one of the SSRIs (Prozac, Paxil or Zoloft), don't use tryptophan at the same time. Agitation, restlessness, aggressiveness, high body temperature, diarrhea and cramping can result.

The Amino Acids

Many alternative health-care practitioners have had great success treating depression with amino acids. Amino acids are the building blocks of protein, and play a vital role in the production and regulation of brain chemicals. Most of the new "personality" drugs have much the same effects on brain chemistry as the amino acids tryptophan, tyrosine, and phenylalanine. These substances affect the brain's production of serotonin, a neurotransmitter that affects our moods. However, please try the simpler solutions such as nutrition and exercise first for treating depression—it's always preferable to begin with the most simple, down-to-earth solutions.

Although amino acids are safe, especially when compared to the prescription drugs, don't take more than the recommended dose unless it's recommended by a health care professional, and monitor yourself carefully to track if and how they affect you (keeping a daily diary of how you're feeling works well). The stimulating amino acids such as tyrosine and phenylalanine can cause irritability in some people.

If you have chronic, recurring depression, work with a health-care professional. Please do *not* take amino acids for depression if you are already taking a prescription drug for it, without consulting your doctor.

If you, your physician or health-care professional want to know about amino acids in detail, read the book *The Healing Nutrients Within* by Eric R. Braverman, M.D. and Carl C. Pfeiffer, M.D., Ph.D. (Keats Publishing, 1987). Your doctor may want to check out some of the 120 pages of references cited. Very few prescription drugs have been so thoroughly tested.

Tyrosine

The amino acid tyrosine is fairly well established through research and the experience of hundreds of alternative health care practitioners as a safe and effective remedy for depression. Tyrosine is the precursor to some of our most important neurotransmitters, so it is an important part of our brain's nutrition. It is also a precursor to adrenaline, thyroid hormones and some types of estrogen. It has been shown to lower blood pressure, increase sex drive and suppress appetite. L-dopa, which is used to treat Parkinson's disease, is made from tyrosine.

Start with 500 mg three times a day with meals. If that doesn't work, try 1,000 mg. The most you should take without consulting a health professional is 1,500 mg a day. Although tyrosine is considered to be one of the safest amino acids, it can trigger a migraine headache in some people and shouldn't be used in conjunction with MAO inhibitors.

Phenylalanine

The amino acid phenylalanine is the precursor to tyrosine and has been used in numerous studies to successfully treat depression. Many supplement manufacturers will combine tyrosine and phenylalanine, but vitamin B6 should be added to this combination for better utilization.

This amino acid should be avoided by people who have PKU (phenylketonuria), a genetic defect in the body's ability to process and use phenylalanine. This defect can cause severe retardation. If it is caught early enough, retardation can be avoided with a phenylalanine-free diet. Some researchers believe that many children who are hyperactive or have learning disabilities are suffering from a mild form of PKU. Because there are a small number of women whose phenylalanine levels fluctuate when they are pregnant, this amino acid should be avoided if you are pregnant, just to be on the safe side.

The most common source of phenylalanine these days is the artificial sweetener aspartame (NutraSweet). Every time you use aspartame you get some phenylalanine and aspartic acid. However, it's better to take phenylalanine in a supplement because we don't know enough about aspartic acid and its side effects, or what it does in combination with phenylalanine.

Phenylalanine has been reported to raise blood pressure, so if you have high blood pressure please monitor it carefully or consult your doctor. Phenylalanine gives some people headaches. A few studies suggest that phenylalanine may promote the growth of cancerous tumors, so if you have cancer this should not be your antidepressant of choice, and please avoid the aspartame! You can take up to 500 mg of phenylalanine three times a day.

Get into the Sunshine

If you tend to get down in the dumps every winter and feel better in the spring, you may have SAD (seasonal affective disorder) and you may want to try light therapy. Relaxing in a room lit at 80 times the brightness of indoor lighting for two hours a day can help to make your hormonal rhythms more pronounced, decreasing your daytime melatonin secretion. You can gain very quick relief with light therapy if you have SAD. If you think this might be for you, check your local health food store for a source of full-spectrum lighting.

CHAPTER 15

Diabetes Drugs and Their Natural Alternatives

IF YOU HAVE adult-onset (Type II) diabetes and your physician isn't working with you to aggressively treat the disease with diet and exercise, then you are being shunted into a money-making pipeline for the medical industry and used as a cash cow. The vast majority of Type II diabetes, especially when it is caught early, can be very successfully treated with diet, exercise and supplements, but most conventional physicians won't take that course. Instead they prescribe drugs that control the symptoms without treating the underlying disease, putting you on a sure road to illness and disability.

A few years ago a slick, full-color, four-page advertisement appeared in a pharmacy magazine that began with the headline, "The Diabetes Consumer: Shops more. Spends more. Shops the whole store." The headline on the following page read, "Maximize Your Profits with Diabetes Category Management." It went on to predict "dramatic growth" in the diabetes market, projected to reach $4 billion by 1998. (The total annual cost of diabetes is estimated to be $92 billion.)

The ad went on to explain that a diabetic customer spends about $2,500 more in a pharmacy each year than the average customer, and listed some 26 products needed by a diabetic, including insulin, syringes, cotton swabs and blood glucose monitors.

Pharmacy costs for a diabetic don't take into account the cost of regular visits to the physician, and the cost of the side effects of diabetes. Diabetics are two to four times as likely to have heart disease or a stroke. They also represent one-third of kidney dialysis patients, and they suffer from impotence, loss of vision, increased susceptibility to infections and loss of sensation in the hands and feet. These costs line the pockets of physicians and hospitals. Any way you look at it, a person with diabetes is a cash cow for physicians, drug companies and pharmacies.

Once you are diagnosed, your physician is pressured from many directions to put you on diabetes drugs to control blood sugar. This guarantees that you will need to visit your physician frequently to renew your prescription, and guarantees the drug company and pharmacy a lifetime customer. All of the diabetes drugs have side effects, and all of them gradually lose their effectiveness, guaranteeing the drug-dependent diabetic the life-threatening side effects of both the drug and the disease.

This wouldn't be such shameful behavior if it weren't for the fact that adult-onset diabetes is one of the most preventable of all chronic diseases, and is highly treatable and reversible through diet and exercise. Taking the right nutritional supplements and herbs improves the picture even more.

Some 90 percent of adult-onset or Type II diabetes, also known as non-insulin dependent diabetes, is caused by poor diet, obesity and lack of exercise. Three-quarters of those diagnosed with Type II diabetes can avoid insulin injections and other drugs by losing weight. But physicians are taught (brainwashed) in medical school that it's too difficult to help patients lose weight and eat properly, so they are most likely to recommend (pay lip service) to weight loss and exercise, while they're writing you out a prescription for a diabetes drug.

WHAT'S SO BAD ABOUT DIABETES DRUGS?

Diabetes is such a profitable business that physicians will put "prediabetic" patients, with only marginally high blood sugar, onto diabetes drugs before even trying weight loss and exercise. In fact a big push now by drug companies and diabetes associations (which are funded by the drug companies) is to "identify" the supposed eight million borderline diabetics so they can get them onto drugs too! The justification for this is that the earlier high blood sugar is controlled, and the more it is controlled, the less likely a person is to suffer from the side effects of diabetes. While this is very true, mysteriously, nutrition and weight loss are rarely mentioned.

Giving a borderline diabetic drugs without lifestyle changes should be considered malpractice. Any physician or health organization that doesn't vigorously, consistently and insistently work with a diabetic patient to lose weight and exercise is not in the business of healing, they are in the business of pushing drugs. Diabetes drugs should never, ever be a substitute for a healthy lifestyle.

But the truth is, in the end it's up to you. Your physician and health care organization can't force you to do anything. Only you can make the changes necessary to avoid the lifetime of ill health created by diabetes. If you get on diabetes drugs and stay on them, without addressing the underlying causes of the diabetes, the disease will inev-

---

ARE PRESCRIPTION DRUGS CAUSING YOUR HIGH BLOOD SUGAR?

How many people have been put on a prescription drug, only to have it cause high blood sugar, precipitating an incorrect diagnosis of diabetes from a physician, and a prescription for diabetes drugs? Here are some prescription drugs that can cause hyperglycemia, or high blood sugar.

Antihypertensives (clonidine, diazoxide, diuretics)
Antituberculosis drugs
(rifampin, isoniazid)
Calcium channel blockers
(nifedipine, nicardipine, diltiazem, verapamil)

Clonidine
Corticosteroids (prednisone)
Diuretics
Epinephrine (bronchodilators, decongestants)
Glucocorticosteroids
Heparin
H2 blockers (Tagamet, Zantac)
Hypothyroid drugs (Levoxine, Synthroid)
Morphine
Nalidixic acid
Nicotine
Oral contraceptives
Pentamidine
Phenytoin (Dilantin)
Sulfinpyrazone

> **Caution!**
>
> If you have diabetes, notify your physician if any of the following occurs:
> Hyperglycemia: excessive thirst or urination.
> Hypoglycemia: fatigue, excessive hunger, profuse sweating or numbness in the extremities.
> Miscellaneous: fever, sore throat, rash, unusual bruising or bleeding.

itably progress, with its serious side effects. The only way to avoid the progression of diabetes is to bring the body back into balance.

In countries where people eat a diet low in fat and sugar and high in whole foods such as unrefined grains and fresh fruits and vegetables, diabetes is almost nonexistent. When they move to the U.S., their diabetes risk skyrockets. Tragically, as Western "nutrition free" processed and fast foods such as McDonalds®, and soft drinks such as Coca-Cola® and Pepsi® are introduced to Third World countries, their rates of diabetes are rapidly rising. It is estimated that by the year 2010, some 40 percent of Americans 65 or older will have adult-onset diabetes.

ARE PRESCRIPTION DRUGS CAUSING YOUR LOW BLOOD SUGAR?

If you are diabetic, or your blood sugar is unstable, and you are suffering from hypoglycemia or hyperglycemia, you should be aware of those substances that can lower your blood sugar:

Alcohol
Allopurinol (Lopurin, Zyloprim)
Ampicillin
Bromocriptine
Chloramphenicol (Chloromycetin)

Clofibrate (Abitrate, Atromid-S)
Fenfluramine (Pondimin) (pulled off the market)
Indomethacin
Lithium
Mebendazole
Monoamine oxidase (MAO) inhibitors
Phenylbutazone (Butatab, Butazolidin)
Probenecid (Benemid, Probalan)
Salicylates (aspirin)
Tetracycline
Theophylline

Diabetes Drugs

Alpha-Glucosidase Inhibitors

Acarbose (Precose)

Acarbose (Precose), the newest type of diabetes drug on the market, works by slowing the digestion of carbohydrates in the small intestine, which reduces the amount of sugar that is released into the blood after eating. The drug works by blocking enzymes that normally break down carbohydrates. These drugs can cause unpleasant stomach and digestive problems such as cramps, gas and diarrhea, and can make existing intestinal problems worse.

What Does It Do in Your Body?

Slows the digestion of carbohydrates in your small intestine, which reduces the amount of glucose (sugar) that is released into your blood after eating.

What Is It Prescribed For?

Lowering blood sugar levels. This drug is intended to be supplemental therapy to diet and exercise.

What Are the Possible Side Effects?

The most common side effects occur in the digestive system, including abdominal pain, diarrhea, and gas.

Acarbose can impair kidney function and has caused cancerous kidney tumors in rats. It can cause hypoglycemia or low blood sugar levels, so if you're taking it, be sure to have a readily available source of dextrose on hand to counteract hypoglycemia.

Caution! Think Twice about Taking This Type of Drug If . . .

- You have kidney problems of any kind.
- You have serious intestinal problems.

- You are exposed to stress such as fever, trauma, infection or surgery.

What Are the Interactions with Other Drugs?

These drugs may increase the effects or prolong the action of acarbose drugs:

↑ Insulin
Sulfonylurea drugs

These drugs may reduce the effects of acarbose drugs:

↓ Digestive enzymes

What Are the Interactions with Food?

Take this drug orally with the first bite of a main meal.

What Nutrients Does It Throw Out of Balance or Interact With?

Vitamin B12.

What Else to Take If You Take This Drug

A supplement of vitamin B12, sublingually.

Insulin

Insulin injection (Insulin, Humulin R)

Insulin injection concentrated (Concentrated Regular)

Insulin zinc suspension, extended Ultralente (Humulin U Ultralente)

Insulin zinc suspension Lente (Humulin L)

Isophane insulin suspension and insulin injection (Humulin 70/30, Humulin 50/50)

Isophane insulin suspension NPH (Novolin N)

Adult-onset diabetes is usually a disease of excess sugar in the blood-stream and an impaired ability to utilize the hormone insulin to carry the sugar out of the blood and into the cells. In rare cases it may be caused by the inability of the pancreas to make insulin. At one time insulin was thought to be the savior of diabetics: Simply inject it into the body to replace what isn't there. But diabetes is always more complicated than a pancreas that doesn't make insulin.

Most people with Type II diabetes actually make plenty of insulin, but have insulin resistance, a condition where their cells are resistant to using it. But the pancreas keeps getting the message that there isn't enough insulin, and keeps producing it. Excess insulin causes its own problems, including high blood pressure and poor cholesterol levels (low HDL and high LDL), increasing the risk of complications as the disease progresses. This is why it is so important that even insulin-dependent diabetics reduce their need for insulin as much as possible through good management of blood sugar levels using diet, supplements and exercise.

WHAT DO THEY DO IN YOUR BODY?

Insulin is taken to replace the insulin that should be produced by the pancreas but is not, or is not produced sufficiently. Insulin regulates blood sugar levels in your body.

WHAT THEY ARE PRESCRIBED FOR?

People who cannot survive without prescribed insulin for blood sugar regulation, which is mostly Type I diabetics.

WHAT ARE THE POSSIBLE SIDE EFFECTS?

Allergic reactions such as rashes, shortness of breath, fast pulse, sweating, a drop in blood pressure resulting in dizziness or lighthead-edness, as well as insulin shock.

If insulin is injected, redness, swelling and itching at the site can occur. Open sores at the site of injection can occur. Also, if injections happen at the same site several times, fat may accumulate at the site and inhibit insulin absorption.

CAUTION! THINK TWICE ABOUT TAKING THESE TYPES OF DRUGS IF . . .

- You have an insulin resistance or allergy. There is almost never a reason to prescribe insulin to a Type II diabetic. Be sure your physician has a good reason if this is the case.

WHAT ARE THE INTERACTIONS WITH OTHER DRUGS?

These drugs may increase the effects or prolong the action of insulin:

↑ Alcohol*   Guanethidine
  Anabolic steroids*   MAO inhibitors*
  Beta-blockers   Salicylates (aspirin)
  Clofibrate   Sulfinpyrazone
  Fenfluramine*   Tetracyclines

These drugs may reduce the effects of insulin:

↓ Corticosteroids   Oral contraceptives
  Diltiazem   Thiazide diuretics
  Epinephrine   Thyroid hormones

WHAT ARE THE INTERACTIONS WITH FOOD?

Coffee decreases the amount of insulin and length of time it is in your system.

WHAT NUTRIENTS DOES IT THROW OUT OF BALANCE OR INTERACT WITH?

Blood sugar, vitamin B12.

WHAT ELSE TO TAKE IF YOU TAKE THIS DRUG

Supplement of sublingual vitamin B12.

---

*Potentially dangerous interaction.

Sulfonylurea Drugs

ACETOHEXAMIDE (Dymelor)

CHLORPROPAMIDE (Diabinese)

GLIMEPIRIDE (Amaryl)

GLIPIZIDE (Glipizide, Glucotrol)

GLYBURIDE (Glyburide)

TOLAZAMIDE (Tolinase)

TOLBUTAMIDE (Orinase)

These oral drugs (taken by mouth) lower the amount of sugar in the bloodstream by stimulating the pancreas to make more insulin. They decrease the liver's production of glucose, a simple sugar, and they make cells more sensitive to insulin, improving the uptake of insulin and sugar for energy. The down side of these drugs is that they increase the risk of dying of heart disease, one of the most common side effects of diabetes, and they tend to cause weight gain, one of the causes of diabetes! They can also cause hypoglycemia (low blood sugar) by removing too much sugar.

Less serious but frequent side effects are digestive upsets such as nausea, vomiting, heartburn, gas, diarrhea and constipation. Some of the older sulfonylurea drugs include tolbutamide (Orinase, Oramide), tolazamide (Tolamide, Tolinase), acetohexamide (Dymelor), chlorpropamide (Diabinese, Glucamide). The new sulfonylurea drugs include glipizide (Glucotrol), glyburide (DiaBeta, Glynase, PersTab) and glimepiride (Amaryl).

WHAT DO THEY DO IN YOUR BODY?

Lower blood glucose.

WHAT ARE THEY PRESCRIBED FOR?

Noninsulin-dependent diabetes mellitus (also called adult-onset or maturity-onset diabetes, ketosis-resistant diabetes and Type II diabetes). In addition, they are sometimes prescribed as temporary adjuncts to insulin therapy to improve diabetic control.

WHAT ARE THE POSSIBLE SIDE EFFECTS?

Digestive system reactions are common. They include nausea, heartburn, diarrhea. They can suppress the immune system and cause anemia, liver and kidney impairment and jaundice.

The effectiveness of these drugs decreases over time, eventually resulting in a complete failure of the drug to control glucose—yet another reason to control your blood sugar with diet, exercise and supplements!

Flushing of the face when taken with alcohol may occur, as can water retention—particularly if you have congestive heart failure or liver cirrhosis. These drugs can also cause weakness, ringing in the ears, fatigue, dizziness and headache.

CAUTION! THINK TWICE ABOUT TAKING THESE TYPES OF DRUGS IF . . .

- You have diabetes complicated with a high count of ketones.
- You are diabetic and pregnant.
- You have heart problems. Diabetic patients using this drug were two-and-a-half times more likely to die from cardiovascular problems.
- You have liver or kidney problems.
- You are elderly, debilitated or malnourished.
- Your adrenal or pituitary glands are not operating sufficiently.

WHAT ARE THE INTERACTIONS WITH OTHER DRUGS?

Sulfonylureas may raise levels or prolong the effects of these drugs:

↑ Alcohol*   Digitalis

These drugs may increase the effects or prolong the action of sulfonylureas:

↑ ACE inhibitors
Androgens
Antibiotics (co-trimoxazole)*
Anticoagulants
Antidepressants*
Chloramphenicol*
Clofibrate
Cortisonelike drugs such as corti-
sone and cortef
Fenfluramine
Fluconazole

Gemfibrozil
H2 blockers
MAO inhibitors*
Methyldopa
Oral contraceptives
Probenecid
Salicylates such as aspirin*
Sulfinpyrazone*
Sulfonamides*
Tricyclic antidepressants

These drugs may reduce the effects of sulfonylureas:

↓ Beta-blockers
Cholestyramine
Diuretics

Hydantoins
Rifampin

WHAT ARE THE INTERACTIONS WITH FOOD?

Food delays absorption of these drugs by about 40 minutes. These drugs are more effective if you take them 30 minutes before eating food.

Do not drink alcohol with these drugs—particularly chlorprop-amide and tolbutamide. Symptoms of this interaction can be dizziness, weakness, mental confusion, collapse and coma.

WHAT NUTRIENTS DO THEY THROW OUT OF BALANCE OR INTERACT WITH?

These drugs lower levels of vitamin B12.

WHAT ELSE TO TAKE IF YOU TAKE THIS DRUG

Sublingual vitamin B12.

---

*Potentially dangerous interaction.

Miscellaneous Diabetes Drugs

METFORMIN (Glucophage)

Metformin (Glucophage) is a fairly new drug in the U.S., and is another oral diabetic drug which lowers blood sugar by suppressing glucose production in the liver and increasing the sensitivity of cells to insulin. Unlike the sulfonylurea drugs, it does not stimulate the production of insulin, so there is less chance of hypoglycemia, and it tends to cause weight loss, not weight gain. Like all of the oral diabetes drugs, digestive discomfort is a common side effect. It can also impair kidney and liver function and shouldn't be used by people who use alcohol excessively.

WHAT IS IT PRESCRIBED FOR?

To lower blood glucose levels in patients with noninsulin-dependent diabetes.

WHAT DOES IT DO IN THE BODY?

It decreases liver glucose (sugar) production, decreases intestinal absorption of glucose, increases uptake and utilization of glucose.

WHAT ARE THE POSSIBLE SIDE EFFECTS?

Low blood sugar if you don't eat enough calories, if you exercise strenuously and don't supplement with additional caloric intake, if you drink alcohol or if you take another glucose-lowering drug with metformin.

Digestive problems can occur with this drug including diarrhea, nausea, vomiting, abdominal bloating, gas, loss of appetite.

Lactic acidosis is a rare but serious metabolic complication where too much of the drug accumulates in the body. It is fatal in 50 percent of the cases. It usually happens in people with kidney impairment.

This drug can increase your chances of dying from cardiovascular problems by two-and-a-half times.

CAUTION: THINK TWICE ABOUT TAKING THESE TYPES OF DRUGS IF . . .

- You have kidney disease or dysfunction.
- You have cardiovascular problems.
- You have inadequate vitamin B12 or calcium intake.

WHAT ARE THE INTERACTIONS WITH OTHER DRUGS?

The following drugs may be reduced in potency or decreased in the amount of time they are effective when combined with metformin:

↓ Furosemide   Glyburide

These drugs may increase the effects or prolong the action of metformin:

↑ Alcohol   Procainamide*
  Amiloride*   Quinidine*
  Cimetidine   Quinine*
  Digoxin*   Ranitidine*
  Furosemide   Triamterene*
  Morphine*   Trimethoprim*
  Nifedipine   Vancomycin*

WHAT NUTRIENTS DOES IT THROW OUT OF BALANCE OR INTERACT WITH?

Vitamin B12.

WHAT ELSE TO TAKE IF YOU TAKE THIS DRUG

Sublingual vitamin B12.

TROGLITAZONE (Rezulin)

This drug lowers glucose by improving cell receptivity to insulin and does not stimulate the pancreas to produce more insulin, like other

---

*Potentially dangerous interaction.

antidiabetic agents. Allergic side effects are more common with this drug, as well as possible heart failure and liver failure.

WHAT DOES IT DO IN YOUR BODY?

It improves your cells' ability to utilize insulin and decreases insulin resistance. It does not stimulate the pancreas to secrete insulin like sulfonylurea drugs.

WHAT IS IT PRESCRIBED FOR?

Blood sugar control for people with Type II diabetes.

WHAT ARE THE POSSIBLE SIDE EFFECTS?

Infection, headache, dizziness, back pain, nausea, inflammation of the interior of the nose, diarrhea, water retention, heart failure, liver poisoning, immune suppression, low blood sugar.

CAUTION! THINK TWICE ABOUT TAKING THIS TYPE OF DRUG IF . . .

- You have heart problems of any kind—particularly if you have been diagnosed as Class III or IV cardiac status.
- You are a Type I or insulin-dependent diabetic.
- You have liver problems.
- You have a suppressed immune system.

WHAT ARE THE INTERACTIONS WITH OTHER DRUGS?

Troglitazone may raise levels or prolong the effects of these drugs:

↑ Sulfonylurea drugs

The following drugs may be reduced in potency or decreased in the amount of time they are effective when combined with troglitazone:

↓ Oral contraceptives (use alternative birth control methods while on this drug)

These drugs may reduce the effects of troglitazone:

↓ Cholestyramine (reduces by 70 percent)
   Oral contraceptives

WHAT ARE THE INTERACTIONS WITH FOOD?

Take this drug with meals.

WHAT NUTRIENTS DOES IT THROW OUT OF BALANCE OR INTERACT WITH?

Vitamin B12.

WHAT ELSE TO TAKE IF YOU TAKE THIS DRUG

Sublingual vitamin B12.

NATURAL ALTERNATIVES TO DIABETES DRUGS

There are many safe, natural and effective ways to help control blood sugar without drugs. The Six Core Principles for Optimal Health are your cornerstone for stable blood sugar, with an emphasis on weight loss, exercise, the reduction of processed foods and sugar and yes!—eat your vegetables, preferably fresh and organic and not overcooked.

The high-carbohydrate diet traditionally recommended by the American Diabetes Association is proving not to be the answer for many diabetics. If you are a Type II diabetic who is overweight and insulin resistant, it may be important for you to cut way back on carbohydrates. When you do eat them, stick to complex carbohydrates with plenty of fiber such as whole grains, vegetables and legumes. Sugar and simple carbohydrates (white flour, pasta, potatoes, corn and bananas for example) create spikes in insulin production, and your goal is to keep both insulin and blood sugar on an even keel. Beans are especially good foods for balancing blood sugar. The book *The Zone* by Barry Sears (HarperCollins, 1995) will give you good, in-depth coverage of a diet for insulin control.

As you read about the supplements that will help stabilize your blood sugar, keep in mind that they *will* affect your blood sugar, so they shouldn't be used without very close monitoring if you have diabetes. You should be able to find all of these supplements at your health food store.

An Ayurvedic, Chinese or naturopathic doctor will work very closely with diabetics, prescribing a variety of herbs and supplements depending on the health of the patient. If you have unstable blood sugar or are diabetic, please work closely with one of these types of physicians, or an M.D. or D.O. willing to use herbs and nutritional supplements. In the Resources section of this book you'll find organizations that will refer you to an alternative health care professional in your area.

Chromium and Niacin: Partners in Blood Sugar Control

Chromium is one of your key supplements when you need better blood sugar control. The people who make those awful bottled "natural" fruit drinks and teas aren't going to like this, but it's possible that the steep rise in our consumption of high fructose corn syrup has contributed to the rise in diabetes by depleting chromium. (As our consumption of high fructose corn syrup has risen 250 percent in the past 15 years, our rate of diabetes has increased approximately 45 percent in about the same time period.) According to studies done at the Agriculture Department's Human Nutrition Resource Center, fructose consumption causes a drop in chromium, raises LDL "bad" cholesterol and triglycerides, and impairs immune system function. Yet another great reason to read labels and avoid processed foods.

According to researchers, giving people with elevated blood sugar a chromium supplement will result in a significant drop in blood sugar in 80 to 90 percent of those people. Please don't be scared away from chromium by recent media reports about it. Taking chromium picolinate supplements of 200 to 600 mcg daily is not the same as giving rats 5,000 to 6,000 times that dose every day, nor is it the same as factory workers breathing chromium dust. It is estimated that 90 percent of Americans are actually deficient in chromium, and at the recommended doses it is very safe and very effective in helping stabilize blood sugar as well as helping burn fat during exercise and producing lean muscle tissue.

The other nutrient necessary to help insulin do its job of ushering sugar into cells is niacin (vitamin B3). Niacin works with chromium, and should be taken in the form of inositol hexanicotinate with enough to give you 100 mg of niacin daily to start with. For example, one brand of 500-mg tablets of inositol hexanicotinate yields 400 mg of inositol and 100 mg of niacin. You can gradually raise the dose if needed, up to 400 mg of niacin daily.

Other Important Supplements for Stable Blood Sugar

Vanadium, a trace mineral taken in the form of vanadyl sulfate, helps insulin work more efficiently. That may be why it also lowers cholesterol and triglyceride levels. Long-term high doses of vanadium are not recommended, but you can use it to help stabilize your blood sugar and then cut back. Start with 6 mg daily and work your way up to 100 mg daily until you get results. Once you begin having results, stay at that dose for up to three weeks and then taper back gradually to 6 to 10 mg daily.

Studies now link a **vitamin D** deficiency with diabetes, immune function and bone loss. It may be that vitamin D deficiency is a factor in the onset of diabetes and that a supplement of vitamin D could help reverse the disease. Take up to 400 IU daily.

Zinc (10 to 15 mg daily), **selenium** (100 to 200 mcg daily) and **manganese** (10 mg daily) all play a role in regulating blood sugar and should be included in your daily multivitamin. Many diabetics are deficient in **magnesium,** which is key to a healthy heart, so be sure you're getting 400 to 800 mg daily in a supplement.

Recent studies have shown that both **vitamin E and vitamin C** significantly improve glucose (sugar) tolerance in Type II diabetics. In fact, two independent studies have shown that low blood levels of vitamin E are correlated with a four times higher risk of diabetes. In a study published recently in the *Journal of Clinical Investigation,* researchers at Harvard who gave diabetic patients intravenous vitamin C found that it significantly improved blood vessel dilation and function. Since impaired blood flow is one of the primary causes of diabetes complications, this is significant information. It's a good idea for almost everyone to take 1,000 to 2,000 mg of vitamin C daily, but if you are diabetic you may want to double that amount. Make sure you're getting your bioflavonoids with it. (Vitamin C can give false readings on some types of glucose tests, so consult with your physician or pharmacist about which form of glucose testing works best with vitamin C.)

The **bioflavonoids** in grapeseed extract and ginkgo biloba help strengthen blood vessels and improve blood flow to the extremities.

Essential fatty acids (EFAs) are especially essential for people with unstable blood sugar, making it very important to cut out the EFA-*blocking* hydrogenated oils found in chips, baked goods and nearly all processed foods. Research has shown that diabetics given evening primrose oil for a year had improved nerve function, while those on a placebo got worse. Other research has shown that diabetics on a high mono-unsaturated oil diet (olive oil, canola oil, avocados, for example) had lower triglycerides and better levels of blood glucose and insulin than those on a primarily high-carbohydrate diet. Eating plenty of fresh, organic vegetables, a variety of whole grains and fish should give you plenty of EFAs over the long term.

Ginseng has been used by the Chinese for centuries to help control diabetes, and recent studies confirm that it can reduce fasting blood glucose as well as improve mood and help in weight reduction. Herbalist Donald Brown recommends a standardized extract with a 5 to 7 percent ginsenoside content. More or less can throw blood sugar off rather than bring it into balance. For this use, ginseng is probably best taken as a liquid extract.

One of the Ayurvedic herbs of choice in India for lowering blood sugar, now available in the U.S., is called **gymenma sylvestre.** There is also some evidence that gymenma sylvestre actually reverses damage to certain cells in the pancreas that can be destroyed by diabetes. You can find it at your health food store. Be sure to tell your healthcare provider that you are taking this herb because if you are taking diabetes drugs, they may need to be adjusted.

Turmeric, a spice often used in the East, and the more familiar spice **cinnamon** have both shown tremendous potential in helping regulate blood sugar. Richard Anderson, Ph.D. tested these spices in a test tube and found that they tripled the insulin's ability to metabo-

Good Foods for Stable Blood Sugar

Apples	Leaf lettuce
Artichokes	Lean, white freshwater fish
Asparagus	Leeks
Basmati rice	Lemons
Beet greens	Lima beans
Broccoli	Limes
Brown rice	Meat
Brussels sprouts	Millet
Buckwheat	Mung beans
Cauliflower	Olive oil (small amounts)
Celery	Olives
Chicken	Onions
Chicory	Papaya
Collard greens	Parsley
Cranberries	Pears
Dandelion greens	Peppers
Endive	Persimmons
Fava beans	Pomegranates
Fish	Rye
Garlic	Rye crisps
Grapefruit	Sunflower seeds, raw
Kale	Swiss chard
Kidney beans	Turkey

lize sugar. Studies indicate that fenugreek is another spice that can aid you in controlling your sugar levels. In addition, **maitake mushrooms** have been found to help maintain correct sugar levels.

Another supplement that shows great potential in helping to stabilize blood sugar is a form of organic sulfur called **methylsulfonylmethane (MSM)**. You can take 1,000 mg two to three times daily.

Drs. Alan Gaby and Jonathan Wright have formulated a vitamin for diabetics called **Glucobalance**, which can be found in most health food stores. To this formula they recommend adding more niacin and essential fatty acids.

Making the Shift to Naturally Stable Blood Sugar

If you are struggling with unstable blood sugar and coping with a physician who just wants to put you on drugs, perhaps you can take some inspiration from a woman named Susan. During an annual checkup to her physician, Susan was told she had high blood sugar and was given a prescription for an oral diabetes drug. She took the drug until she went on a lengthy vacation and ran out. Remembering the advice she had read in one of Dr. Mindell's books to cut out sugars, processed foods, and get plenty of exercise, she did just that while on vacation. She felt so great that she continued this regimen when she got back home and never renewed her prescription for the drug. A few months later she went back to her physician and her blood sugar was perfectly normal. When she wrote to me, her blood sugar had been normal for nearly a year and she was in great health. Congratulations to Susan, and to all of you who have taken charge of your health and are feeling better for it!

Ideally I'd like you to go off any drug under the supervision of a health-care professional. As you change your diet, begin to exercise and take the recommended supplements, your blood sugar will go down and it will stabilize. It is very important for you to track it daily and adjust any medications you're taking accordingly.

Exercise: An Essential Part of Managing Diabetes

You cannot properly control adult-onset diabetes without a good exercise program. There's no getting around it. One of the most devasta-

Foods That Raise Blood Sugar	
Carrots	Raisins
Oatmeal	Refined grains (white bread, pasta)
Oranges	Sugar, molasses
Potatoes	Sweet corn
Processed cereals	Yams

CARING FOR YOUR FEET

Because of poor circulation in the extremities, diabetics need to take care of their feet conscientiously to avoid severe complications. Open sores on feet are very common. At least 15 percent of diabetics eventually get a foot ulcer and six out of every 1,000 will lose an arm or leg to infection.

To avoid these severe complications, check with a podiatrist and do the following:

- Examine your feet and toes every day for any injuries or abnormalities like cuts, bruises, sores, infections or bumps.
- Wash your feet every day with a mild soap and warm water. Don't soak too long or you'll lose the protection of the calluses on your feet. Use a soft towel to dry your feet carefully, particularly between your toes.
- If your feet are dry, apply an oil-based lotion to them before putting on your socks and shoes. This will protect your skin from cracking and creating a sore which could progress into an infection later.
- Thick, soft cotton socks are the best choice. Stockings with seams or mended areas may rub away protective skin, creating a sore.
- Only wear shoes that allow your toes to move and that fit your foot snugly but not too tight. Make sure your shoes don't have any sharp edges or tears.
- Always clip your toe nails straight and check corners to avoid creating a cut on a neighboring toe.
- Don't ever remove protective calluses or cut off any growths yourself. Go to a professional.
- Don't take extremely hot baths.
- Avoid going barefoot—including by the pool or beach.
- Sit with your legs uncrossed to allow optimal circulation.
- Use socks to warm your feet at night.

ting side effects of diabetes over time is failing circulation to the extremities, causing numbness, tingling, loss of sensation and sometimes even the loss of a limb. Exercise is essential for keeping circulation strong.

You don't have to run a marathon or pump iron for hours to get the exercise you need. A brisk, 20-minute walk every day will do the trick. If you can walk longer, do it. If you can't walk briskly or get aerobic exercise, try stretching exercises, yoga or qi gong. If you are housebound by weather and want to get some aerobic exercise, find an exercise program on TV or put on your favorite dancing music. The best exercise is whatever is fun and easy for you to do *every day*.

CHAPTER 16

Drugs for Eye Diseases and Their Natural Alternatives

YOUR EYES ARE a window to more than your soul. Unhealthy eyes can reveal ill health before signs of illness emerge in other parts of the body. The condition of the tiny blood vessels that nourish the eye is a good indicator of the health of the blood vessels throughout the rest of your body. For example, if the tiny blood vessels in your eyes are broken or leaking, you can be sure the process is underway in your larger arteries. If your eyes are dry enough to require rewetting drops, chances are the rest of your body is low on important nutrients needed to make lubricating tears, or you have an allergy caused by an overstressed immune system. Vision-stealing diseases like glaucoma, cataracts, macular degeneration and diabetic retinopathy are often caused or precipitated by a combination of exposure to toxins and poor nutrition.

WHAT CAUSES EYE DISEASE?

Glaucoma can be caused by long-term use of steroid drugs or by overconsumption of optic nerve toxins like aspartame and MSG (monosodium glutamate). Drugs used to treat glaucoma are designed to lower pressure in the eyeball. Much like the medical approach of bombarding the body with cholesterol-lowering or blood pressure-lowering medication at the cost of general health and well-being, this tactic doesn't always help more than it hurts.

Macular degeneration is the most common cause of blindness in

USING EYE DROPS EFFECTIVELY

Using eye drops properly can make the difference between an eye drug that works and one that doesn't. If you don't get enough of the medication into your eye, or if it all runs out onto your cheeks before it can be absorbed, you won't get the benefits of the medication. If the dropper becomes contaminated with bacteria and you touch it to your eyeball, you can cause an eye infection.

Here are some tips for using eye drops effectively:

1. Wash your hands thoroughly before using any kind of eye medication.
2. With some kinds of drops you may also need to remove your contact lenses.
3. Never use drops that have changed color or look as though they've separated.
4. Tilt your head back, or lie down and look upward.
5. Pull your lower eyelid away from the eye, creating a pouch.
6. Hold the dropper directly over the eye, being careful not to touch it to the eyeball, fingers or any other surface.
7. Be sure to roll your eyes upward before applying a drop. Just after the drop falls into your eye, roll your eyes downward for several seconds.
8. Release the eyelid and close the eyes gently. Put a small amount of pressure on the inside corners of

the eye with your fingertips. This blocks the duct at the inner corner of the eye, so that medication doesn't drain through it too quickly. The longer the medicine stays on your eyeball, the more effective it will be.

9. Don't rub the eye, squeeze the eyelid or blink. If you need to use more than one drop in the eye, wait five or more minutes before applying the next drop.
10. Don't rinse the dropper.
11. If you have shaky hands or poor aim, you can try the closed-eye method: Drops can be placed on the inner corner of the closed eye so that they fall into the eye when it's opened. Once you've done this, follow steps six through eight above.

When using eye drugs in ointment form, follow these guidelines:

1. Hold the tube of ointment between your palms for a few minutes to warm it, so that it can flow more easily out of the tube.
2. Wash your hands thoroughly.
3. Tilt your head backwards or lie down and roll your eyes upward.
4. Pull out the lower eyelid to make a pouch.
5. Squeeze one-quarter to one-half inch of ointment along the lower lid.
6. Close the eye for one to two minutes and roll the eyeball around to distribute the medication.

7. Your vision may be blurry for a few minutes; don't immediately drive or try to perform activities that require you to see clearly.

If you are using more than one kind of drop, or both drops and ointment, don't use them within five minutes of one another.

With any multi-dose container of eye drops or ointment there is risk of contamination of the tip by bacteria. If you begin to have symptoms of eye infection while using these drugs, contact your eye physician right away. You may need to stop using the medication for awhile.

adults over 50. Unlike glaucoma, macular degeneration doesn't result in complete blindness, but instead causes loss of central vision. In advanced stages of this debilitating eye disease, most of the visual field is blurred beyond recognition, rendering the person legally blind. The macula is a part of the retina that's particularly vulnerable to damage from sun and poor nutrition. Because darker eyes have more dark pigment to filter out ultraviolet rays, brown-eyed people are at lower risk than those with blue, green or hazel eyes. There's no medical treatment that stops this disease from progressing, no drugs to take. Laser surgery is a last resort, but is only done on people with very advanced disease because it carries the risk of making vision worse. Fortunately there's a lot that can be done nutritionally to prevent and control macular degeneration.

Cataracts are another very common vision problem. Clouding of the lens of the eye can be caused by too much sun exposure, an unhealthy diet over the years, heavy smoking or diabetes. The lens loses its flexibility as we age, and focusing gets more difficult. (Ever notice how many people who never needed glasses in their adult lives are suddenly wearing them when they hit 40?) The lens yellows and becomes very cloudy, blurring vision and causing uncomfortable glare from bright light.

Diabetic cataracts result from an accumulation of excess sugar in the lens. Cataracts make seeing color accurately impossible. Faces may become difficult to recognize and family members may mistakenly think the person has become senile. Elderly people who fall and break a hip may have missed seeing the step they tripped on because of cataracts. There aren't any drugs for the treatment of cataract; surgical removal of the clouded lens is the treatment of choice. It's a very simple surgery that yields excellent results, especially when a new, synthetic lens implant replaces the old lens.

Diabetic eye disease is common in both Type I (insulin-dependent) and Type II (noninsulin-dependent) diabetes. Blood vessels throughout the body are more prone to clogging with fatty deposits in diabetics. Their risk of heart disease, peripheral vascular disease and stroke is considerably higher than in the rest of the population. The blood vessels that feed the retina are especially at risk. When these vessels are unhealthy, the retina can't get the nourishment it needs. The body tries to get blood to the area by actually sprouting new blood vessels to bypass the clogged ones. Unfortunately, they grow over the retina, causing blindness. Laser surgery and vitrectomy (where blood that has leaked into the eyeball is "vacuumed" out) are the only medical treatments available for diabetic retinopathy, and by the time these are needed, the disease is advanced. Good nutrition and the right supplements can do a great deal to keep things from going that far.

WHAT CAUSES IRRITATED EYES?

Itchy, runny, allergic, bloodshot, dry, gritty or burning eyes are common complaints for which we tend to buy over-the-counter eye drops. It's estimated that over 30 million Americans complain of dry eyes.

PRESERVATIVES COMMONLY USED IN EYE DROPS

A preservative used in glaucoma and other eye drops, *benzalkonium chloride*, has been shown to worsen dry eyes and to actually be toxic to the cells of the cornea. Look for preservative-free artificial tears. If you have to use glaucoma eye drops, you'll be exposed to benzalkonium chloride; they aren't made without preservatives.

Thimerosal is another eye drop preservative that can cause problems. It isn't hard to find thimerosal-free drops, but again, if you have to use a certain prescription eye drug you may not have an alternative. If your eyes become dry while using these drugs, try our nutritional and lifestyle prescriptions to relieve dry eye symptoms.

Smog, chemical irritants, contact lenses (which can pull moisture off of the eyes), low humidity, cigarette smoke, dust, wind, sun, air conditioning, heaters, chronic crying (which dilutes the viscous tear film that keeps moisture in), and droopy lower eyelids (which can allow tears to evaporate too quickly) are common causes of dry eye. People who suffer from arthritis tend to have dry eyes. In Sjogren's syndrome, which affects mostly women over the age of 40, the eyes and mouth become very dry. Tooth decay and severe eye discomfort can result.

A long list of medicines can cause dry eyes, and benzalkonium chloride, a preservative used in most eye drops, may make dry eyes worse. If you are taking any type of medication and are suffering from dry eyes, be sure to check the package insert to find out if one of the drug's side effects is dry eyes or vision problems. Aspartame (NutraSweet) has also been shown to cause dry eyes.

If you have any of these eye diseases, or are at risk for them, read the book *Save Your Sight* (Warner Books, 1998) by Drs. Marc and Michael Rose, twin brothers and eye doctors who have made good nutrition and supplements a primary part of their prescription for good eye health.

PRESCRIPTION DRUGS FOR THE EYES

Glaucoma Drugs: Sympathomimetics

APRACLONIDINE (Iopidine)

BRIMONIDINE (Alphagan)

DIPIVEFRINE (Propine)

EPINEPHRINE (Epifrin, Glaucon)

WHAT DO THEY DO IN THE BODY?

These drugs increase the outflow of fluid (aqueous humor) from the eyeball. They also reduce the production of aqueous humor.

WHAT ARE THEY USED FOR?

Decreasing eye fluid pressure in people with ocular hypertension or glaucoma.

WHAT ARE THE POTENTIAL SIDE EFFECTS/ADVERSE EFFECTS?

Alphagan: Ten to 30 percent of those who use this drug have dry mouth, blood congestion in the eyes, burning and stinging, headache, blurred vision, feeling of having something stuck in the eye, fatigue or drowsiness, inflamed eyelash follicles or eyelids, eye allergy symptoms and itching of the eye.

Other side effects include staining or erosion of the cornea, increased sensitivity to light, redness or swelling of the eyelids or conjunctiva, aching or dry eyes, eye irritation, tearing, upper respiratory problems, dizziness, gastrointestinal problems, weakness, whitening or hemorrhage of the conjunctiva, abnormal vision, muscle pain, lid crusting, abnormal sense of taste, insomnia, depression, high blood pressure, anxiety, palpitations, nasal dryness and fainting.

Epinephrine: These drops tend to cause a lot of stinging and burning, which may lessen over time. Other side effects include eye pain or ache, headache, allergic reaction on eyelid, swelling or change in color of the conjunctiva, change in color of the cornea, eye irritation, deposits on the conjunctiva or cornea (with long-standing use), headache, palpitations, rapid heartbeat or other cardiac arrhythmias, high blood pressure and faintness.

Dipivefrin: This is turned into epinephrine in the body and has most of the same adverse effects, but is less irritating to the eyes.

Apraclonidine: blood congestion in the eyes, eye itching, discomfort and tearing, swelling of the eyelids, and feeling of having something stuck in the eye. Many other side effects have been reported, but they are rare.

CAUTION!

- Most of these drops contain a preservative called benzalkonium chloride which can be absorbed by soft contacts. Take out lenses before using glaucoma drops and wait at least 15 minutes before putting them back in.

- If you have clinical depression, Buerger's disease, Raynaud's phenomenon, orthostatic hypotension (drastic dips in blood pressure when you sit up from lying or stand up from sitting), diabetes, hyperthyroidism, bronchial asthma or kidney or liver impairment, you should be cautious when using any sympathomimetic eye drop.
- Those with high blood pressure, cerebrovascular disease (clogging of blood vessels in the brain which can lead to stroke) or heart disease should use caution, as these drugs can cause blood pressure to rise slightly.
- Elderly people are especially vulnerable to side effects from these drugs.
- Sympathomimetic drugs can cause fatigue or drowsiness, and most of these drugs alter vision temporarily; be careful while driving.

Brimonidine (Alphagan) may lose its pressure-lowering effect over time, so your eye pressure should be checked regularly.

Epinephrine can cause attacks of narrow-angle glaucoma. Your eye doctor should check to be sure you are not at risk for this before starting you on epinephrine.

If you have had a lens removed from one of your eyes due to cataract, epinephrine can cause damage to the tiny spot on the retina called the macula. If you have a rapid loss of vision in that eye, stop using epinephrine right away.

Don't wear soft contacts while using epinephrine. Your lenses could change color.

If you are using **dipivefrin (Propine)** and miss a dose, don't try to "catch up" on a missed dose by taking two at once.

You should not use **apraclonidine (Iopidine)** if you are taking monoamine oxidase inhibitors (MAO inhibitors). Iopidine's effectiveness may decrease over a month's time. Some people who take iopidine are hypersensitive and suffer from blood congestion in the eye, itching, general discomfort, tearing, feeling of having something stuck in the eye and swelling of the eyelids and conjunctiva. If you have these problems, you need to try a different drug.

WHAT ARE THE INTERACTIONS WITH OTHER DRUGS?

Brimonidine: Central nervous system depressants such as alcohol, barbiturates, opiates, sedatives or anesthetics can have additive effects with Alphagan. You may not be able to tolerate your usual number of drinks, or your sleep or pain pills may really knock you out.

Beta-blockers (both ophthalmic and systemic) and other high blood pressure drugs, as well as cardiac glycosides such as digoxin, can add to the reductions in pulse and blood pressure that can occur with brimonidine.

Tricyclic antidepressants can shorten the duration of action or decrease the effectiveness of this drug in the body.

Epinephrine: The following drugs may increase potency or prolong the actions of epinephrine:

↑ Alpha-adrenergic blockers such as phentolamine
　Antihistamines
　Bretylium may result in arrhythmias
　Cardiac glycosides may result in arrhythmias
　Guanethidine may result in severe hypertension
　Halogenated hydrocarbon anesthetics
　Levothyroxine
　Other sympathomimetic drugs may lead to toxicity and serious
　　arrhythmias
　Tricyclic antidepressants

The following drugs may reduce potency or shorten the actions of epinephrine:

↓ Some beta-blockers (propanolol, nadolol, timolol, penbutolol, carteolol,
　　sotalol and pindolol)
　Diuretics
　Ergot alkaloids and phenothiazines

Apraclonidine: This drug may reduce pulse and blood pressure, and many cardiovascular drugs also have this effect. Pulse and blood pressure should be checked frequently if these drugs are combined. Apraclonidine and MAO inhibitors should not be used together.

Beta-Blocker Eye Drops

BETAXOLOL (Betoptic, Betoptic S)

CARTEOLOL (Ocupress)

LEVOBUNOLOL (AKBeta, Betagan Liquifilm)

METIPRANOLOL (OptiPranolol)

TIMOLOL (Timoptic, Timoptic-XE)

WHAT DO THEY DO IN THE BODY?

When used as eye drops, these drugs decrease the rate of production of aqueous humor (fluid) in the eyeball.

WHAT ARE THEY USED FOR?

Lowering of intraocular pressure in glaucoma.

WHAT ARE THE POTENTIAL SIDE EFFECTS/ADVERSE EFFECTS?

Headache, depression, heart rhythm irregularities, fainting, stroke or cerebral ischemia (insufficient oxygen going to parts of the brain), and cardiovascular effects such as heart rhythm changes, heart attack, stroke, heart failure, cardiac arrest (usually in elderly people who already are at risk for heart attack, stroke, heart failure and other cardiovascular problems), palpitations, nausea, bronchospasm, respiratory failure, masking of low blood sugar in those with insulin-dependent diabetes, inflammation of the cornea, drooping of the upper eyelid, visual disturbances and double vision have occurred with all of the ophthalmic beta-blockers.

Carteolol (Ocupress): eye irritation, burning, tearing, blood congestion in the conjunctiva, swelling, blurred or cloudy vision, sensitivity to light, decreased night vision, eyelid inflammation, abnormal staining or sensitivity of the cornea, decreased blood pressure, shortness of breath, weakness, dizziness, insomnia, sinus inflammation, changes in sense of taste.

Metipranolol (OptiPranolol): eye irritation, eyelid dermatitis or inflammation, blurred vision, tearing, brow ache, abnormal vision, sensitivity to light, swelling, allergic reaction, weakness, high blood pressure, heart attack, heart rhythm irregularities, angina, nausea, runny nose, shortness of breath, nosebleed, bronchitis, coughing, dizziness, anxiety, depression, sleepiness, nervousness, arthritis, muscle pain, rash.

Levobunolol (AKBeta, Betagan): burning and stinging, eyelid inflammation, decreased corneal sensitivity.

Timolol (Timoptic, Timoptic-XE): eye irritation, conjunctivitis, eyelid inflammation, decreased corneal sensitivity, visual disturbances such as double vision, dizziness, fatigue, lethargy, hallucinations, confusion, shortness of breath, aggravation of myasthenia gravis, hair loss, change in color of fingernails, hypersensitivity resulting in rash, itching, weakness, impotence, decreased libido, electrolyte imbalances, diarrhea and tingling of the extremities.

CAUTION! DON'T USE THESE DRUGS IF . . .

- You have bronchial asthma or chronic obstructive pulmonary disease.
- You have a heart rhythm disorder called sinus bradycardia (very slow heart rate), or if you have second-degree or third-degree atrioventricular block.
- You have congestive heart failure or have ever had cardiogenic shock.

These eye drops can be absorbed in large enough amounts to cause the systemic reactions seen with beta-blocker pills. Fatal asthma attacks in asthmatics and cardiac failure in those with heart disease have been reported with use of beta-blocker eye drops.

Beta-blockers can increase the risks of surgical anesthesia, potentially causing pronounced dips in blood pressure during surgery. If you are having heart surgery, beta-blockers can make it harder to restart your heart.

If you are diabetic, please remember that beta-blockers may mask the symptoms of dangerously low blood sugar. Symptoms of hyperthyroidism (including very rapid heartbeat) may also be masked.

If your physician has ever told you that you have cerebrovascular insufficiency (too little blood flowing to parts of the brain), beta-blockers can worsen the problem.

WHAT ARE THE INTERACTIONS WITH OTHER DRUGS?

The accepted wisdom used to be that eye drops and other topical medications wouldn't enter the bloodstream enough to affect the rest of the body, but we now know that's not true. If you're taking any type of drug that interacts with the beta-blockers (see Chapter 9), you should be watchful for adverse reactions.

Oral (usually given to lower blood pressure) and topical beta-blockers (for glaucoma) used together can become overwhelming to the body. Dangerous adverse side effects become much more likely.

Ophthalmic epinephrine used together with ophthalmic beta-blockers may not be a good combination. Increased blood pressure can result.

Don't combine these drugs with the heart medication verapamil. Timolol and verapamil together have caused very slow heartbeat and cardiac arrest.

The heart drug quinidine can raise levels of timolol to dangerous levels.

WHAT ELSE TO DO WHILE TAKING THIS DRUG

Take 200 to 600 mg of chromium to help boost "good" HDL cholesterol while using beta-blocker eye drops.

Direct-Acting Miotics

CARBACHOL (Miostat)

PILOCARPINE (Isopto Carpine, Pilocar, Piloptic, Pilostat, Adsorbocarbine, Akarpine, Pilopine HS)

WHAT DO THEY DO IN THE BODY?

When applied to the eye, they cause the pupils to constrict. This allows more aqueous humor (fluid) to flow out of the back of the eyeball.

WHAT ARE THEY USED FOR?

Lowering of intraocular pressure in glaucoma.

WHAT ARE THE POTENTIAL SIDE EFFECTS/ADVERSE EFFECTS?

Carbachol: transient stinging and burning, clouding of the cornea, blisters on the cornea, inflammation of the iris after cataract extraction, retinal detachment, inflammation of the ciliary bodies and conjunctiva, spasm of the ciliary bodies (which makes vision less acute), headache, salivation, gastrointestinal cramps, vomiting, diarrhea, asthma, fainting, heart rhythm irregularities, flushing, sweating, stomach distress, a feeling of tightness in the bladder, low blood pressure, frequent need to urinate.

Pilocarpine: transient stinging and burning, tearing, spasm of the ciliary bodies (which makes vision less acute), blood congestion of the conjunctiva, headache, inflammation of the cornea, nearsightedness (especially in younger people when first starting with this drug), blurred vision, difficulty adapting to darkness, and poor dim light vision (especially in those with cataracts), hypertension, very fast heartbeat, airway tightening, fluid in the lungs, excessive salivation, sweating, nausea, vomiting.

CAUTION! DON'T USE THESE DRUGS IF . . .

- You have acute iritis, acute or anterior uveitis, secondary glaucoma (with some exceptions), pupillary block glaucoma, or acute inflammatory disease of the anterior chamber.
- You have an abrasion on your cornea. This makes excessive penetration of the medication carbachol more likely.
- You have recently had a heart attack, or if you have heart failure, asthma, stomach ulcer, hyperthyroidism, gastrointestinal spasm, urinary tract obstruction, Parkinson's disease, hypertension or hypotension. Use caution when using direct-acting miotics.

Before starting to use these drugs, you should be sure your ophthalmologist gives you a thorough eye examination. Some people are more susceptible to retinal detachment than others, and miotics can cause this to happen in those people.

Use caution while driving at night. Miotics affect your ability to see in the dark.

In susceptible people, miotics can bring on attacks of angle-closure glaucoma.

WHAT ARE THE INTERACTIONS WITH OTHER DRUGS?

Carbachol and topical nonsteroidal anti-inflammatory drugs (NSAIDs) may cancel out each other's actions in the eye so that neither has the desired effect.

WHAT ELSE TO DO WHILE TAKING THESE DRUGS

Take 1000 to 3000 mg a day of the bioflavonoids quercetin and rutin.

Cholinesterase-Inhibiting Miotics

DEMECARIUM (Humorsol)

ECHOTHIOPHATE (Phospholine Iodide)

PHYSOSTIGMINE (Eserine Sulfate)

WHAT DO THEY DO IN THE BODY?

Cause complete, rapid shrinking of the pupil of the eye.

WHAT ARE THEY USED FOR?

Lowering of intraocular pressure in ocular hypertension or glaucoma.

WHAT ARE THE POTENTIAL SIDE EFFECTS/ADVERSE EFFECTS?

Iris cysts, burning, watering of the eyes, twitching of the eyelid, redness of the conjunctiva and ciliary bodies, headache, nearsightedness and blurring, retinal detachment, cataract, nausea, vomiting, abdominal cramps, diarrhea, urinary incontinence, fainting, sweating, excessive salivation, difficulty breathing, heart problems, and thickening of the conjunctiva. Deterioration of the nasal canals and tear ducts can occur with long-term use.

Cysts may grow on the iris of the eye treated with these drugs. These can grow large enough to interfere with vision. They usually shrink or disappear when the drug is stopped. You should have regular eye exams to be sure you aren't developing any iris cysts.

CAUTION! DON'T TAKE THESE DRUGS IF . . .

- You have active uveal inflammation or any inflammatory disease of the iris or ciliary body.
- You have glaucoma associated with iridocyclitis.
- You have any kind of angle-closure glaucoma. Don't use echothiophate. The other drugs in this class can also aggravate angle-closure glaucoma.
- You have myasthenia gravis. If you are taking cholinesterase inhibitors to control it, using topical cholinesterase inhibitors puts you at greater risk for adverse effects.

Overexcitability of the vagus nerve (vagotonia), asthma, gastrointestinal spasm, stomach ulcer, very slow heartbeat or low blood pressure, recent heart attack, epilepsy and Parkinson's disease all put you at greater risk of problems with cholinesterase-inhibitor eye drops.

The shrinking of the pupil (miosis) caused by this drug limits your ability to adapt to darkness. Use caution while driving at night.

You should discontinue these drugs three to four weeks before having eye surgery.

WHAT ARE THE INTERACTIONS WITH OTHER DRUGS?

Avoid contact with carbamate or organophosphate insecticides and pesticides while using cholinesterase inhibitors. (Avoid them no matter what!)

Succinylcholine, a general anesthetic, can cause respiratory and cardiovascular collapse in people using these drugs.

Systemic and topical cholinesterase inhibitors have additive effects and can be a dangerous combination.

WHAT ELSE TO DO WHILE TAKING THESE DRUGS

Take 1000 to 3000 mg a day of the bioflavonoids quercetin and rutin.

MISCELLANEOUS GLAUCOMA DRUGS

DORZOLAMIDE (Trusopt)

WHAT DOES IT DO IN THE BODY?

Trusopt is a carbonic anhydrase inhibitor. Inhibition of this enzyme system causes the eye to make less aqueous humor (fluid).

WHAT IS IT USED FOR?

Lowering of intraocular pressure in ocular hypertension or glaucoma.

WHAT ARE THE POTENTIAL SIDE EFFECTS/ADVERSE EFFECTS?

Bitter taste in the mouth and burning, stinging and discomfort in the eye right after medication is used, inflammation of the cornea, symptoms of eye allergy, blurred vision, tearing, dryness, increased sensitivity to light, headache, nausea, skin rashes and calcium deposits in the urinary tract (urolithiasis).

CAUTION!

- Dorzolamide is a sulfa drug, similar to sulfa antibiotics. Enough is absorbed into the bloodstream when it's used topically to bring on the same adverse reactions that can occur with sulfa antibiotics. Some people have severe reactions to these drugs, which have in a few cases been fatal. Look out for any signs of hypersensitivity, including itching, rash, swelling of the eye sockets, difficulty breathing and blood congestion in the conjunctiva or sclera (part of the tough covering over the eyeball).

- If you have any kind of kidney impairment, you should not use dorzolamide. Those with less than full liver function should use with caution.
- Don't use these drops while wearing soft contact lenses. They contain benzalkonium chloride which can be absorbed into lenses.

LATANOPROST (Xalatan)

WHAT DOES IT DO IN THE BODY?

Latanoprost resembles chemicals made in the body called prostaglandins. The body's natural prostaglandins increase the outflow of fluid from the eyeball, and this drug enhances this effect.

WHAT IS IT USED FOR?

Lowering of elevated intraocular pressure in ocular hypertension or glaucoma. It's used in cases where other medications don't work or are not as effective as they need to be.

WHAT ARE THE POTENTIAL SIDE EFFECTS/ADVERSE EFFECTS?

Blurred vision, burning and stinging, blood congestion in the conjunctiva, feeling of having something stuck in the eye, itching, darkening of the iris, inflammation of the cornea, dry eye, excessive tearing, eye pain, crusting over the eyelid, swelling and redness of the eyelid, eyelid discomfort and pain, increased sensitivity to sun, upper respiratory infection, cold, flu, muscle pain, rash, allergic reaction.

CAUTION!

- Latanoprost may cause a permanent change of eye color from blue, green or hazel to brown. The change happens gradually, with pigment darkening from the pupil outward.

- Don't use latanoprost while wearing contact lenses. Benzalkonium chloride, a preservative used in many eye drops, can accumulate on lenses.

WHAT ARE THE INTERACTIONS WITH OTHER DRUGS?

Don't use latanoprost within five minutes of any eye drop containing thimerosal.

EYE DROPS FOR ALLERGIES AND OTHER TYPES OF EYE IRRITATION

Ophthalmic Vasoconstrictors

NAPHAZOLINE (Allerest Eye Drops, Clear Eyes, Degest 2, Naphcon, Allergy Drops, VasoClear, Comfort Eye Drops, Maximum Strength Allergy Drops, AK-Con, Albalon, Nafazair, Naphcon Forte, Vasocon Regular)

OXYMETAZOLINE (OcuClear, Visine L.R.)

PHENYLEPHRINE (Paredrine)

TETRAHYDROZOLINE (Collyrium Fresh, Eyesine, Geneye, Mallazine Eye Drops, Murine Plus, Optigene 3, Tetrasene, Visine)

WHAT DO THEY DO IN THE BODY?

In low concentrations sold over the counter, these drugs cause the blood vessels in the eyes to constrict. They stimulate the sympathetic nervous system and so are sometimes called sympathomimetics.

WHAT ARE THEY USED FOR?

Relief of eye redness and irritation.

WHAT ARE THE POTENTIAL SIDE EFFECTS/ADVERSE EFFECTS?

Stinging when first instilled, blurred vision, pupil dilation, increased redness, irritation, discomfort, inflammation of the cornea, tearing, increased intraocular pressure, palpitations, heart arrhythmias, high blood pressure, heart attack, burst blood vessels in the lungs or brain, stroke, headache, blanching, trembling, sweating, dizziness, nausea, nervousness, drowsiness, weakness and high blood sugar. (The more serious of these tend to happen with prescription-strength doses, not the over-the-counter varieties.)

CAUTION!

- Don't use these drugs if you have narrow-angle glaucoma or a predisposition to this problem.
- Overuse of these drugs can cause eye redness or rebound congestion.
- If you have high blood pressure, diabetes, hyperthyroidism, cardiovascular problems or hardening of the arteries, you are at greater risk for side effects.
- Phenylephrine can cause floaters in the aqueous humor of elderly people. It can also temporarily blur or destabilize vision, so be cautious when driving or performing other hazardous tasks.

WHAT ARE THE INTERACTIONS WITH OTHER DRUGS?

The following drugs may increase levels or prolong the effects of ophthalmic vasoconstrictors:

↑ Beta-blockers
  Monoamine oxidase (MAO) inhibitors

As with any eye drop, if used long enough or in high enough doses, other side effects and drug interactions usually only seen in those using the drug internally can occur. See Chapter 11.

Ophthalmic Corticosteroids

DEXAMETHASONE (AK-Dex, Decadron Phosphate, Maxidex)

FLUOROMETHOLONE (Fluor-Op, Flarex, FML, FML Forte, FML S.O.P.)

MEDRYSONE (HMS)

PREDNISOLONE (Pred Mild, Econopred, AK-Pred, Inflamase Mild, Econopred Plus, Pred Forte)

RIMEXOLONE (Vexol)

TOBRADEX, a combination steroid and antibiotic

WHAT DO THEY DO IN THE BODY?

Decrease inflammation.

WHAT ARE THEY USED FOR?

Allergic conjunctivitis, corneal inflammation (keratitis) including herpes zoster keratitis, iris inflammation (iritis), inflammation of the ciliary bodies that control pupil size (cyclitis), treatment of injuries to the cornea and some forms of eye infection.

WHAT ARE THE POTENTIAL SIDE EFFECTS/ADVERSE EFFECTS?

Raising of intraocular pressure with optic nerve damage (glaucoma), loss of some visual ability, formation of cataracts, eye infections including ocular herpes simplex, perforation of the eyeball, worsening of fungal infections of the eye, stinging or burning when drops are instilled, blurred vision, discharge, discomfort, eye pain, feeling of having something stuck in the eye, blood congestion, itching.

With longtime use or high doses of steroid eye drops, enough can be absorbed into the bloodstream to cause systemic side effects.

Corticosteroid drugs can also cause an outbreak of intestinal or vaginal candida (see Chapter 10).

CAUTION! DON'T USE THESE DRUGS IF . . .

- You are having an outbreak of herpes virus of the cornea (herpes simplex keratitis).
- You have any fungal eye disease.
- You have ocular tuberculosis.
- You have just had a foreign object removed from your cornea.

While using steroid eye drops, you should have frequent exams to be sure you aren't developing elevated eye pressure or cataracts.

Any steroid drug can mask signs of infection. See your eye physician regularly to nip dangerous infections in the bud.

WHAT ARE THE INTERACTIONS WITH OTHER DRUGS?

No specific interactions of steroid eye drops with other eye medications have been reported.

Over-the-Counter Antihistamine Eye Drops

ANTAZOLINE (Vasocon-A)

PHENIRAMINE MALEATE (Naphcon-A, AK-Con-A, Opcon-A)

WHAT DO THEY DO IN THE BODY?

Block the actions of histamine in the eye. All products containing these drugs also contain the decongestant naphazoline.

WHAT ARE THEY USED FOR?

Temporary relief of itchy, watering eyes caused by allergies.

WHAT ARE THE POTENTIAL SIDE EFFECTS/ADVERSE EFFECTS?

Burning, stinging and discomfort when instilled. Ophthalmic antihistamines may also cause pupils to dilate.

CAUTION! DON'T USE THESE DRUGS IF . . .

- You are at risk for angle-closure glaucoma.

NATURAL ALTERNATIVES TO EYE DRUGS

First let's talk about your eyes and the sun. Despite all the bad press it's getting lately, sunshine is a nutrient essential for the health of your eyes and the rest of your body. Sunlight striking the retina keeps it active, much like exercise keeps your body fit. It stimulates the glands to produce hormones that regulate our waking and sleeping cycles, fluid balance and mood. Vitamin D is made by your body and stored in your liver when you go out in the sun. If there's a shortage of vitamin D, calcium metabolism in your body is thrown off, and bones begin to deteriorate.

On the other hand, too much sunlight can do you harm. Ultraviolet rays are invisible to our eyes but can cause cataracts, skin cancer, temporary blindness from glare off sand, snow or water, growths on the eyes called *pterygia*, macular degeneration and melanoma on the back of the eyeball. Sunlight causes an increase in the rate at which harmful free radicals are produced in the eye, which can contribute to getting eye diseases that can make you go blind.

Put on Your Shades

The first step to take in prevention of cataracts and macular degeneration is to invest in a pair of sunglasses that block 100 percent of ultraviolet rays. You can also buy sun goggles that fit over your prescription glasses. The best sunglasses also filter out some blue light. A hat with a brim should also accompany you out into the sunshine. You don't have to be fanatical about it unless you already have severe eye disease, because your eyes need some ultraviolet light. The majority of the time you spend outdoors, however, you should be wearing these sun-protection accessories.

Nutrition for Healthy Eyes

People with eye diseases such as glaucoma, cataracts and macular degeneration can often prevent or slow the disease with some dietary changes and the right supplements. The mainstay of an eye-healthy diet is a wide variety of fresh vegetables (especially the deep green, leafy variety), fruits and whole grains, complemented by good protein sources such as deep-water fish, eggs, chicken and turkey. Red meat is okay, but not every day.

Eggs are loaded with sulfur, a mineral your body needs to make glutathione, an antioxidant substance essential for eye health. Asparagus, onions and garlic are also good sources of sulfur.

Deep-water fish is rich in vitamins D and A, and in DHA, an essential fatty acid. Fish oils improve circulation in the tiny blood vessels of the eye. Whatever you can do to keep your blood vessels healthy will insure that the retina and optic nerve cells get plenty of oxygen and nourishment.

Of course, the more you avoid refined, processed foods loaded with sugar, white flour, hydrogenated oils, artificial flavorings and colorings, the healthier your whole body will be.

Especially good foods for healthy eyes include berries, watermelon and carrots for their bioflavonoids and carotenoids, any foods rich in vitamin C such as citrus fruits and kiwi, as well as foods rich in essential fatty acids such as almonds, olive oil and avocados. While you replace "bad" fats like artery-clogging hydrogenated vegetable oils with the "good" fats listed, try to keep daily fat intake below 30 percent of total calories.

Avoid optic nerve toxins like aspartame, MSG (monosodium glutamate), steroid drugs, tranquilizers, the antidepressants lithium and monoamine oxidase (MAO) inhibitors, antibiotics and cigarettes.

Vitamins for Healthy Eyes

Certain nutrients are more important to good eye health than others. If you have an eye disease, or are at risk for one, please supplement your daily vitamins with the following:

- Vitamin C, at least 1000 mg of vitamin C a day, with bioflavonoids
- A mixed carotenoid supplement
- Vitamin E, 400 IU
- Vitamin A, 10,000 IU a day
- Quercetin and rutin are bioflavonoids that help keep your retinas healthy; try 1000 to 1,500 mg a day.
- Magnesium at bedtime, between 300 to 400 mg
- Coenzyme Q10 is a great circulation booster, 90 to 200 mg a day
- Carnitine can help boost the heart's pumping power and get more nourishment to your optic nerves and retinas.
- Selenium, a mineral with powerful antioxidant and antiviral potential, protects cell membranes from being destroyed by free radicals.
- N-acetyl cysteine, an amino acid, helps to keep your body's antioxidant defenses strong and increases the production of glutathione, 500 mg two to three times a day.
- Those with macular degeneration or cataract should get 10 to 15 mg of zinc a day, either in a multivitamin or a separate supplement.

NATURAL REMEDIES FOR EYE DISEASES

Glaucoma

If you have glaucoma, you can try an herbal remedy that's been used in India for centuries. Derived from the coleus plant, forskohlin relaxes blood vessel walls to relieve high blood pressure and high intraocular pressure. Look for capsules of *forskohlhii* and take 200 to 400 mg per day.

You can supplement omega-3 fish oils in capsules or liquid form; the DHA, an essential fatty acid found in fish oil, is an important component of the optic nerve lining. Take care to ensure that fish oil supplements haven't gone rancid. Keep them in the fridge and use a brand that contains a natural preservative such as vitamin E.

Vitamin B12, 1,000 to 2,000 mcg taken intranasally or sublingually, can help slow vision loss from glaucoma.

Macular Degeneration

If you have been diagnosed with macular degeneration, start taking a lutein/zeaxanthin supplement right away. Lutein and zeaxanthin are protective yellow pigments that cover the macula and protect it from light damage. These carotenoids are found naturally in foods like spinach, collard greens and kale. Supplements are usually derived from marigold petals. Make an effort to take them at different times than your multivitamin if it contains beta-carotene, because they can block each other's path into the body. Also eat beta-carotene rich foods and lutein/zeaxanthin-rich foods at different meals.

Diabetic Eye Disease

Diabetics should use 1000 to 1,500 mg of quercetin and 200 mcg of chromium a day. Quercetin inhibits an enzyme that may be directly responsible for the formation of sugar cataracts, while chromium helps to balance blood sugar.

To slow the progression of cataracts, include plenty of tofu, eggs, asparagus, onions, garlic, carrots, cantaloupe, yams, corn and leafy greens in your diet. Make sure you're getting 50 mg of riboflavin in your multivitamin, or add an extra riboflavin supplement. Please don't hesitate to have cataracts extracted if you feel your quality of life is being compromised. These days it's a relatively risk-free surgery.

For control of diabetic retinopathy, control of diabetes is essential. Check blood sugars at least four times a day and keep levels in the range your physician has recommended. A diet rich in colorful vegetables, fruits and whole grains, moderation in the drinking of alcohol and intake of sugar and refined flour, daily exercise and maintenance of a healthy weight are all important for the diabetic.

See Chapter 15 for details on natural alternatives to diabetes drugs.

Diabetics shouldn't use a multivitamin with iron, because iron can increase the formation of free radicals. (I don't recommend daily iron for any adult over the age of 30 or for men at any age.)

Eye Allergies

Those who see a doctor with the complaint of itchy, watery, allergic eyes are generally prescribed antihistamine, decongestant or steroid eye drops. An eye doctor can distinguish eye allergy from dry eye by checking for small bumps along the lower eyelid. These drugs can be useful for temporary symptom relief, but it's important to support your body nutritionally with the goal of reducing or eliminating the need for eye drops. These drugs have too many side effects to justify their use for more than a couple of days at a time. See the chapter on allergy drugs for details on natural remedies.

Aside from supporting your body nutritionally, your best strategy for avoiding allergies is to determine what irritates your eyes and try your best to avoid exposure. Women may need to change to a different kind of eye makeup or stop using it altogether. Hair sprays, certain eye drops or contact lens solutions can cause allergic reactions in some people. Fumes from copy machines and laser printers can have a strongly irritating effect too.

Quercetin can be very helpful in decreasing allergic inflammation. Take 1,000 to 2,000 mg a day and eat plenty of red onions, Brussels sprouts, red apples, bell peppers, asparagus and kale. Vitamin B6 taken with omega-6 essential fatty acids (found in evening primrose oil) can also take the edge off of eye allergies. Vitamin C (1000 to 2,000 mg a day) also helps relieve allergic inflammation.

Dry Eyes

Before you turn to constant use of artificial tears to relieve dry eyes, try to improve your eyes' ability to keep themselves moist. Here are some tips for treating dry eyes:

- Buy a humidifier and use it whenever you turn on the heater or air conditioner in your home.
- Avoid smog, ozone and fumes.
- Don't use products that contain aspartame (NutraSweet).
- Wear wraparound sunglasses outside to keep tears from evaporating.

- Soft contacts can cause dry eyes, so keep glasses around to wear when your eyes feel uncomfortable.
- Try to blink more.
- If you work at a computer, arrange your workspace so that you are looking slightly downward at the screen, lids lowered.
- Don't use a lot of eye makeup.
- Check to be sure your glasses aren't pulling your lower lids away from your eyes.
- Use only preservative-free eye drops (preservatives can actually worsen dry eyes).
- Eat more fruit, vegetables, walnuts and cold-water fish.
- Evening primrose oil capsules (500 to 1500 mg per day), 1,000 to 2,000 mg of vitamin C and 50 mg of B6 can also help relieve eye dryness.

DRUGS THAT CAN CAUSE DRY EYES

Antihistamines	Diuretics
Atropine	Isotretinoin
Benzodiazepine tranquilizers (Valium, Xanax)	Methotrexate and other cancer drugs
Beta-blockers (taken by mouth or as eye drops)	Morphine
Codeine	Scopolamine
Decongestants (taken by mouth or as eye drops)	Some glaucoma eye drops
	Tricyclic antidepressant (Elavil)

CHAPTER 17

Drugs for the Prostate and Their Natural Alternatives

OVER 20 PERCENT of all American men over the age of 50 will develop prostate problems of some kind, and one in 11 will develop prostate cancer. By the time they are 70, over 50 percent of American men will have an enlarged prostate gland, and by the time they are 80, the number goes up to 85 percent. This amounts to an epidemic of prostate problems, and once again it looks like bad fats and excessive estrogen in the environment may be the biggest culprits. Nutritional deficiencies also play a role, but you'll find out more about that later. What "modern" medicine has to offer you if you have prostate troubles are drugs and surgery that are only sometimes effective and often have side effects such as impotence and urinary dysfunction (for surgery, these side effects are permanent).

If you have been following the Six Core Principles for Optimal Health, which include a low-fat diet, a daily supplement of zinc, and six to eight glasses of clean water daily, you are probably free of prostate problems.

WHAT IS THE PROSTATE GLAND?

The prostate is a gland in men located at the neck of the bladder and urethra (the tube through which urine and semen pass on the way out of the body). It's about the size of a grain of rice when you are born, and by the time you're in your twenties it's about the size and shape of a chestnut. Starting at puberty, the gland produces a milky fluid that mixes with semen during ejaculation.

The prostate stays about the same size until you reach the age when some male hormones begin to decline (in most men, their fifties), and the prostate begins to grow again. This is called benign prostatic hypertrophy (BPH). If the gland grows too much, it begins to pinch the urethra, interfering with urination. Symptoms of an enlarged prostate can include dribbling, a decrease in the size of the stream during urination, frequent or difficult urination, and chronic discomfort in the abdominal area.

WHAT CAUSES PROSTATE ENLARGEMENT?

Some scientists believe that when testosterone production declines, other male hormones synthesized from testosterone not only decline, but are thrown out of balance, causing prostate enlargement. Unfortunately the answer is not as simple as giving men testosterone supplementation—we learned the hard way that this not only causes the prostate to enlarge even more, it can also cause the growth of prostate tumors. However, it's not clear whether those effects are caused by the synthetic testosterones only or an excessively high dose of testosterone. Few studies have been done with real testosterone in small doses.

Dihydrotestosterone (DHT) is a hormone synthesized from testosterone that is thought to contribute to prostate enlargement. The drug Proscar (finasteride) is supposed to keep testosterone from producing DHT. However this drug has only been partially successful in treating prostate enlargement and has side effects (including a high price, about $2 a pill, one daily). Adverse reactions may include impotence, decreased libido and decreased volume of ejaculate (which most men don't think are minor problems!). The most frequent adverse effect of Proscar is breast enlargement, which is also not a minor problem.

Many studies suggest that a high-fat diet is a major culprit in prostate troubles in men. We only have theories as to why this happens, but one of the most likely is that animal fat contains estrogens that lower testosterone levels and stimulate cell growth. Estrogen is the female hormone, and one of its primary jobs in the body is to stimulate cell growth in reproductive areas. It's perfectly plausible that it would stimulate the growth of the prostate.

Estrogens are also everywhere in our environment these days, hiding mostly in plastics and pesticides that mimic estrogen's action in the body. We are also exposed to estrogens when we eat most supermarket meat. Estrogen is widely used in the livestock industry for fattening up before market. In the future the epidemic of prostate enlargement in men will most likely be found to be caused by excessive estrogen in the environment. We hope somebody will research estrogen and prostate disease in the near future.

Among Japanese men who traditionally eat a diet low in fat and high in soy products, prostate problems are rare, as they are in other cultures that favor low-fat diets. However, a study of Japanese men who moved to Hawaii and presumably began eating a typically high-fat American diet showed that they had prostate problems at the same rate as Americans.

A study of 51,000 American men ages 40 to 75 who were followed for two to four years showed that prostate cancer was directly related to total fat consumption, with red meat showing the strongest association with advanced cancer.

Another study in Italy comparing 271 men with prostate cancer to 685 men who did not have the disease concluded that a high dietary consumption of milk was a significant indicator of prostate cancer risk, even in men who also ate a lot of whole grains and fresh vegetables.

Other studies have linked prostate cancer to exposure to herbicides which are typically used in agriculture, forestry and in cities and suburbs to control weeds. Many pesticides are potent estrogen mimics.

DRUGS FOR TREATING AN ENLARGED PROSTATE

FINASTERIDE (Proscar)

WHAT DOES IT DO IN YOUR BODY?

Inhibits an enzyme that converts testosterone to dihydrotestosterone, lowering levels of DHT in the blood serum.

WHAT IS IT PRESCRIBED FOR?

Benign prostatic hypertrophy (enlarged prostate).

WHAT ARE THE POSSIBLE SIDE EFFECTS?

Liver damage, impotence, decreased libido, decreased volume of ejaculate, breast tenderness and enlargement, rash.

CAUTION: THINK TWICE ABOUT TAKING THIS DRUG IF . . .

• You are having sex with a woman who might become pregnant. Any exposure to this drug, even in minute amounts, can cause abnormalities in the male fetus; do not use. Give the natural remedies a good try before resorting to finasteride.

WHAT ARE THE INTERACTIONS WITH OTHER DRUGS?

The following drugs may be reduced in potency or decreased in the amount of time they are effective when combined with finasteride:

↓ Theophyllines

TERAZOSIN (Hytrin)

WHAT DOES IT DO IN YOUR BODY?

Terazosin is a drug normally used to lower blood pressure, that is also prescribed to treat BPH. It doesn't work very well and the side effects certainly aren't worth it. See Chapter 9 for details on terazosin.

NATURAL REMEDIES FOR PROSTATE ENLARGEMENT

There are nutrients and herbs that can dramatically improve the symptoms of prostate enlargement in men over time. Your best bet is to find a formula that combines these ingredients.

Zinc

Zinc is necessary for the proper function of the prostate gland. In men, higher concentrations of this mineral are found in the prostate than anywhere else in the body. A recent study looked at zinc supplementation in young men, and found that when plasma zinc levels were low, there was a corresponding drop in testosterone. There have been many clinical studies showing that zinc supplementation can reduce the size of the prostate gland, along with troublesome symptoms.

It's a good idea for all men to take 10 to 15 mg of zinc daily, and include zinc-rich foods in the diet such as oysters (well-cooked, please!), lamb chops and wheat germ. Pumpkin seeds are a good source of zinc, and are also rich in the amino acids alanine, glycine and glutamic acid, which seem to have a positive effect in reducing the size of the prostate. A handful of dried pumpkin seeds a day is plenty. Please don't get pumpkin seeds that have been roasted in oil and salted—the oil is probably rancid and you don't need the extra salt. Plain roasted pumpkin seeds have a pleasant, nutty flavor. Pumpkin seed oil capsules are also available.

Selenium

Selenium is another important mineral in male hormone regulation that is found in large amounts in the prostate. Blood levels of both zinc and selenium are low in men who have prostate cancer. Men who live in areas where the soil is rich in selenium tend to have lower rates of prostate cancer. Rich sources of selenium are garlic, shellfish, grains and chicken. If you're over the age of 50 you can supplement your diet with up to 400 mcg of selenium daily.

Soy Products

Soy products such as miso, tofu and tempeh may help reduce the risk of prostate enlargement and cancer. The products contain *phytoestrogens* which take up estrogen receptor sites in the body, but only have a weak estrogenic effect on the body. This connection is only speculation at this point, but it may explain why the Japanese diet, which is heavy in soy products, is protective against prostate enlargement and tumors. There are soy supplements available that isolate the active ingredients in soy called isoflavones.

Pygeum Africanum

Pygeum Africanum, an evergreen tree from Africa, is an important part of your healthy prostate program. The bark of pygeum helps balance hormone levels and reduce prostate inflammation. Pygeum also improves the quality and quantity of prostate secretions.

Saw Palmetto

Saw palmetto is your most important prostate herb. An extract made from the berry of saw palmetto (*Serena repens*), also called sabal, a palm tree native to Florida, Texas and Georgia, has been shown in numerous studies to reduce the urinary symptoms caused by prostate enlargement. Although the exact action of saw palmetto hasn't been pinpointed, it is theorized that it inhibits the production of dihydrotestosterone (DHT). This is the same thing Merck was trying to accomplish with its drug Proscar, but as tends to happen, the herb shows no side effects, seems to be more effective, and is significantly less expensive! It's also possible that it opposes or blocks estrogen.

THE HEALTHY PROSTATE PROGRAM

The Six Core Principles for Optimal Health have all the elements of a healthy prostate diet. Here is where the special emphasis should be if you're a man over the age of 50:

Eat More . . .

Fiber
Fish oils or other sources of omega-3 fatty acids
Garlic
Hormone-free chicken (a good source of selenium)
Oysters or lamb chops every other week (a good source of zinc)
Pumpkin seeds
Soy products such as miso, tofu and tempeh (or take in capsule form)

Drink More . . .

Clean water (at least six to eight glasses daily)

Avoid . . .

Red meat (unless it is organic)
Vegetable oils and hydrogenated oils
Whole milk (yogurt is okay)

Supplements to Take

Selenium: 200 to 400 mcg daily
Zinc: 15 to 30 mg daily

Herbs to Use

Saw Palmetto: Follow directions on the bottle.

CHAPTER 18

Synthetic Hormones and Their Natural Alternatives

HORMONES ARE A hot topic these days and for good reason. Anti-aging researchers believe they are one of the keys to slowing age-related physical deterioration. The theory is that if you supplement hormones that decline with age, your body will age more slowly. Although hormones are not the fabled fountain of youth, hormone levels are directly related to aging. Your goal in hormone supplementation isn't immortality, but to maintain as high a quality of life as possible for as long as possible.

THE IMPORTANCE OF HORMONE BALANCE

Hormones play innumerable roles in the everyday workings of your body. Lack of a single hormone can make the difference between well-being and life-threatening illness. Hormonal pathways and interactions are so complex that we have only a weak grasp of exactly how they work. The body uses hormones as one way to maintain *homeostasis* (balance) in all of its systems despite drastic changes in the environment. For example, your body goes from sleep in a toasty warm bed to rising, bathing, and cooking and eating an assortment of foods. On that same day you might engage in vigorous exercise, have an emotional conflict with a loved one, relax in the sunshine, and see a sad movie. If you are working in a stressful profession, you might have to work capably while under considerable pressure. All of these activities in some way put a demand on the body to maintain balance.

You're probably most familiar with the steroid hormones progesterone, dehydroepiandrosterone or DHEA, the cortisones, the estrogens and testosterone. All of these hormones are made from a hormone called pregnenolone, which is made from cholesterol. This is why the myth that all cholesterol is bad is a dangerous one. While your body can manufacture 75 percent of its own cholesterol, the remaining 25 percent comes directly from cholesterol that you eat. Cut out all cholesterol and you're asking for a hormone imbalance.

When you drink a glass of juice, your blood sugar rises, and the hormone insulin, secreted by the pancreas, is required to bring it back down. Thyroid hormones, which regulate how the body uses energy, are secreted by the thyroid gland in the neck. Adrenaline, the cortisones and DHEA are a few of the hormones secreted by the adrenal glands. Your brain secretes the hormone melatonin in response to darkness, but it's also found in larger quantities in your intestines. Believe it or not, vitamin D is really a hormone which regulates (among other things) how your bones take up minerals.

Your hormone or *endocrine* system is actually a group of systems which work via the circulation. Hormones are secreted by glands into the bloodstream as the body demands them. For example, when you exercise, you use glucose, which your body can replace by activating *cortisol*, a hormone that allows you to manufacture more glucose in your liver. As these specialized molecules pass through the body, they are recognized by receptors on cells which fit them like a lock and key. Once the hormone locks on to the receptor it causes the cell to behave in a generally predictable way. For example, some estrogens can stimulate cell growth and testosterone can stimulate the growth of facial hair.

There are many ways your hormone systems can be thrown out of balance, which will automatically throw your health out of balance. Symptoms may be subtle or blatant. Chronic stress can cause the constant release of cortisol and adrenaline, hormones that were originally designed for occasional use only, such as hunting a woolly mammoth or fighting a bear for a cave. Routine exposure to bright lights late into the night has most likely thrown our melatonin levels out of balance. Environmental pollution is contributing to hormone imbalance thanks to thousands of plastics and pesticides with molecules that resemble estrogen and fit into estrogen receptors, stimulating an estrogen-like response in the body. The millions of women who have undergone hysterectomies are plunged into instant hormone imbalance even if their ovaries are intact. Nutritional deficiencies, which are widespread in the U.S., especially among the elderly, can cause glands to atrophy and malfunction.

In an ideal universe, we wouldn't need supplemental hormones. The systems developed over millions of years of evolution could continue to do the job just fine. Our universe being less than ideal, small amounts of natural hormone supplements can be safely used to help our bodies function optimally. *Physiologic* dosages of hormones are very small, only enough to restore balance. They are approximations of what the body itself would secrete under ideal conditions, and are much safer and work better than *pharmacologic* doses of many times what the body would make itself.

The typical medical model advocates the "more is better" philosophy. In the case of hormones, this approach is not only ineffective, but can be counterproductive. Hormones are powerful agents designed for very specific use. The use of pharmacologic dosing (often with synthetic versions of the natural hormones our bodies make) has a lot to do with the negative outcomes in many medical studies of hormone replacement. The following recommendations for hormone supplementation only involve physiologic doses of the natural hormone.

What's Wrong with Synthetic Hormones?

Physicians in the U.S. seem to have completely forgotten that synthetic, not-found-in-nature hormones are not the same as the real thing. A synthetic drug isn't one that was made in a lab, because they all are (vitamins are too), it is one that is not found in nature. Drug companies prefer that you take synthetic hormones not because they are better for you, but because they can be patented, so they can charge you more for them.

A natural substance cannot be patented, so drug company scientists take a perfectly good natural substance, take it into the lab, and add a methyl group here, an acetate group there, and *voila*! They have created a drug that has many of the same effects as the natural substance, but can be patented. Nowhere is there a better example of how tragically awry this practice has gone in our country than in hormones.

John R. Lee, M.D., a pioneer in the use of natural progesterone cream, tells a great story about a package he received in the mail from a woman who sent him copies of her medical charts and a letter pleading for help. Her physician had put her on a progestin (a synthetic progesterone) and then a few months later taken her blood and measured her progesterone levels. According to her blood test, her progesterone levels hadn't risen at all, so he increased the dose of progestins and a few months later a lab test still didn't measure any progesterone. Meanwhile the woman was suffering terribly from the side effects of the progestin. Dr. Lee pointed out to her that her physician was giving her a progestin and measuring for progesterone, and they aren't the same, so of course it didn't show up on her blood tests! This confusion is rampant throughout the medical literature, where even in the most prestigious medical journals the terms progesterone and progestin are used interchangeably, and whole theories are advanced on the basis that testing one is the same as testing the other. The real victims of this mistaken identity are the women who are prescribed progestins.

In case your physician wants to argue with you that progestins and progesterone are the same, you might remind him or her that progesterone is the first and foremost hormone necessary for a healthy pregnancy, while progestins taken during pregnancy cause birth defects. Progestins almost universally make women feel awful, while progesterone almost universally makes women feel great.

Synthetic estrogens aren't any better. For awhile the makers of Premarin were trying to convince women that the synthetic Premarin is a natural estrogen because part of it is made from the urine of pregnant mares. Horse estrogen is natural if you're a horse, but it's not natural if you're a human, and the combination is certainly not found in nature. Marla Alghrimm, R.Ph., a pharmacist who specializes in providing individualized natural hormone combination creams, has noticed that women taking Premarin suffer more from breast tenderness, water retention and high blood pressure than those taking natural estrogen.

Methyltestosterone, a synthetic version of testosterone, has a long list of side effects that natural testosterone doesn't have.

When it comes to hormone replacement therapy, there doesn't seem to be any reason why anybody, anytime, would use synthetic hormones instead of natural hormones. It just doesn't make sense if you're going for optimal health.

If at all possible, please avoid long-term use of birth control pills. They are made from synthetic hormones, they suppress your body's ovulation, and they increase the risk of strokes and breast cancer. It's just not worth it when there are so many other forms of birth control available.

Although most of the natural hormones are available by prescription, and some are available over the counter, in the prescription drugs section of this chapter only the most commonly used synthetic hormones are listed. More important is the natural hormones section of this chapter where you can find out more about taking natural hormones.

SYNTHETIC HORMONES

Synthetic Estrogens

CONJUGATED ESTROGEN (Premarin)

CONJUGATED ESTROGEN WITH A PROGESTIN (Prempro)

ESTERIFIED ESTROGENS (Estratab, Menest)

ESTROGEN COMBINATIONS (PMB 200, Menrium)

ESTROPIPATE (Ortho-Est, Ogen)

WHAT DO THEY DO IN YOUR BODY?

Natural estrogens have dozens of effects on the body, including the development and maintenance of female sex characteristics such as the ovaries, uterus and breasts. Estrogens given as hormone replacement therapy during menopause may relieve hot flashes, night sweats and vaginal dryness. The claims made for estrogens in preventing heart disease, osteoporosis and Alzheimer's are grossly exaggerated. They appear to have a beneficial effect on the skin because they cause water retention, which smoothes out wrinkles, but they have no other beneficial effect on the skin.

WHAT ARE THEY PRESCRIBED FOR?

For hormone replacement therapy, both for menopausal women and women who have had a hysterectomy. Estrogens are prescribed for the symptoms of menopause, including hot flashes, night sweats and vaginal dryness. However, these days physicians prescribe them to any woman near the age of 50 as a matter of course, a practice which should be called malpractice.

WHAT ARE THE POSSIBLE SIDE EFFECTS?

Natural estrogens given in small amounts and in balance with progesterone to menopausal women have few, if any side effects. However, the synthetic estrogens, estrogens in high doses, and estrogens without progesterone can cause: water retention, headaches (including migraines), irritability, mood swings, depression, fatigue, lack of libido, breast tenderness, breast and uterine cancer, gallbladder disease, strokes (they reduce vascular tone and strength), increased blood pressure, low thyroid function, cervical dysplasia, breakthrough bleeding, vision problems, asthma, PMS and low cellular oxygen levels.

CAUTION!

Please avoid the synthetic estrogens altogether and use natural estrogens. You should absolutely *not* take them if you have a history of breast cancer or uterine cancer in your family, if you have a history of stroke in your family, gallbladder disease or if there is any chance of getting pregnant.

WHAT ARE THE INTERACTIONS WITH OTHER DRUGS?

Estrogens may raise levels or prolong the effects of these drugs:

↑ Amitryptyline (Elavil)   Tricyclic antidepressants
  Corticosteroids

The following drugs may be reduced in potency or decreased in the amount of time they are effective when combined with estrogens:

↓ Acetaminophen (this combina-   Anticoagulants*
   tion can also increase harm   Beclomethasone
   to the liver)

These drugs may reduce the effects of estrogens:

↓ Barbiturates   Hydantoins

WHAT NUTRIENTS DO THEY THROW OUT OF BALANCE OR INTERACT WITH?

Excess estrogens and synthetic estrogens can block the action of thyroid hormone, leading to low thyroid symptoms with normal thyroid test results. Excess estrogens and synthetic estrogens also increase sodium retention, which causes water retention or bloating.

Excess estrogens and synthetic estrogens cause depletion of the B vitamins in general, but especially folic acid and vitamin B6, which can lead to elevated homocysteine levels, a major risk factor for heart disease; cervical dysplasia; and carpal tunnel syndrome. They also cause vitamin C to be cleared from the body more rapidly.

There is also some evidence that some types of birth control pills deplete the mineral zinc.

WHAT ELSE TO TAKE IF YOU TAKE THIS DRUG

If you're taking small amounts of natural estrogens to treat menopausal symptoms, you should be fine. If for some reason you're not, it's important to take supplements of vitamin B6 (50 mg daily), folic acid (400 mcg daily) and vitamin C (500 mg three times daily). You should also be taking vitamin E to offset the risk of blood clots and strokes that comes with taking estrogens. Make sure you're getting at least 5 mg of zinc in your daily multivitamin.

---

*Potentially dangerous interaction.

The Progestins

MEDROXYPROGESTERONE ACETATE (Cycrin, Provera, Amen, Curretab)

MEGESTROL ACETATE (Megace, Enovid)

NORETHINDRONE ACETATE (Aygestin)

WHAT DO THEY DO IN YOUR BODY?

The progestins are mainly used as pseudo-progesterones in hormone replacement therapy to offset the cancer-causing effects of estrogens, but these strange hybrid hormones also behave a little like androgens (male hormones) and steroids, which natural progesterone does not. For a more detailed explanation of what natural progesterone does in the body, turn to the section at the end of this chapter on using natural hormones.

WHAT ARE THEY PRESCRIBED FOR?

In addition to being used in hormone replacement therapy for menopausal women, progestins are used to stop abnormal uterine bleeding, to regulate irregular menstrual periods, in birth control pills and to control endometriosis.

WHAT ARE THE POSSIBLE SIDE EFFECTS?

The side effects of the progestins are so severe that many women refuse to take them, preferring the risks of unopposed estrogen to the unpleasantness of progestin side effects. Most doctors don't seem to realize that women can use natural progesterone, which has none of the side effects of the progestins. First and foremost, progestins can cause birth defects. Like excess or synthetic estrogens, they increase the risk of some types of strokes, they can cause loss of vision, migraine headaches, fluid retention, depression, weight gain, fatigue, tender breasts, and they are hard on the liver. They can also cause insomnia, nausea, breakthrough bleeding, and amenorrhea (no menstruation). Like testosterone and other androgens, they can cause excessive hair growth where women *don't* want it, hair loss where they *do* want it, and a variety of skin problems and rashes, including acne.

Progestins can also cause high blood sugar, reduced HDL ("good") cholesterol, raised LDL ("bad") cholesterol, and photosensitivity.

Like the cortisones, megestrol acetate actually increases appetite, can increase your risk of respiratory infections, and may suppress your adrenal function.

CAUTION!

Please don't use the progestins at all, either as hormone replacement therapy or in birth control pills. In rare cases they may be useful to stop excessive breakthrough bleeding, but otherwise it's difficult to imagine why any physician who wanted to do the right thing would prescribe this horrible drug when he or she could prescribe natural progesterone.

WHAT ARE THE INTERACTIONS WITH OTHER DRUGS?

Progestins may raise levels or prolong the effects of these drugs:

↑ Amitryptyline (Elavil)   Sulfonylurea drugs
Benzodiazepines   Theophyllines*
Beta-blockers

The following drugs may be reduced in potency or decreased in the amount of time they are effective when combined with progestins:

↓ Beclomethasone   Insulin
Clofibrate

These drugs may increase the effects or prolong the action of the progestins:

↑ Cholesterol-lowering statins   Troglitazone

*Potentially dangerous interaction.

These drugs may reduce the effects of progestins:

↓ Aminoglutethimide   Rifampin
  Antibiotics   Troglitazone

Oral Contraceptives

BIPHASIC (Jenest, Nelova, Ortho-Novum)

LEVONORGESTREL (Progestasert)

MEDROXYPROGESTERONE ACETATE (Depo-Provera)

MONOPHASIC (Loestrin FE, Demulen, Desogen, Genora, Levora, Norethin, Norinyl, Ortho-Cept, Ortho-Novum, Ovcon, Ovral)

PROGESTIN ONLY (Micronor Nor-Q.D., Ovrette)

TRIPHASIC (Ortho-Novum, Tri-Levlen, Tri-Norinyl, Triphasil)

WHAT DO THEY DO IN YOUR BODY?

Oral contraceptives are either a combination of a synthetic estrogen, usually ethinyl estradiol combined with a progestin, or a progestin alone.

WHAT ARE THEY PRESCRIBED FOR?

Birth control and to regulate menses.

WHAT ARE THE POSSIBLE SIDE EFFECTS?

Oral contraceptives can cause all of the side effects of the synthetic estrogens and the progestins, and have their own unique profile of negative effects on the body. One of their most frequent side effects is breakthrough bleeding and spotting.

Oral contraceptives increase the risk of blood clots, stroke, heart attacks, liver cancer and gallbladder disease, especially in women already susceptible to those diseases. This includes women with high blood pressure, high cholesterol, obese women and diabetic women.

Women who smoke absolutely should not use oral contraceptives—it is a deadly combination, especially in women over the age of 35. Oral contraceptives also increase the risk of arterial disease and vision loss, and controversial studies suggest they increase the risk of breast and cervical cancer, especially when taken long term. Oral contraceptives can cause candida overgrowth, breast tenderness and lumpiness, and nausea.

Women going off them may be infertile, usually for a few months, but in older women it can be permanent.

CAUTION!

Please avoid these drugs altogether and use an alternative form of birth control. If the only other choice is an unwanted pregnancy, then perhaps birth control pills should be an option, but they absolutely cannot be considered a safe drug.

WHAT ARE THE INTERACTIONS WITH OTHER DRUGS?

(Also see drug interactions for estrogens and progestins.)
Oral contraceptives may raise levels or prolong the effects of these drugs:

↑ Anticoagulants   Beta-blockers
  Antidepressants   Corticosteroids
  Benzodiazepines   Theophyllines

The following drugs may be reduced in potency or decreased in the amount of time they are effective when combined with oral contraceptives:

↓ Acetaminophen   Benzodiazepines
  Aspirin   Clofibrate
  Anticoagulants

These drugs may reduce the effects of oral contraceptives:

↓ Antibiotics   Barbiturates

WHAT NUTRIENTS DO THEY THROW OUT OF BALANCE OR INTERACT WITH?

Primarily vitamins B6 and folic acid. See the sections on synthetic estrogens and progestins for details.

WHAT ELSE TO TAKE IF YOU TAKE THESE DRUGS

Vitamin B6 (50 mg daily), folic acid (400 mcg daily), vitamin C (2,000 mg daily).

SYNTHETIC TESTOSTERONE

FLUOXYMESTERONE (Halotestin)

METHYLTESTOSTERONE (Android, Oreton Methyl, Testred, Virilon)

WHAT DO THEY DO IN YOUR BODY?

The synthetic testosterones tend to have more of the muscle-building properties of testosterone, and less of the effects such as deepening of the voice and the growth of body hair.

WHAT ARE THEY PRESCRIBED FOR?

A deficiency of testosterone, which may be caused by genetics, environment or disease. They are used in women to treat metastatic breast cancer and postpartum breast pain.

WHAT ARE THE POSSIBLE SIDE EFFECTS?

Although the effects of the synthetic testosterones are hard to separate out from the effects of real testosterone, you can probably safely assume that most of the side effects are caused by the synthetic testosterones or by excessive doses of real testosterone. Side effects can include hypercalcemia (too much calcium in the blood), liver damage, reduced ejaculatory volume, fluid retention, abnormal swelling of the breast in men, masculinization and menstrual irregularities in women, worsening of prostate enlargement and prostate cancer, acne, baldness, nausea, headache, aggressiveness, anxiety, and increased or decreased libido. They may also raise the risk of some types of cancer in women.

CAUTION!

Please don't use synthetic testosterone. If you need testosterone, use the real thing. See the section on testosterone under the natural hormones section of this chapter.

WHAT ARE THE INTERACTIONS WITH OTHER DRUGS?

Synthetic testosterones may raise levels or prolong the effects of these drugs:

↑ Anticoagulants

Glucocorticoids (Adrenal Hormones)

CORTISONE

DEXAMETHASONE (Decadron, Dexameth, Dexon)

HYDROCORTISONE/CORTISOL (Cortef)

METHYLPREDNISOLONE (Medrol)

PREDNISOLONE (Delta-Cortef, Prelone)

PREDNISONE (Deltasone, Orasone, Panasol, Meticorten)

TRIAMCINOLONE (Aristocort, Atolone, Kenacort)

WHAT DO THEY DO IN YOUR BODY?

They are potent anti-inflammatory drugs that also play a role in regulating the immune system, appetite and sodium balance in the cells. They play literally dozens of roles in the body having to do with metabolism and inflammation. Cortisone and hydrocortisone are the natural versions of these drugs. See the section in this chapter on natural hormones for more information.

WHAT ARE THEY PRESCRIBED FOR?

Adrenal insufficiency, arthritis, lupus, psoriasis, allergies, eye inflammations, respiratory diseases such as bronchial asthma, Crohn's disease, multiple sclerosis and other diseases that involve severe, chronic inflammation or overactive immune response.

WHAT ARE THE POSSIBLE SIDE EFFECTS?

The glucocorticoids have many very dangerous and destructive side effects, but many are due to the use of the synthetic versions of the drug and excessively high doses.

Side effects and adverse reactions can include weight gain, osteoporosis, increased blood pressure, peptic ulcers, adrenal suppression, immunosuppression, increased susceptibility to bacterial and fungal infections, masking of bacterial and fungal infections, water retention, weight gain, increased appetite, cataracts, glaucoma, steroid psychosis, muscle weakness, blood clots, pancreatitis, heartburn, thin fragile skin, scaly lesions, headaches, dizziness, menstrual irregularities, increased sweating, and blood sugar imbalances.

People who are taking these drugs over a long period of time should never stop taking them abruptly. See your health-care provider.

CAUTION: THINK TWICE ABOUT TAKING THESE TYPES OF DRUGS IF . . .

- You have high blood pressure.
- You have osteoporosis.
- You have ulcers, eye disease, kidney or liver disease.
- You have a fungal infection.
- You are obese, elderly or pregnant.

WHAT ARE THE INTERACTIONS WITH OTHER DRUGS?

Glucocorticoids may raise levels or prolong the effects of these drugs:

↑ Anticoagulants   Diuretics
  Cyclosporine   Theophyllines
  Digitalis drugs

The following drugs may be reduced in potency or decreased in the amount of time they are effective when combined with glucocorticoids:

↓ Anticoagulants   Salicylates
  Anticholinesterase drugs Somatrem
  Isoniazid   Theophyllines

These drugs may increase the effects or prolong the action of glucocorticoids:

↑ Oral contraceptives   Ketoconazole
  Estrogens   Macrolide antibiotics

These drugs may reduce the effects of glucocorticoids:

↓ Aminoglutethimide   Hydantoins
  Barbiturates   Rifampin
  Cholestyramine

Thyroid Hormones

LEVOTHYROXINE, T4 (Synthroid, Levo-T, Levoxyl, Eltroxin)

LIOTHYRONINE, T3 (Cytomel, Triostat)

LIOTRIX, T3 and T4, synthetic (Euthroid, Thyrolar)

THYROGLOBULIN, dessicated beef or pork, T4 and T3 (Proloid)

USP THYROID, dessicated beef or pork, T3 and T4 (Armour)

WHAT DO THEY DO IN YOUR BODY?

Thyroid hormones regulate many types of metabolism in the body, including heart rate and strength of heartbeat, respiratory rate, oxygen consumption, body temperature, metabolism of food, growth, maturation and enzyme activity.

WHAT ARE THEY PRESCRIBED FOR?

Thyroid deficiency. (See the section in this chapter on natural hormones for more details on thyroid.)

WHAT ARE THE POSSIBLE SIDE EFFECTS?

Side effects of a physiologic dose of USP thyroid in someone who is thyroid deficient are rare. Excessive thyroid can cause heart palpitations, rapid heartbeat, irregular heartbeat, angina, heart attack, tremors, headache, nervousness, insomnia, diarrhea, weight loss, menstrual irregularities, sweating and intolerance to heat.

CAUTION: THINK TWICE ABOUT TAKING THESE TYPES OF DRUGS IF . . .

- You have diabetes. Work very carefully with your doctor.
- You have Addison's disease. Work very carefully with a doctor.

WHAT ARE THE INTERACTIONS WITH OTHER DRUGS?

Thyroid may raise levels or prolong the effects of these drugs:

↑ Anticoagulants   Theophyllines

The following drugs may be reduced in potency or decreased in the amount of time they are effective when combined with thyroid:

↓ Beta-blockers   Digitalis drugs

These drugs may reduce the effects of thyroid:

↓ Cholestyramine   Estrogens
  Colestipol

WHAT ELSE TO TAKE IF YOU TAKE THESE DRUGS

If you have hypothyroidism it's a good idea to eat iodine-rich foods regularly such as dried seaweeds (dulse, kelp).

USING NATURAL HORMONES

Pregnenolone

Pregnenolone is a steroid hormone made from cholesterol. All of the other steroid hormones, including progesterone, DHEA, the cortisols, the estrogens and testosterone are made from pregnenolone. Like progesterone, pregnenolone is not a sex steroid, meaning it doesn't have masculinizing or feminizing effects on the body, and it seems to be safe even in very high doses.

There was a flurry of research done on pregnenolone in the 1940s, but the only clear effect it had was in relieving symptoms of rheumatoid arthritis. You can try 10 to 200 mg divided into three doses daily for arthritis and see if it helps. Give it at least three weeks to work.

More recent studies show that pregnenolone improves memory after learning, which makes sense because it has an excitatory effect on the brain and blocks GABA receptors, which play a role in blocking memory. Studies in rats and humans suggest that giving pregnenolone enhances the ability to learn and enhances memory. Other studies suggest that it improves sleep and reduces anxiety.

Even though pregnenolone is a precursor to all of the other steroid hormones, taking a pregnenolone supplement will not necessarily raise the levels of other hormones in the body. It might, but so far the evidence isn't in that this happens reliably.

Pregnenolone needs to be studied much more closely, but it is clearly of benefit for people who complain that they aren't retaining information when they learn something new. You can take up to 100 mg daily between meals for improving memory.

Progesterone

Progesterone is a steroid hormone with important effects nearly every-where in the body. It is a precursor to all of the other steroid hor-mones except pregnenolone, and is made by the adrenal glands in both sexes, and in a woman's ovaries. There is some evidence that pregnenolone and progesterone are also made in the peripheral ner-vous system. They are known to be an essential part of the Schwann cells that form the myelin sheath that protects nerves. Studies done with progesterone and pregnenolone on rats with spinal cord injuries showed that those given these steroid hormones had better recovery.

One of progesterone's biggest roles in a woman's biochemistry is opposing or balancing estrogen in the uterus and probably elsewhere. While estrogen stimulates cell growth, progesterone signals cells to mature and differentiate, an effect that progesterone expert John R. Lee, M.D. likens to the ripening of an apple.

Women only produce progesterone in their ovaries when they ovu-late. During months when they don't ovulate but still have a men-strual period, they may be estrogen dominant, a condition where estrogen levels aren't necessarily high, but there is no progesterone to balance its effects. This can cause PMS, and over time, according to Dr. Lee, it can also cause fibroids, fibrocystic breasts and cervical dys-plasia. In women going through menopause, it can cause symptoms such as weight gain, irritability, mood swings and headaches.

A woman's ovaries normally produce 20 to 30 mg of progesterone daily during the middle part of the menstrual cycle. Progesterone is made by the placenta in pregnant women in relatively huge quantities (as much as 300 mg daily in the last trimester). Dr. Lee speculates that much of postpartum depression may be caused by the plunge in progesterone levels.

At menopause, progesterone production in a woman drops even more than estrogen does, and women can often relieve menopausal symptoms using only a natural progesterone cream. In a bizarre twist of conventional medicine working hand in hand with drug company marketing and advertising, progesterone has been all but forgotten in the rush to prescribe estrogen, and yet it is equally if not more impor-tant than estrogen in hormone replacement therapy.

There is convincing evidence from Dr. Lee and others that progesterone stimulates bone growth, making it important in preventing osteoporosis. Premenopausal and menopausal women who use progesterone cream also report that their hair becomes thicker, their libido comes back and their vaginal dryness disappears.

Progesterone should never be confused with its synthetic cousins the progestins such as Provera, which have many negative side effects. Natural progesterone is made in a laboratory, but it is the exact same molecule found in your body. The progestins have been altered to produce not-found-in-nature molecules that can be patented and sold at high prices. Women who take them generally report feeling awful and their risk of dangerous side effects is very real. In contrast, women who use natural progesterone tend to be very healthy, and there are no known negative side effects at prescribed doses.

If you are using hormone replacement therapy or contemplating it, please use natural progesterone and natural estrogens. The book *What Your Doctor May Not Tell You About Menopause* by John R. Lee, M.D. and Virginia Hopkins (Warner Books, 1996) is a classic that is recommended for all premenopausal and menopausal women. It will give you a very good sense of how your hormones work and how to balance them in a safe, natural way.

Progesterone cream works wonders for the majority of postmenopausal women; most feel dramatically better physically, mentally and emotionally. It also works well for women of any age suffering from premenopause symptoms such as weight gain, mood swings, fibroids and fibrocystic breasts.

In general, the best way to use progesterone is as a cream, in a dose of 15 to 20 mg daily. We know that physicians prefer to give pills, but in this case the cream probably gives a more accurate dose. When taken orally, as much as 80 percent of the progesterone is processed by the liver and excreted, so you have to take 100 mg or more to get the dose you need. Depending on how your liver is working, you may get far more or far less than you need.

In a two-ounce jar of progesterone containing 800 mg of progesterone, a physiologic dose would work out to ¼ to ⅓ teaspoon per day. Only progesterone USP is natural progesterone.

Please avoid "wild yam" products, and be sure to read the information on diosgenin/wild yam/dioscorea creams in the section in this chapter on DHEA. Your body will not convert them to progesterone.

Use the real thing. In Dr. Lee's book you will find a list of progesterone creams and the amount of progesterone they contain. It's best to stick with those containing 400 mg or more per ounce.

Don't think that more is better when it comes to dosing with hormones. If the recommended dose doesn't help your symptoms, then you need to do more detective work to find out what's causing the problem.

You can buy a variety of progesterone creams over the counter, but if you don't understand how to use them, work with a health-care professional. At the very least, read Dr. Lee's book before using progesterone or estrogen.

Dehydroepiandrosterone (DHEA)

Dehydroepiandrosterone (DHEA) is a steroid hormone manufactured in the adrenal glands. These prune-sized glands sit on top of the kidneys and are responsible for the secretion of over 150 hormones. The adrenal hormones are our major stress buffers, allowing us to adapt to whatever stresses our environment brings.

DHEA is the most abundant steroid hormone in the body. It acts as a precursor from which several other steroid hormones are made, including estrogens and testosterone, but not progesterone or the cortisols. It is an androgenic or male hormone. Only 5 percent of the body's circulating DHEA is in the active form; the remainder is joined to sulfur molecules (DHEAS) and serves as a reserve of the hormone which can be easily converted back to the active form.

DHEA production peaks between the ages of 20 and 25, with men having a higher peak than women. There is about a 2 percent decrease in blood levels for each year of life that follows. A large body of research, particularly on men, shows a clear relationship between this progressive drop in DHEA levels and diseases of aging, such as cardiovascular disease, diabetes and some cancers. In other words, sick people have less DHEA in their bodies than well people do. Elderly people have less than young people, and elderly people with higher DHEA levels are healthier than those with low levels.

Several studies have shown that when DHEA is given to elderly subjects who started out with low levels, there is a sizeable improvement in their sense of well-being. Both men and women with some types of cancer, allergies, Type II diabetes or autoimmune diseases (such as rheumatoid arthritis) have low blood levels of DHEA. This has led researchers to guess that raising DHEA levels can help to prevent or treat these diseases. Some clinicians have reported success in treating patients who have lupus with DHEA.

DHEA may help prevent heart disease in men, but its effect on heart disease risk in women is much less promising. Most studies on this topic indicate that risk may even increase somewhat in women if it is supplemented in too high a dose. Here again, it's important to use a physiologic dose, or one close to what the body would produce naturally. In a woman that would be less than in a man.

DHEA aids in the body's immune defenses against unwelcome invaders. One mechanism for this may involve DHEA's opposing actions to *cortisol*, a "fight or flight" hormone secreted by the adrenal glands when we are under stress. Cortisol suppresses some parts of the immune system. This makes sense if you're a caveman. If your body thinks you are in some kind of immediate danger, it wouldn't waste energy on building up the immune system during the crisis. This would be like deciding to cook dinner for the family in the kitchen of a house that's burning down. Modern life resembles the house at a slow burn, too dangerous to relax and cook a nourishing meal in, but not such an emergency that you have to escape immediately. Chronic stress (an almost inescapable part of life these days) leads to chronically elevated cortisol levels, which lessen our immunity against illness. The result of many years of constantly high cortisol levels can exhaust your adrenal glands, causing output of cortisol and DHEA to drop to unhealthy lows. This seems to be particularly true of women.

DHEA supplementation appears to enhance the youth-preserving effects of growth hormone, which will be addressed in detail later in this chapter. This may be one reason for DHEA's remarkable effect on well-being.

In one study, a large dose of DHEA given before sleep to 10 healthy young men increased the amount of REM (rapid eye movement) sleep. REM sleep is the most restorative kind of sleep, and is reduced in the elderly.

In a study of pregnant women, intravenous DHEAS (the same form as the body's reservoir of DHEA) dilated a major eye artery, increasing blood flow. This points to a possible use of DHEAS as a blood vessel dilator that can improve circulation to the eyes.

It follows that raising DHEA levels could have powerful health-enhancing and youth-preserving effects. However, straightforward assumptions rarely work with hormones, and we can't assume that DHEA levels appropriate for a 25-year-old will be safe for a 75-year-old. That might be like putting a jet engine on an old biplane; it might fly really fast for a little while but a crash is inevitable. We do recommend DHEA, especially for older men, but again, in moderate doses and with regular measurement of hormone levels.

If you are a man over 40 years old and want to try DHEA, start out with 25 mg daily. If you are a woman, take 10 mg daily or every other day. Men can take up to 50 mg daily, but if you're taking that much, please get your blood or saliva levels tested at least every six months to make sure you're not overdoing it.

Because the end products of DHEA in women are primarily androgens (male hormones), women should monitor themselves carefully for any masculinizing effects of supplementation. If you notice loss of hair on the head and/or growth of hair on the face, acne, or weight gain around the midsection, cut back significantly on the dosage. Chances are good that if you are experiencing these side effects, you will also begin to develop insulin resistance, a first step towards adult-onset diabetes. In men, DHEA has the opposite effect, actually improving insulin uptake.

Women can experience benefit from DHEA supplementation with doses as low as 5 mg a day, or 25 mg every other day or every third day. Don't take more than 25 mg daily.

One of the reasons the medical establishment may be so cautious about DHEA is because in many of the studies, the doses given were quite high. The likelihood of negative side effects is much greater with higher dosing.

You should avoid DHEA altogether if you have or have had a hormone-sensitive cancer such as breast, ovarian, testicular or prostate cancer. DHEA is a precursor to estrogen and testosterone, meaning that the body can manufacture those hormones from DHEA. Reproductive cancers in women and men seem to be largely driven by the sex hormones estrogen and testosterone, so it makes sense not to boost hormone levels when you have these types of cancer.

Keep in mind that these recommendations are based on theory and guesswork derived from what seems to be common sense and logic. In truth we have a long way to go before we really understand how the steroid hormones interact with each other and their effects on cancer.

DHEA is not recommended for people under the age of 40 unless your levels are measurably low, as it can suppress your own natural hormone production. (Remember, more isn't necessarily better when it comes to hormones.)

For anyone using DHEA, a check of salivary levels of this hormone every six months is a good idea. Ask your health-care professional about this, and be sure he or she knows you are using it.

Please don't take supplements derived from Mexican yam (*Dioscorea mexicana*) or wild yam (*Dioscorea villosa*) thinking that you're getting DHEA, progesterone or any other hormones. These products are often billed as DHEA or progesterone "precursors" which is patently false information.

While it is true that pharmaceutical grade steroid hormone drugs are made from the diosgenin extracted from wild yam or soybeans, this all goes on in the laboratory, not in your body. As far as we can tell, our bodies simply do not have the enzymes necessary to break diosgenin down into the steroid hormones. Many studies have been done trying to prove that diosgenin raises steroid hormone levels, using both blood and salivary hormone level testing, and not one has shown an effect. Don't waste your money on these products. If you want DHEA, take DHEA. If you want progesterone, take progesterone. It's also wise to purchase DHEA that says "pharmaceutical grade" DHEA on the label.

The Estrogens

Estrogens are the female hormones, produced in the ovaries, adrenal glands and fat cells of women, and in much smaller amounts in the adrenal glands and fat cells of men. There are three predominant types of estrogens: estriol, estradiol and estrone. These are the only natural estrogens on the market. Accept no substitutes! The natural estrogens used by conventional physicians include estrone (Aquest, Kestrone) and estradiol (Vivelle, Climara, Estraderm, Estrace). They come in oral, cream and patch form. Currently there is no conventional estriol available, but you can find sources for it in the Resources section of this book.

Estrogens stimulate the growth of breasts and the maturing of a girl's other reproductive organs. They are central to the menstrual cycle, and stimulate the growth of tissue in the uterus each month. In excess, or without progesterone, they can cause weight gain, fluid retention, mood swings and depression and can block thyroid function. They increase the risk of strokes and the risk of reproductive cancers.

The estrogens' value as an anti-aging hormone has more to do with advertising and marketing by big drug companies than it does with biochemical reality. The truth is that all those studies supposedly showing that estrogen cures everything from osteoporosis to heart disease would have been laughed out of the physician's office if they had been nutrition studies. The first study showing benefit in Alzheimer's disease had only 12 patients and yet it was widely disseminated by the media.

In thin postmenopausal women whose fat cells and adrenal glands aren't producing much, if any, estrogen, some supplementation with a natural estrogen cream might be justified. Women who are having menopausal symptoms such as night sweats, hot flashes and vaginal dryness may also benefit from some estrogen, but it's only needed in tiny amounts once or twice a week. Taking small amounts of estrogen right around the time of menopause can also help prevent the large drop in bone density seen around that time, so if you are at risk for osteoporosis it might be worth supplementing it for a few years. But it's more important to also use progesterone cream, which will actually build bone. Please don't think of estrogen as a long-term replacement hormone unless you're very thin. Your fat cells and adrenal glands will make what you need, and you're getting dosed with it every time you're exposed to pesticides and plastics, which for most of us is many times daily.

There is a myth among physicians that women who have had their ovaries removed don't need progesterone along with their estrogen.

What they don't realize is that estrogen alone frequently makes women feel as if they have permanent PMS. You'll feel dramatically better if you use both, or even just progesterone cream.

The first approach for menopausal symptoms should be the Six Core Principles for Optimal Health. Exercise alone will often diminish or eliminate menopausal symptoms. A next step is to try eating soy products and plenty of fresh vegetables. Soy and many vegetables contains compounds called *phytoestrogens* because they behave like weak estrogens. Tofu, miso soup and tempeh are easily available soy products.

Estrogen is available by prescription only. If you decide you need some estrogen, use the smallest dose possible that will alleviate your symptoms. Dr. Lee's book (mentioned under progesterone) will give you a lot of helpful and eye-opening information on estrogen.

Tri-Est is an estrogen cream containing estrone, estriol and estradiol, developed by Jonathan Wright, M.D. that attempts to replicate the levels and balance of estrogen naturally found in the body. This is a good choice if you're going to try some estrogen. See the Resources section in the back of the book for information on how to order it.

Testosterone

This steroid hormone is produced in relatively large amounts in the testes of men and in much smaller amounts in the ovaries of women and the adrenal glands of both sexes. The typical male secondary sex characteristics of men (deeper vocal tone, more abundant body hair, thicker skin, greater muscle mass, higher metabolism and pattern baldness) are attributable to testosterone. There is a significant drop in both male and female testosterone levels in late life.

Studies of testosterone replacement in elderly men have shown increased libido and musculoskeletal mass and strength. In men, testosterone builds bone. Men who have had their testicles removed, or who are using anti-androgenic drugs to treat prostate cancer, have a much higher rate of osteoporosis.

Testosterone replacement is worth trying in men if levels are measurably low or if there are symptoms of deficiency such as muscle wasting. In cases of unexplained weight gain, thinning skin, fatigue or loss of muscle tone with aging, testosterone replacement could help. All forms of supplemental testosterone are only available by prescription. Ask your physician to give you a natural form, which is best used with a patch or a cream. Please avoid the synthetic forms of testosterone such as methyltestosterone, as they have unpleasant and potentially dangerous side effects. Stick to the natural form, which means that the testosterone molecule looks identical to those produced in your own body.

Testosterone is a very potent hormone that can cause undesirable side effects in doses that are even slightly elevated. It's generally recommended that you try DHEA first, since it is an androgen and theoretically can be converted to testosterone in the body. If symptoms don't improve after three months or so, then you could try a very low-dose testosterone patch.

It would be a mistake to try to achieve the testosterone levels you had as a young man or woman. The body of a 50-year-old is simply no longer equipped to handle such a hormone load. The goal is to have the symptoms of testosterone deficiency go away, not to feel like a 20-year-old again.

Thyroid Hormone

In every cell in your body, thyroid hormone plays a major role in regulating metabolic rate, your body's rate of energy production. The thyroid gland is located in the neck, with half of its 20 gram mass lying on each side of the trachea (windpipe). Lack of thyroid hormone causes a precipitous drop in your ability to expend energy, while too much of the hormone expends more energy than is necessary.

More thyroid tells the body to speed things up, causing you to breathe faster, use more oxygen, raise body temperature, have a faster heartbeat, have more blood pumping through the circulatory system, have quicker burning of calories and a higher production of enzymes. Symptoms of too much thyroid (*hyperthyroidism*) include rapid heartbeat, intolerance to heat, headache, irritability, nervousness and sweating.

Symptoms of low thyroid hormone (*hypothyroidism*) are low energy, cold intolerance, especially cold feet and hands, unexplained weight

gain, depression, dry skin, recurrent infections, headaches and constipation. Although excess thyroid is relatively rare, thyroid deficiency
affects up to 25 percent of American adults. Aging is one explanation,
as the thyroid gland shrinks and becomes less active with age. Ten
to 24 percent of cases of thyroid deficiency are missed by the blood
test commonly used to screen for it. This is because blood tests measure *thyroxine*, or T4, which makes up 90 percent of thyroid gland
secretion. Another form, *triiodothyronine* (T3), is a derivative of T4 and
is the most active form. There are many people whose thyroid function would appear normal according to blood tests but who have
trouble making the T4 to T3 conversion. Functionally, these people
are thyroid deficient and their symptoms clear up when they are given
thyroid supplementation. Sometimes a deficiency that doesn't show
up when T4 and T3 are measured will show up when thyroid stimulating hormone (TSH) is measured. Elevated levels may indicate
hypothyroidsim.

If you want to know more about thyroid and hypothyroidism, read
the classic book by Broda Barnes, *Hypothyroidism: The Unsuspected Illness* (Harper and Row, 1976). Barnes believed that the most accurate
way to detect a thyroid deficiency was simply by taking your temperature. The Barnes Basal Temperature Test can give you a good idea
of whether you should be concerned about your thyroid function:

1. Shake down a basal thermometer (you can get it at your drugstore) to below 95 degrees Fahrenheit and leave it by your bedside when you go to sleep.
2. When you wake in the morning, put the thermometer in your
   armpit for 10 full minutes. Try to move as little as possible, keeping your eyes closed, until the 10 minutes are up.
3. After 10 minutes, record the temperature and date of the
   measurement.
4. Repeat the test for three mornings, at the same approximate time
   of day. If you are a premenopausal woman, perform the test on
   the second, third and fourth days of your menstrual cycle (days
   two through four of your period), because your temperature will
   go up slightly when you're ovulating in mid-cycle. Men and
   postmenopausal women can perform the test at any time.

If the average measurement is below 97.2 degrees Fahrenheit, and you have the symptoms mentioned above, you may want to first try some natural methods for increasing thyroid function.

NATURAL METHODS FOR INCREASING THYROID PRODUCTION

Deficiencies of zinc, copper, iron, selenium and the amino acid tyrosine can prevent the thyroid from functioning properly. The absence of these nutrients also causes problems with the T4 to T3 conversion. Tyrosine is found plentifully in soy and in chicken, fish, and beef or you can take it in supplement form, following directions on the container.

Chronic high cortisol levels due to excessive stress block the conversion of T4 to T3.

Iodine is an essential component of the thyroid hormones. Goiter, a disease that was once common in peoples living too far from the ocean to get fresh fish, manifests itself in the form of a swollen thyroid gland. This swelling occurs due to lack of iodine. Today most salt is iodized and salt water fish are readily available. You can also get iodine by eating sea vegetables (seaweed) such as dulse, wakame, kombu and nori. You can take supplemental iodine (no more than 1,000 mcg a day should be used without a physician's prescription) if you think your thyroid gland needs extra help.

If stress relief and nutritional interventions don't work to relieve your symptoms or raise your basal temperature, see your physician. Thyroid hormone replacement may be necessary and can only be done by prescription. The closest thing you'll find to a natural thyroid is USP thyroid (Armour, for example) which is a combination of T3 and T4 from cows or pigs in the ratios naturally found in the body.

Hydrocortisone (Natural)

This hormone is another classic example of drug company profits taking precedence over your health. When prednisone and the other synthetic, patentable and much more profitable synthetic cortisone-type drugs were invented some 50 years ago, hydrocortisone was all but forgotten and research on it came to a standstill.

Prednisone and the other synthetic cortisones are renowned for their nasty, life-destroying side effects. And yet, for many people who need them, low doses of cortisone or hydrocortisone, the natural forms of glucocorticoids, cause few or minimal side effects. If you are taking a synthetic cortisone and want a wonderful source of good information on cortisones, read the book *The Safe Uses of Cortisone* by William McK. Jefferies, M.D., FACP (Charles C. Thomas Publisher, 1981).

Cortisone and cortisol are important glucocorticoid adrenal hormones that regulate dozens of functions in the body, but especially inflammation and immune response. They are widely used to treat autoimmune diseases such as lupus and arthritis, because of their immune-suppressing properties, and severely inflammatory diseases such as Crohn's disease and psoriasis. They are also used to treat adrenal insufficiency, a condition of "tired" adrenal glands that aren't producing enough hormones. People with transplanted organs usually take cortisone-type drugs for life to suppress their body's rejection reaction.

A lot of low-level adrenal insufficiency, especially in women, is diagnosed as chronic fatigue. It's not severe enough to show up as Addison's disease, a severe deficiency of cortisone, but it is enough to cause chronic fatigue, low blood pressure and chronic allergies. Again, if you think you might fall into that category, read Jefferies' book.

Taking hydrocortisone drugs can suppress your own adrenal function if you take too much over a long period of time. It should be used with great care, in the smallest possible dose to alleviate symptoms, over the shortest possible period of time.

Chronic stress over a long period of time is what usually causes tired adrenal glands and rest is the best medicine. Licorice root in a tea or tincture form can also be helpful, as it supports glucocorticoid function. Some of the nutrients important to adrenal function include vitamin C, vitamin B6 and vitamin E.

For more information on glucocorticoids, see the prescription drug section of this chapter.

Human Growth Hormone

The use of human growth hormone (HGH) as an anti-aging hormone is very controversial and at the time of publication of this book it is very expensive to use. However the price is dropping rapidly, and within the next decade we'll probably be using as much growth hormone for anti-aging purposes as we do estrogen, natural progesterone and DHEA.

The pituitary gland lies at the base of the brain. One of the many hormones it secretes is *somatotropin,* more commonly known as growth hormone. Some of its effects are:

- Increase in lean muscle mass.
- Decrease in fat mass.
- Increase in size and functional capacity of organs.
- Growth of endplates of bones, increasing their length (this is how children grow to adult stature) and with it, the growth of collagen, a component in skin and other tissues.
- Synergistic stimulation of thyroid hormone and DHEA.

The physical transformation of tiny infant to small child to adult happens in large part due to plentiful growth hormone stimulation of the body's tissues. In the years since growth hormone was isolated, it has been used to help children with malfunctioning pituitary glands grow to normal size. Adults who are growth-hormone deficient because of pituitary tumors or other diseases have been helped a great deal with growth hormone replacement.

For each decade of adult life, growth hormone secretion drops 14 percent. People over the age of 60 are, for all intents and purposes, deficient in this hormone relative to youthful levels. As a result, as we age, organs shrink and work less effectively and lean mass is replaced by fat. Thyroid and DHEA production dwindle. It's no wonder scientists have begun to think that supplemental growth hormone might be one key to eternal youth.

Excess cortisol (due to stress) and excess insulin (seen in most cases of adult-onset diabetes) hamper growth hormone production. Lack of quality sleep also robs us of growth hormone's benefits: The most pronounced surge in growth hormone production occurs during deep sleep.

Giving growth hormone, GHRH (growth hormone releasing hormone), and IGF-1 (insulin-like growth factor 1) to older adults has been shown to restore growth hormone blood levels to those of younger people. The expected positive changes in body composition are seen. In people with growth hormone deficiency caused by pituitary disease, administration of growth hormone had beneficial effects on bone, heart, thyroid and psychological health.

At high doses, growth hormone can cause side effects, including fluid retention, carpal tunnel syndrome, worsening of adult-onset diabetes and increased risk of heart failure. Since tumors use growth hormone to fuel their growth just as do other cells within the body, there is some concern that supplementation might increase the rate of growth of cancers. On the other hand, the evidence that growth hormone stimulates and strengthens the immune system may mean it can help fight cancer.

Growth hormone may be a good choice for those who are deficient, in small, physiologic doses that mimic what the body would produce naturally. Because it needs to be taken by injection and is financially out of reach for many, it is fortunate that there are several things you can do to enhance your body's own production of this youth-preserving hormone.

Growth hormone secretion is stimulated after a meal rich in dietary protein. Especially powerful in this regard are the amino acids *arginine* and *ornithine*. Any source of complete protein (eggs, milk, and meat) is rich in these amino acids. Supplements containing arginine and ornithine are available. You can start by taking 1 gram (1,000 mg) twice a day of arginine (2 grams total) or 500 mg twice a day of ornithine (1 gram or 1,000 mg total). This is a relatively large dose and is probably best taken in powder form and mixed with juice or in a shake. If you have oral or genital herpes or shingles you may want to use arginine with caution as it can stimulate an outbreak.

Growth hormone secretion can be stimulated during a fast. Naturopathic doctor Leon Chaitow, N.D., D.O. suggests periodic short fasts to boost growth hormone production.

Growth hormone secretion can be stimulated during and following a bout of exercise. It appears that to significantly increase growth hormone secretion you need to exercise regularly and hard enough to see a noticeable improvement in endurance and/or strength.

Within a few months, a moderate program of weightlifting can produce increases in lean muscle mass equal to those produced by growth hormone injections.

Growth hormone secretion can be stimulated during deep sleep.

CHAPTER 19

Drugs for Osteoporosis and Their Natural Alternatives

ALTHOUGH CARDIOVASCULAR DISEASE is the leading cause of death among American women, osteoporosis is the disease they are most likely to develop as they age. Four out of 10 white women in the U.S. will fracture a hip, spine or forearm due to osteoporosis. As many as five out of 10 will develop small fractures in their spine, causing great pain and a shrinking in height. This amounts to 15 to 20 million people affected by a crippling and painful disease that is almost entirely preventable and reversible.

Osteoporosis is a gradual decrease in bone mass and density that can begin as early as the teen years. Bone mass should be at its peak in our late twenties or early thirties, but thanks to a poor diet and lack of exercise, many women are already losing bone in their twenties. Bone loss occurs more rapidly in women than in men, especially right around the time of menopause, when an abrupt drop in estrogen and progesterone accelerates bone loss.

When you think of your bones you may imagine a dead skeleton, but your bones are living tissue, just like the rest of your body, and they need a good supply of nutrients and regular exercise. New bone is constantly being made, while old bone is being reabsorbed and excreted by the body. Our larger long bones, such as our arm and leg bones, are very dense, and they are completely replaced about every 10 to 12 years. Our less dense bones, such as our spine and the ends of our long bones, are less dense and turn over every two to three years. Thus, as you can see, we always have the opportunity to be creating better bone for ourselves.

We all hear about how having enough calcium in the diet and taking estrogen can help prevent osteoporosis, but there is a much bigger nutritional and lifestyle picture to look at when we are talking about preventing this bone-robbing disease.

The most important element of bones is minerals. Without minerals we don't have bones. The most important bone minerals are calcium, magnesium, potassium, phosphorous and fluoride. Equally important is the balance between the minerals. Too much phosphorous or fluoride will create poor bone structure.

Without enough magnesium, the calcium can't be absorbed onto the bone. Vitamins are also involved. For example, vitamin B6 works with magnesium to get calcium onto your bones.

The hormones testosterone, estrogen and progesterone are also actively involved in the making and unmaking of bone. Testosterone and progesterone build bone, while estrogen slows bone loss.

In osteoporosis, the old bone is being reabsorbed faster than new bone is being made, causing the bones to lose density and become thinner and more porous. The integrity and strength of our bones is related to bone mass and density. The bones of a woman with osteoporosis gradually become thinner and more fragile. A progressive loss of bone mass may continue until the skeleton is no longer strong enough to support itself. When that happens, bones can spontaneously fracture. As bones become more fragile, falls or bumps that would not have hurt us before can cause a fracture. Bone loss seems to be most severe in the spine, wrists and hips. Unfortunately there are usually no signs or symptoms of osteoporosis until a fracture occurs.

SHOULD YOU TAKE HORMONE REPLACEMENT THERAPY TO PREVENT OSTEOPOROSIS?

There is a misconception that osteoporosis begins at menopause. In reality, bone mass begins declining in most women in their mid-thirties, accelerates for three to five years around the time of menopause, and then continues to decline at the rate of about 1 to 1.5 percent per year. Because bone loss accelerates at menopause, and because estrogen levels decline at menopause, conventional medicine has adopted

---

EARLY SIGNS OF OSTEOPOROSIS

Gradual loss of height   Nightly leg and foot cramps
Gum disease, loose teeth   Persistent low back pain
Sudden insomnia and restlessness

---

the belief that osteoporosis is an estrogen deficiency disease that can be cured with estrogen replacement therapy. This is only partly true. The missing piece of this puzzle is diet and lifestyle, plus the bone-building hormone progesterone, which drops much more precipitously at menopause than estrogen does. (Progesterone refers to the natural hormone, not the synthetic progestins. See chapter 18 for more detailed information on natural hormones.)

There is no question that estrogen can slow bone loss around the time of menopause, but the scientific evidence is very clear that after five to six years, bone loss continues at the same rate, with or without estrogen. A very large study, published in the *New England Journal of Medicine* in 1995, studied risk factors for hip fractures in white women. After following over 9,500 women for eight years, researchers found no benefit in estrogen supplementation in women over the age of 65.

In the *NEJM* study, risk factors for hip fractures included:

- Being tall (they fall farther).
- Poor overall health.
- Previous hyperthyroidism (high thyroid, which would make them thin, with less bone).
- Treatment with long-acting benzodiazepines or anticonvulsant drugs (which made them dizzy and drowsy and more likely to fall).
- Heavy coffee drinking (which depletes calcium).
- Lack of exercise.
- Poor depth perception (which would naturally increase the tendency to fall).

PRESCRIPTION DRUGS FOR OSTEOPOROSIS

There are a number of pharmaceutical drugs being used to treat osteoporosis, none of which work very well, and all of which have unpleasant side effects.

The big drug companies know that with millions of baby boom generation women entering their fifties, whoever finds a drug to prevent, reverse or even halt osteoporosis would be onto a financial gold mine. Merck has teamed up with the Premarin-producing giant American Home Products to "promote" osteoporosis to American women and sell their new osteoporosis drug, called Fosamax.

According to an article in the *Wall Street Journal*, the two companies plan to work as a team to get more X-ray machines measuring bone density into the marketplace, and to "educate" physicians about giving menopausal women a combination of Premarin and Fosamax for osteoporosis.

Before you let your physician prescribe Fosamax, tell him or her it's just another version of failed osteoporosis drugs such as etidronate (Didronel) that appear to build bone density for awhile. However, while the bone is denser, it is of poor quality, and after three to six years the rate of bone fractures in women taking these medications is

---

YOUR RISK OF OSTEOPOROSIS IS HIGHER IF YOU:

Are a woman.

Have a family history of osteoporosis.

Are white.

Are thin.

Are short.

Went into menopause early.

Have a low calcium intake.

Don't exercise.

Smoke cigarettes.

Drink more than two alcoholic drinks daily.

Are on chronic steroid therapy (e.g., prednisone).

Are on chronic anticonvulsant therapy.

Are taking drugs which can cause dizziness.

Have hyperthyroidism.

Eat too much animal protein.

Use antacids regularly.

Drink more than two cups of coffee daily.

increased. The Fosamax studies didn't go on long enough to show this kind of damaging side effect, and yet it is well known in the other drugs. You can once again thank the FDA for looking the other way while a damaging drug is marketed to millions of unsuspecting women.

Biphosphonates

ALENDRONATE (Fosamax)

ETIDRONATE (Didronel)

WHAT DO THEY DO IN YOUR BODY?

They slow bone loss by inhibiting the mechanism by which old bone is reabsorbed.

WHAT ARE THEY PRESCRIBED FOR?

They are prescribed for osteoporosis. Unfortunately, the old bone which is saved by using biphosphonates is structurally unsound, and after three to six years tends to *increase* the rate of hip fracture.

WHAT ARE THE POSSIBLE SIDE EFFECTS?

Severe heartburn that can cause permanent damage to the esophagus, stress on the kidneys, impaired fertility, diarrhea, low calcium, vitamin D deficiency, magnesium deficiency, flatulence, rash, headache, muscular pain. Rats given high doses of these drugs developed thyroid and adrenal tumors.

CAUTION!

Please don't use these drugs. There are too many other safe, effective alternatives.

WHAT ARE THE INTERACTIONS WITH OTHER DRUGS?

Biphosphonates may raise levels or prolong the effects of this drug:

↑ Aspirin

This drug may increase the effects or prolong the action of biphosphonates:

↑ Ranitidine

These drugs may reduce the effects of biphosphonates:

↓ Antacids   Calcium supplements

WHAT NUTRIENTS DO THEY THROW OUT OF BALANCE OR INTERACT WITH?

These drugs can cause a deficiency in just about every nutrient important to healthy bones, including calcium, magnesium and vitamin D.

WHAT ELSE TO TAKE IF YOU TAKE THESE DRUGS

A good mineral supplement.

MISCELLANEOUS OSTEOPOROSIS DRUGS

CALCITONIN-SALMON (Calcimar, Salmonine, Osteocalcin, Miacalcin)

WHAT DOES IT DO IN YOUR BODY?

This is a hormone made by the thyroid gland that can temporarily slow bone loss. The long-term side effects are not well-known, and its effectiveness diminishes rapidly after a few years.

WHAT IS IT PRESCRIBED FOR?

Osteoporosis.

WHAT ARE THE POSSIBLE SIDE EFFECTS?

Flu-like symptoms, back pain, respiratory problems such as cough and bronchitis, high blood pressure, angina, rapid heartbeat, irregular heartbeat, hyperthyroidism, dizziness, numbness, insomnia, anxiety, dizziness, headaches, vision disturbances, swollen lymph glands, nausea, loss of appetite or increased appetite, dry mouth, diarrhea, rash, increased sweating, tinnitus (ringing in the ears).

CAUTION!

This is an outdated drug that doesn't work. Please don't use it.

NATURAL REMEDIES FOR OSTEOPOROSIS

Now that we know the process of preventing osteoporosis begins early in life, we are hearing about sugary drinks fortified with calcium for teenagers, antacids with calcium, and calcium supplements. Osteoporosis is not a calcium deficiency disease, it is a disease of excessive calcium loss. In other words, you can take all the calcium supplements you want, but if your diet and lifestyle choices are unhealthy, or you're taking prescription drugs that cause you to lose calcium, you will still lose more calcium from your bones than you can take in through diet.

In fact, getting adequate calcium is only a small part of the prevention picture. Please pass up the sugary drinks and antacids. The dam-

HOW AWARE OF OSTEOPOROSIS ARE YOU?

A Gallup poll sponsored by the National Osteoporosis Foundation found that:

- 75 percent of women believed they were familiar with osteoporosis, but
- 80 percent were not aware that it was responsible for disabling fractures,
- 90 percent were surprised to learn that osteoporosis frequently causes death, and
- 60 percent could not identify the risk factors of osteoporosis.

age that refined sugar does to a growing teenage body or even an adult body far outweighs any benefit that might come from a little calcium supplementation. There is even some evidence that sugar depletes calcium, so the added calcium in these drinks may only be balancing out the damage done by the sugar. The same goes for antacids containing calcium. Since antacids tend to cause you to lose calcium, the added calcium may only offset that damage.

Although osteoporosis is not a calcium deficiency disease, you can rest assured that getting adequate calcium *is* an important factor in preventing osteoporosis. Some good food sources of calcium are snow peas, broccoli, leafy green vegetables such as spinach, kale, beet and turnip greens; almonds, figs, beans (soybeans are the best), nonfat milk, yogurt and cottage cheese. Please don't depend on milk to get your calcium. This is because milk has a poor calcium-to-magnesium ratio. Your body needs a certain amount of magnesium in order to get the calcium into your bones—without magnesium, calcium can't build strong bones.

In fact, magnesium deficiency may be more common in women with osteoporosis than calcium deficiency. Although many fruits and vegetables have some magnesium in them, especially good sources of magnesium are whole grains, wheat bran, leafy green vegetables, nuts (almonds are a very rich source of magnesium and calcium), beans, bananas and apricots.

Trace minerals are also important in helping your body absorb calcium. Eating plenty of green leafy vegetables gives you calcium along with these helpful trace minerals. Boron and manganese are especially important. Foods that contain boron include apples, legumes, almonds, pears and green, leafy vegetables. Foods that include manganese include ginger, buckwheat and oats. Be sure you're getting 1 to 5 mg of boron in your daily multivitamin or osteoporosis formula.

The organic matter in our bones consists mainly of collagen, the "glue" that holds together skin, ligaments, tendons and bones. Zinc, copper, beta-carotene and vitamin C are all important to the formation and maintenance of collagen in the body. If you're following the Six Core Principles for Optimal Health, you'll be getting plenty of these vitamins.

Japanese women have a significantly lower rate of osteoporosis than American women do, and it's likely that their high consumption of soy products is a factor. Adding soy products such as miso, tempeh and tofu to your diet will contribute to better overall health and stronger bones.

Progesterone and Osteoporosis

John Lee, M.D., an internationally known expert on women's hormones, has suggested that the most important factor in osteoporosis is a lack of progesterone, which causes a decrease in new bone formation. He and others have extensive clinical experience showing that using a natural progesterone cream will actively increase bone mass and density and can *reverse* osteoporosis. These patients consistently show as much as a 29 percent increase in bone mineral density in three years or less of progesterone therapy. After treating hundreds of patients with osteoporosis over a period of 15 years, Dr. Lee found that those women with the lowest bone densities experienced the greatest relative improvement, and those who had good bone density to begin with maintained their strong bones.

Postmenopausal women using a transdermal (on the skin) progesterone cream or oil should use the equivalent of 15 to 20 mg daily for three weeks out of the month, with a week off each month to maintain the sensitivity of the progesterone receptors.

NUTRITIONAL SUPPLEMENTS FOR OSTEOPOROSIS

Calcium

Everyone should have at least 1,200 mg of easy-to-absorb calcium daily. Although you can easily get that much with a healthy diet, taking a calcium/magnesium supplement is an excellent form of health insurance. In fact, calcium supplements can help slow bone loss in some women. To be incorporated into bone, calcium requires the help of enzymes, which require magnesium and vitamin B6 to work properly. We tend to be more deficient in magnesium and B6 than we do in calcium.

THESE DEPLETE CALCIUM OR MAGNESIUM

Alcohol

Lack of exercise

Lack of the hormone progesterone or
  testosterone

Phosphorus (found in soda)

Sugar

Too much protein

TO ABSORB CALCIUM AND BUILD BONES WE NEED . . .

Exercise

Hydrochloric acid in the stomach

Magnesium

Progesterone (women) or testosterone
  (men)

Vitamin D

All calcium supplements are not the same. The best absorbed form is called calcium citrate. Avoid the oyster shell calcium, as it can be contaminated with heavy metals. If you're female and over the age of 12, you should be taking 1,200 mg of calcium, combined with 600 to 800 mg of magnesium every day. If you can find a formula that also includes vitamin B6, so much the better.

Sunshine Is the Best Medicine: Vitamin D

Vitamin D is another important ingredient in the recipe for strong bones because it stimulates the absorption of calcium. A deficiency of vitamin D can cause calcium loss. The best way to get vitamin D is from direct sunlight on the skin. Sunlight stimulates a chain of events in the skin leading to the production of vitamin D in the liver and kidneys. (This is why liver and kidney disease can produce a vitamin D deficiency.) Going outside for just a few minutes a day can give us all the vitamin D we need, and yet many people don't even do that. They go from their home, to their car, to their office, and back home, without spending more than a few seconds outdoors. Many elderly people are unable to get outside without assistance, but this should be a priority for their caretakers.

Stomach Acid: Betaine Hydrochloride

As we age, we tend to produce less stomach acid. To be absorbed, calcium requires vitamin D *and* stomach acid. For this reason, it's important to avoid antacids and the H2 blockers such as Tagamet and Zantac, which block or suppress the secretion of stomach acid. Contrary to what the makers of heartburn and indigestion remedies would have you believe, the last thing in the world most people need is *less* stomach acid. Heartburn and indigestion are caused by poor eating habits and a *lack* of stomach acid. Ulcers are caused by a bacteria, not by too much stomach acid. (See Chapter 10 for more information on preventing heartburn and indigestion.) A simple way to improve your calcium absorption may be to take a betaine hydrochloride supplement just before or with meals, to increase your stomach acid. You can find betaine hydrochloride at your health food store.

The Collagen Vitamins and Minerals: Zinc, Vitamins A and C

Collagen is the tissue that makes up your bone. To build collagen you need vitamin A (or beta-carotene), zinc and vitamin C. Vitamin C is especially important, as it is the primary ingredient in the collagen matrix. An esterfied vitamin C—2,000 mg daily—is good preventive medicine for nearly everyone.

WHAT TO AVOID TO PREVENT OSTEOPOROSIS

There's a good chance that one of the leading contributors to osteoporosis in the U.S. is carbonated soft drinks containing phosphorus. Research has shown a direct link between too much phosphorus and calcium loss. If you're guzzling down a couple of fizzy soft drinks a day, you're most likely creating bone loss.

Our other source of excessive phosphorus in the U.S. is eating too much meat. The average American gets more than enough protein, so for most of us it can only help to cut down on our meat consumption. A recent trend among those who love food but don't love the consequences of too much fat and protein is to use meat as a garnish or flavoring in a meal, rather than as a major portion. Fill up on vegetables and complex carbohydrates (whole grains, potatoes, rice, corn, beans), and use meat to enrich your meals. Beans are an excellent and nutritious source of protein and contain many important vitamins and minerals.

Coffee, Alcohol and Cigarette Smoking

Here's yet another good reason to either give up coffee and alcohol or use them in moderation. And do you need to be told how important it is to stop smoking now? (It's *never* too late to reap the benefits of quitting smoking.) Each of these substances creates a negative calcium balance in the body. Substances called phytates and oxylates bind with calcium in the large intestine and form insoluble salts, rendering the calcium useless. The bone mineral content of smokers is 15 to 30 percent lower in women and 10 to 20 percent lower in men. Cigarette smoking is a significant risk factor for osteoporosis. Twice as many women with osteoporosis smoke as compared with women who do not have osteoporosis.

Aluminum

Don't take antacids with aluminum and don't use aluminum cooking pots. It has been shown that small amounts of aluminum-containing antacids increase the urinary and fecal excretion of calcium, inhibit absorption of fluoride, and inhibit absorption of phosphorus, creating a negative calcium balance. The calcium is excreted instead of being utilized. Aluminum is also found in tap water, processed cheese, toothpastes, white flour.

Diuretics

Diuretics are medicines that cause water loss in the body. Along with the water you lose minerals, most notably calcium, magnesium and potassium. They are commonly used in conventional medicine to treat high blood pressure, swelling of the lower legs and congestive heart disease. People who use diuretics have a higher risk of fracture. If you need to use a diuretic, try a gentle herbal one such as dandelion root in a tincture, capsule or tea.

High-Dose Cortisone

A well-known risk for osteoporosis is long-term treatment with the synthetic cortisones such as prednisone. Since the cortisones are closely related to progesterone in their molecular structure, the theory is that they compete for the same receptor sites on bone-building cells. However, while progesterone gives bones the message to grow, the cortisones give bones the message to stop growing. If you must be on a cortisone, talk to your physician about using a low-dose natural cortisone called hydrocortisone rather than the synthetic cortisones. You can refer him or her to the book *The Safe Uses of Cortisone* by William Jefferies, M.D., FACP (Charles C. Thomas Publisher, 1981).

Fluoride Is Bad for Your Bones

The common and seemingly irrefutable wisdom is that the number of cavities has been greatly decreased by the addition of fluoride to our drinking water and our toothpaste. But it's not true, and that fluoride is most likely doing a great deal of harm.

Here's the story behind the story. During World War II we learned how to manufacture things from aluminum: airplanes, buildings, pots and pans, to name a few. We also greatly increased our production of chemical fertilizers. The down side of both these manufacturing processes was a byproduct called fluoride. Although fluoride is a trace mineral naturally occurring in our food, in anything but those trace amounts it's a more potent poison than arsenic. Disposing of the thousands of pounds of fluoride by-product became a major problem in American manufacturing. The manufacturers tried blowing it out their smokestacks, dumping it into rivers and burying it in the ground, but the immediate result was dead and deformed cows and other animals within miles of the smokestacks, rivers full of dead fish, and poisoned water aquifers. In fact its primary use was as a rat poison. Finally the U.S. Public Health Service did a study that claimed to show that one part per million of fluoride in water reduced tooth decay by 60 percent, and thus began the trickling of fluoride into our water supply.

The price of fluoride went up 1,000 percent almost overnight, and the problem of how to dispose of a potent toxin was solved. The practice of water fluoridation was further justified by more glowing studies claiming to show that communities using fluoridated drinking water had a much lower rate of tooth decay than those using unfluoridated water. The fluoride and cavity myth has been perpetuated by the fact that the rate of dental cavities has dropped steadily in the past 30 years, approximately the amount of time that our water has been fluoridated. So it must be good for us, right? Wrong.

The studies that were supposed to show how well fluoridated communities did are highly suspect. The original U.S. Public Health study on fluoridation was supposed to compare hundreds of communities, but the final study only included a few dozen, presumably those that fit the desired pro-fluoridation profile. And even those were flawed. For example, two towns in Michigan were compared for dental cavities, but those children studied in the fluoridated community had higher incomes, received regular dental checkups, and agreed to brush their teeth twice a day. It wouldn't seem strange that they would have a lower rate of cavities, with or without fluoride! "But," you may be protesting, "I had lots of cavities when I was a kid, and my kids hardly have any. It must be due to fluoride." Not so. In both fluoridated and unfluoridated areas in North America and Europe the decline in tooth decay has been the same for 30 years. This even holds true for entire countries in Europe that have not had fluoridated water or toothpaste.

What has changed is that dental hygiene has improved, nutrition has improved, and access to dental care has improved. Studies do show a strong correlation between higher rates of tooth decay and lower economic status.

Japan and all of continental Europe either rejected the fluoride concept from the beginning or have stopped the practice. Most of Great Britain has also discontinued the practice, and Australia and New Zealand are in the process of reversing the trend. A 1994 study of virtually all New Zealand schoolchildren showed no benefit in dental health in fluoridated communities.

What's so bad about fluoride? There is good, solid evidence in eight reputable studies that fluoridated drinking water increases your risk of hip fractures by 20 to 40 percent. For awhile it was thought that fluoride might actually help prevent osteoporosis. But long-term studies with hundreds of thousands of people proved the wisdom of checking things out thoroughly. There is a clear correlation between bone fractures and fluoridation. It turns out that while fluoride does create denser bone, it is poor quality, structurally unsound bone that is actually more prone to fracture over the long term.

So much fluoride has been put into our water and toothpaste over the past 30 years that levels in our food chain are very high. While eating a normal diet, the average person *exceeds* the recommended dose. Fluoride is a potent enzyme inhibitor that interferes with enzymes in the body, particularly in the lining of your intestines, causing stomach pain, gas and bloating. This enzyme-inhibiting effect also interferes with thyroid gland function. Some studies indicate that fluoride damages the immune system, leading to autoimmune disorders and arthritis. There is also evidence that communities with fluoridated water have a higher incidence of heart disease, and higher rates of bone cancer in young men. Some 30 percent of children in fluoridated communities have fluorosis, a malformation of tooth enamel that causes discoloration (usually chalky white patches) and brittleness. This is a permanent change in the teeth that has also been associated with abnormal bone structure.

Advocates of putting fluoride in toothpaste and mouthwash argue that it is not swallowed, and therefore not ingested. However, fluoride is absorbed through the mucous membranes of the mouth, and young children do not have control over their swallowing reflex. There have been numerous reports of children poisoned by ingesting high levels of fluoride through school fluoride mouthwash programs, or fluoridated toothpastes full of sweeteners that kids want to swallow. Who knows how many stomachaches, in kids and adults alike, have been caused by unknowingly ingesting too much fluoride?

Please avoid fluoride, in all forms including toothpastes. This substance has crept into every link in our food chain, and the evidence is that even without fluoridated water and toothpaste we're getting a higher dose than is safe or recommended in our daily diets.

Avoiding Fluoride in Your Water

You can be thankful if you live in an unfluoridated community because it's not easy to get rid of fluoride in your tap water. Distillation and reverse osmosis are the only two reliable methods for removing fluoride. Other water filters may work at eliminating fluoride for a short period of time, but fluoride binds so strongly and quickly to filter materials such as charcoal, that the binding sites become fully occupied after a short time. The best ways to avoid fluoride are to stay away from toothpastes and mouthwashes that contain it. (You can also become politically active and begin to educate your community about the harmful effects of fluoride.)

If you are at a high risk for osteoporosis, it's worth spending the money on a reverse osmosis water purification system.

BONE MINERAL DENSITY (BMD) TESTING

One of the best ways to find out if you're losing bone is to have someone measure your height, and then check it every six months or so. If you start losing height, that's a sure sign that you're losing bone on your spine. It's a good idea for women at risk for osteoporosis to get a bone mineral density measurement as they're going into menopause. That way you'll have a baseline with which to compare later bone density tests, to measure your progress. The safest and most accurate ways to measure bone are with Photon Absorptiometry and Dual Energy X-ray Absorbtiometry (DEXA), which is 96 to 98 percent accurate and uses very low-dose X-rays. CAT scans use too high a level of X-rays. A newer technique for measuring bone loss is called Urinary Excretion of Pyridinium, which measures a substance in the urine that can indicate rapid bone turnover rate.

EXERCISE FOR STRONG BONES: USE 'EM OR LOSE 'EM

Lack of exercise is one of the primary causes of osteoporosis. Using your bones keeps them strong and healthy. Weight-bearing exercise is the only thing besides progesterone found to actually *increase* bone density in older women. Weight-bearing means exercise that uses your bones. Brisk walking counts as weight-bearing exercise, but add some hand-held weights and it's even better. Pushing a vacuum cleaner or lawn mower, gardening, dancing and aerobic exercise also qualify.

Your exercise plan should include a minimum of 20 minutes of weight-bearing exercise three to four times a week. An hour is even better. In contrast to women who exercise, those who don't continue to lose bone, regardless of what else they are doing. Studies of elderly people who fall and break a bone show that these people had poor flexibility, poor leg strength, instability when first standing, and difficulty getting up and down in a chair. Exercise can help increase flexibility, strength and coordination. A weightlifting program of just half an hour three to four times a week can significantly improve bone density. You don't need to go to the gym to do a weightlifting program. You can lift a can of peas or a small carton of milk. Women with advanced osteoporosis should work with a physical therapist to create a safe, effective program to reduce the risk of fracture. The Asian movement exercises such as yoga, tai chi and qi gong can also be excellent for improving strength, flexibility and coordination.

In a recent study on bone density and exercise, older women who did high-intensity weight training two days per week for a year were able to increase their bone density by 1.0 percent, while a control group of women who did not exercise had a bone density *decrease* of 1.8 to 2.5 percent. The women who exercised also had improved muscle strength and better balance, while both decreased in the nonexercising control group.

CHAPTER 20

Drugs for Herpes and Their Natural Alternatives

COLD SORES (TYPE 1 herpes), genital herpes (Type 2 herpes) and shingles (herpes zoster) affect many millions of Americans with painful, burning and itching blisters. The herpes virus is in the same strain as the chicken pox virus, and we know that shingles has its origin in chicken pox, which hides out in the nerves for decades, usually reappearing in the elderly as extremely painful blisters around the rib cage. We don't know where cold sores and genital herpes originated, but we do know that genital herpes is a highly contagious sexually transmitted disease. Some researchers have implicated cold sores with Bell's Palsy, which causes facial paralysis.

Having oral sex with a partner who has a cold sore on the lips can also cause a genital herpes outbreak, and vice versa. No herpes virus ever completely goes away that we know of; it just retreats back into the nerves.

Genital herpes is a virtual epidemic among the baby boomers, affecting an estimated 20 million people. The first outbreak of blisters is usually the most painful and lasts the longest. After that the progression of the disease is very individualized. In a lucky 40 percent of people who are infected it retreats completely, never appearing again. In others it reappears only occasionally. Others are plagued by constant outbreaks that can have a negative impact on self-esteem and sexuality.

Like all sexually transmitted diseases, herpes carries with it the burden of shame, guilt and the risk of passing it on to somebody else. The first thing you can do is drop the shame and guilt (it will reduce emotional stress, which will help prevent the next outbreak), and be extremely careful about passing it on to somebody else. This is not a gift that keeps on giving, it's a curse that keeps on cursing! And although it may be an embarrassment to pass it on to another adult, it can be dangerous when passed on to a newborn baby during a vaginal birth.

Although the virus can theoretically be present and thus contagious when there are no symptoms, if you're in touch with your body you can usually feel it coming on. That's the time to abstain or use a condom—abstention is the safest.

DRUGS FOR TREATING HERPES

ACYCLOVIR (Zovirax)

FAMCICLOVIR (Famvir)

PENCICLOVIR (Denavir)

WHAT DO THEY DO IN YOUR BODY?

Inhibit the herpes virus.

WHAT ARE THEY PRESCRIBED FOR?

Treatment of herpes virus infections.

WHAT ARE THE POSSIBLE SIDE EFFECTS?

Acyclovir has caused testicular atrophy in rats. It can cause kidney damage, liver damage, electrolyte (mineral) balance disturbances. Adverse reactions to acyclovir have included fatigue, nausea and vomiting, headaches, dizziness, skin rash, loss of appetite, water retention, swollen lymph glands, numbness, tingling.

Famciclovir has caused cancer, mutated cells and impaired fertility in rodents. Adverse effects include a high incidence of headaches as well as dizziness, insomnia, fatigue, itching, fever, sinus infections, back and joint pain, numbness, nausea, diarrhea, constipation, vomiting and appetite loss.

Penciclovir is a topical cream approved for treating cold sores. It has caused headaches, rash and numbness.

CAUTION: THINK TWICE ABOUT TAKING THESE TYPES OF DRUGS IF . . .

- You have kidney or liver disease.

WHAT ARE THE INTERACTIONS WITH OTHER DRUGS?

Famciclovir may raise levels or prolong the effects of this drug:

↑ Digoxin

These drugs may increase the effects or prolong the action of famciclovir and/or acyclovir:

↑ Famciclovir/cimetidine
Famciclovir and acyclovir/
probenecid

Famciclovir/theophylline
Acyclovir/zidovudine

NATURAL ALTERNATIVES FOR HERPES DRUGS

Your best preventive strategy for preventing a herpes outbreak is to keep your immune system strong. That means following the Six Core Principles for Optimal Health. You can also take extra vitamin A for up to two weeks (10,000 IU daily), an extra 10 to 15 mg of zinc daily for up to two weeks, and the herbs astragalus and echinacea, which both stimulate and support the immune system. Naturopath and author Michael Murray recommends thymus extracts derived from young calves and standardized (follow the directions on the container).

With both drug and natural treatments, it's important to begin treatment in the earliest possible stages of the outbreak. Shingles doesn't recur very often, but when it does it is generally preceded by fatigue and an aching or sharp pain in the area of the first outbreak.

Most people know when an outbreak of cold sores or genital herpes is coming. The area around the mouth where cold sores occur is usually tingly or numb for a day or two before the outbreak. Genital herpes may be preceded by fatigue, sore or tired muscles, a fever, pain in the groin, hips or legs, swollen lymph glands in the groin area and then shortly before the outbreak, numbness and tingling in the area where the blisters will appear.

Some of the factors that we know can bring on an outbreak of cold sores or genital herpes are stress, infections, fevers, colds and flus, sun exposure, and menstruation. Women have noticed that sexual conflict or ambivalence (a form of stress) can aggravate herpes.

Arginine and Lysine

We also know that chocolate, nuts, grains, beans and other foods containing high levels of the amino acid arginine can precipitate a herpes outbreak. (It's possible that for some people it's only peanuts that aggravate herpes—you'll have to experiment for yourself.) Too much acidic food such as tomatoes, and in some people, vitamin C, can also aggravate an outbreak.

Lysine is the amino acid that opposes arginine, so taking a lysine supplement, 500 mg three times daily between meals at the first sign of an outbreak, can help reduce symptoms. If you have chronic herpes outbreaks you can take 500 mg of lysine daily as a preventive. Foods that are high in lysine include fish, turkey, chicken, beef and dairy products.

The Antiviral Duo: Selenium and Elderberry

Two recent new additions to your antiviral natural medicine cabinet are elderberry extracts and selenium. Both are powerful antiviral agents. See Chapter 11 on colds and flus for details on elderberry. There are anecdotal reports that a combination of elderberry and selenium at the first signs of an impending genital herpes outbreak stopped the outbreak altogether. Follow the directions on the container for elderberry dosage.

For some people, taking a preventive dose of 200 mcg of selenium daily has noticeably reduced the incidence of outbreaks. If you feel an outbreak coming on, or have one, you can increase the dosage for a week. By the way, you can try this dynamic duo of elderberry and selenium for any type of viral infection.

Lemon Balm

It's nice to have lemon balm (*Melissa officinalis L.*) around the garden because it smells so good. This member of the mint family is also an herbal remedy for herpes, and a lemon balm cream is the best-selling cold sore remedy in Germany, where it has been well-studied. Some reports are that when the cream is applied to cold sores regularly, eventually they don't recur. At the very least, lemon balm cream speeds up the healing process. You should be able to find it at your health food store.

RESOURCES

For a Referral to an Alternative Medicine Health Care Professional in Your Area
American College for Advancement in Medicine
P. O. Box 3427
Laguna Hills, CA 92654
(800) 532-3688
In California: (714) 583-7666

To Report an Adverse Drug Reaction to the FDA
Call (800) FDA-1088

National Clearinghouse for Alcohol and Drug Abuse Information
(800) 729-6686

Narcotics Anonymous
(818) 780-3951

For referrals to local meetings call: (212) 870-3400

RECOMMENDED READING

ALTERNATIVE MEDICINE

Bland, John H., M.D., *Live Long, Die Fast*, Fairview Press, Minneapolis, 1997.

Bland, Jeffrey, Ph.D., *The 20-Day Rejuvenation Diet Program*, Keats Publishing, New Canaan, Conn., 1997.

Blaylock, Russell, *Excitotoxins: The Taste That Kills*, Health Press, Santa Fe, New Mex. 1994.

D'Adamo, Peter, N.D., *Eat Right 4 Your Type*, Putnam, New York, 1996.

Fallon, Sally, *Nourishing Traditions*, ProMotion Publishing, San Diego, 1995.

Galland, Leo, M.D., *The Four Pillars of Healing*, Random House, New York, 1997.

Golan, Ralph, M.D., *Optimal Wellness*, Ballantine Books, New York, 1995.

Jahnke, Roger, *The Healer Within*, HarperCollins, San Francisco, 1997.

Mindell, Earl, Ph.D., and Hopkins, Virginia, *Dr. Earl Mindell's What You Should Know About . . . Series*, Keats Publishing, New Canaan, Conn., 1996.

Morton, Mary and Michael, *Five Steps to Selecting the Best Alternative Medicine*, New World Library, Novato, Calif., 1996.

Pizzorno, Joseph N., *Total Wellness*, Prima Publishing, Berkeley, Calif., 1996.

Robbins, John, *Reclaiming Our Health*, HJ Kramer, Tiburon, Calif., 1996.

Sears, Barry, *The Zone*, Harper Collins, New York, 1996.

Todd, Gary Price, M.D., *Nutrition, Health and Disease*, Whitford Press, West Chester, Penn., 1985.

HORMONES

Barnes, Broda, *Hypothyroidism: The Unsuspected Illness*, Harper and Row, New York, 1976.

Colborn, Theo, *Our Stolen Future*, Penguin Books, New York, 1997.

Khalsa, Dharma Singh, M.D., *Brain Longevity*, Warner Books, New York, 1997.

Klatz, Ronald and Goldman, Robert, *Stopping the Clock*, Bantam Books, New York, 1996.

——————, with Kahn, Carol, *Grow Young with HGH*, Harper-Collins, New York, 1997.

Lee, John R., M.D., and Hopkins, Virginia, *What Your Doctor May Not Tell You About Menopause: The Breakthrough Book on Natural Progesterone*, Warner Books, New York, 1996.

Sahelian, Ray, *Melatonin: Nature's Sleeping Pill*, Avery Publishing, Garden City Park, N.Y., 1995.

——————, *DHEA: A Practical Guide*, Avery Publishing, Garden City Park, N.Y., 1996.

DRUGS

Breggin, Peter, *Talking Back to Prozac*, St. Martin's Press, New York, 1994.

Lappe, Marc, *When Antibiotics Fail: Restoring the Ecology of the Body*, North Atlantic Books, Berkeley, Calif., 1995.

Schmidt, Michael, and Smith, Lendon, M.D., and Sehnert, Keith, *Beyond Antibiotics*, North Atlantic Books, Berkeley, Calif., 1994.

CHILDREN

Lappe, Marc, *When Antibiotics Fail: Restoring the Ecology of the Body*, North Atlantic Books, Berkeley, Calif., 1995.

Schmidt, Michael, and Smith, Lendon, M.D., and Sehnert, Keith, *Beyond Antibiotics*, North Atlantic Books, Berkeley, Calif., 1994.

Smith, Lendon, M.D., *How to Raise a Healthy Child*, M. Evans & Co., New York, 1996.

Zand, Janet, O.M.D., and Walton, Rachel, R.N., and Rountree, Robert, M.D., *A Parent's Guide to Medical Emergencies*, Avery Publishing, Garden City Park, N.Y., 1997.

REFERENCES

CHAPTER 1: CHANGING THE PILL-POPPING MINDSET

Classen, D., "Adverse Drug Events in Hospitalized Patients," *JAMA*, 1197;277:301–306.

Johnson, J., et al., "Drug Related Morbidity and Mortality—A Cost of Illness Model," *Arch Intern Med.;* 155, Oct. 9, 1996.

Nelson, K., et al., "Drug-Related Hospital Admissions," *Pharmacotherapy,* 16(4):701–707, 1996.

Soumerai, S. B., et al., "Effects of Medicaid drug-payment limits on admissions to hospitals and nursing homes." *N Engl J Med* 325:1072–1077, 1991.

CHAPTER 2: HOW TO AVOID PRESCRIPTION DRUG ABUSE

Tanouye, Elyse, "Antidepressant Makers Study Kids' Market," *Wall Street Journal,* April 4, 1997.

Weber, Tracy, "Tarnishing the Golden Years with Addiction," *Los Angeles Times,* Dec. 20, 1996.

CHAPTER 3: HOW YOUR BODY PROCESSES DRUGS

Logsdon, B. A., "Drug Use During Lactation," *Journal of the American Pharmaceutical Association,* vol. NS37, No. 4, July/August 1997.

Tschanz, C., et al., "Interactions Between Drugs and Nutrients," *Advances in Pharmacology,* vol. 35, 1996.

CHAPTER 4: HOW DRUGS INTERACT WITH FOOD, DRINK AND SUPPLEMENTS

Kirk, J. K., "Significant Drug-Nutrient Interactions," *American Family Doctor,* April 1995;51(5):1175–1182.

Tschanz, C., et al., "Interactions Between Drugs and Nutrients," *Advances in Pharmacology,* vol. 35, 1996.

CHAPTER 8: THE SIX CORE PRINCIPLES FOR OPTIMAL HEALTH

Antioxidants

Aruoma, O. I., et al., "Nutrition and Health Aspects of Free Radicals and Antioxidants," *Fd. Chem. Toxic.,* 32(7):671–683, 1994.

Costanzo, L. L., et al., "Antioxidant Effect of Copper on Photosynthesized Lipid Peroxidation," *Journal of Inorganic Biochemistry*, 57:115–125, 1995.

Elson, "Cholesterol- and Tumor-Suppressive Actions of Fruits and Vegetables," *The Nutrition Report*, April 1995;13(4):17, 24.

Fuller, Cindy J., et al., "Effects of Antioxidants and Fatty Acids on Low-Density-Lipoprotein Oxidation," *American Journal of Clinical Nutrition*, 60(supp):1010S-3S, 1994.

Gaziano, J. Michael, et al., "Natural Antioxidants and Cardiovascular Disease: Observational Epidemiologic Studies and Randomized Trials," *Natural Antioxidants in Human Health and Disease*, Academic Press, 13:387–409, 1994.

Gilligan, David J., M.D., et al., "Efect of Antioxidant Vitamins on Low Density Lipoprotein Oxidation and Impaired Endothelium-Dependent Vasodilation in Patients with Hypercholesterolemia," *Journal of the American College of Cardiology*, Dec. 1994;24(7):1611–1617.

Hoffman, Richard M., M.D. and Garewal, Harinder S., "Antioxidants and the Prevention of Coronary Heart Disease," *Archives of Internal Medicine*, Feb. 13, 1995; 155:241–246.

Kanter, Mitchell M., "Free Radicals, Exercise, and Antioxidant Supplementation," *International Journal of Sports Nutrition*, 4:205–220, 1994.

Oliver, Michael F., "Antioxidant Nutrients, Atherosclerosis, and Coronary Heart Disease," *British Heart Journal*, 73:299–301, 1995.

Rautalahti, Matti, et al. "Antioxidants aned Carcinogenesis," *Annals of Medicine*, 25:435–441, 1993.

Regling, G., et al., "The Biological Role of Oxygen Radicals, Lipid Peroxidation and Antioxidative Therapy in Connective Tissue Regulation," *Wolffs Law and Connective Tissue Regulation*, 231–241, 1993.

Singh, R., et al., "Diet, Antioxidant, Vitamins, Oxidative Stress and Risk of Coronary Artery Disease: The Purzuda Prospective Study," *Acta Cardiology*, 49(5):453–467, 1995.

Stavric, Bozidar, "Role of Chemopreventers in Human Diet," *Clinical Biochemistry*, 27(5):319–332, 1994.

Todd, Susan, et al., "An Investigation of the Relationship Between Antioxidant Vitamin Intake and Coronary Heart Disease in Men and Women Using Logistic Regression Analysis," *Journal of Clinical Epidemiology*, 48(2):307–316, 1995.

Tribble, Diane L., Ph.D., et al., "Dietary Antioxidants, Cancer, and Atherosclerotic Heart Disease," *Western Journal of Medicine*, 161:605–613, 1994.

Wei, Qingyi, et al., "Vitamin Supplementationi and Reduced Risk of Basal Cell Carcinoma," *Journal of Clinical Epidemiology*, 47(8):829–836, 1994.

Grapeseed Bioflavonoids

Chang, W. C., et al., "Inhibition of Platelet Aggregation and Arachidonate Metabolism in Platelets by Procyanidins," *Prostagland Leukotri Essential Fatty Acids* 38:181–8,1989.

Frankel, E. N., et al., "Inhibition of Oxidation of Human Low-density Lipoprotein by Phenolic Substances in Red Wine," *Lancet* 341:454–7, 1993.

Gomez Trillo, J. T., "Varicose Veins of the Lower Extremities. Symptomatic Treatment with a New Vasculotrophic Agent," *Prensa Med. Mex.*, 38:293–6, 1973.

Harmand, M. F., et al., "The Fate of Total Flavonolic Oligomers (OFT) Extracted from 'Vitis vinifera L.' in the Rat," *Eur. J. Drug Met. Pharmacokin* 1:15–30, 1978.

Henriet, J. P., "Veno-lymphatic Insufficiency. 4,729 Patients Undergoing Hormonal and Procyanidol Oligomer Therapy," *Phlebolgie* 46:313–25, 1993.

Hertog, M. G., et al., "Dietary Antioxidant Flavonoids and Risk of Coronary Heart Disease: The Zutphen Elderly Study," *Lancet* 342:1007–11, 1993.

Lagrue, G., et al., "A Study of the Effects of Procyanidol Oligomers on Capillary Resistance in Hypertension and in Certain Nephropathies," *Sem. Hosp. Paris* 57:1399–401, 1981.

Masquelier, J., "Procyanidolic Oligomers," *J. Parfums Cosm. Arom.* 95:89–97, 1990.

————, "Pycnogenols: Recent Advantages in the Therapeutical Activity of Procyanidins," *Natural Prod. Med. Agents* 1:243–56, 1981.

————, et al., "Stabilization of Collagen by Procyanidolic Oligomers," *Acta Therap.* 7:101–5, 1981.

Meunier, M. T., et al., "Inhibition of Angiotensin I Converting Enzyme by Flavenolic Compounds: In Vitro and In Vivo Studies," *Planta Med.* 54:12–5, 1987.

Schwitters, B., et al., "OPC in Practice: Bioflavanols and Their Application," *Alfa Omega*, Rome, Italy, 1993.

Tixier, J. M., et al., "Evidence by In Vivo and In Vitro Studies That Binding of Pycnegols to Elastin Affects Its Rate of Degradation by Elastases," *Biochem. Pharmacol.* 3:3933–9, 1984.

Wegrowski, J., et al., "The Effect of Procyanidolic Oligomers on the Composition of Normal and Hypercholesterolemic Rabbit Aortas," *Biochem. Pharmacol.* 33:3491–7, 1984.

Green Tea Bioflavonoids

Apostolides, Z., et al., "Screening of Tea Clones for Inhibition of PhIP Mutagenicity," *Mutat. Res.*, Feb. 1995, 326(2):219–25.

Bu-Abbas, A., et al., "Marked Antimutagenic Potential of Aqueous Green Tea Extracts: Mechanism of Action," *Mutagenesis*, July 1994, 9(4):325–31.

Burr, Michael L., et al., "Antioxidants and Cancer," *Journal of Human Nutrition and Dietetics*, 7:409–416, 1994.

"Foods That May Prevent Breast Cancer: Studies Are Investigating Soybeans, Whole Wheat and Green Tea Among Others," *Primary Care and Cancer*, Feb. 1994, 14(2):10–11.

Gao, F. M., et al., "Studies on Mechanisms and Blockade of Carcinogenic Action of Female Sex Hormones," *Sci. China B.*, April 1994, 37(4):418–29.

Graham, H. N., "Green Tea Composition, Consumption, and Polyphenol Chemistry," *Prev. Med.* May 1992, 21(3): 334–50.

Hirose, M., et al., "Inhibition of Mammary Gland Carcinogenesis by Green Tea Catechins and Other Naturally Occurring Antioxidants in Female Sprague-Dawley Rats Pretreated with 7,12-demethylbenz[alpha]anthracene." *Cancer Lett.* 83(1–2):149–56, 1994.

Ikigai, H., et al., "Bactericidal Catechins Damage the Lipid Biolayer," *Biochem. Biophys Acta* 1147(1):132–6, Apr. 8, 1993.

Imai, K. et al., "Cross Sectional Effects of Drinking Tea on Cardiovascular and Liver Diseases," *British Medical Journal* 310(6981):693–6, Mar. 18, 1995.

Katiyar, S. K., et al., "Inhibition of Spontaneous and Photo-enhanced Lipid Peroxidation in Mouse Epidermal Microsomes by Epicatechin Derivatives from Green Tea," *Cancer Lett.* 79(1):61–6, April 29, 1994.

————, et al., "Protection Against Malignant Conversion of Chemically Induced Benign Skin Papillomas to Squamous Cell Carcinomas in SENCAR Mice by a Polyphenolic Fraction Isolated from Green Tea," *Cancer Res.* 53(22)5409–12, Nov. 15, 1993.

————, et al., "Protective Effects of Green Tea Polyphenols Administered by Oral Intubation Against Chemical Carcinogen-induced Forestomach and Pulmonary Neoplasia in A/J Mice," *Cancer Lett.* 73(2–3):167–72, Sept. 30, 1993.

Kawaguchi, M., et al., "Three Month Oral Repeated Administration Toxicity Study of Seed Saponins of Thea Sinensis L. (Ryokucha Saponin) in Rats," *Food Chem. Toxicol.,* 32(5):431–42, May 1994.

Kimura, R., et al., "Effect of theanine on norepinephrine and serotonin levels in rat brain," *Chem. Pharm. Bull.,* July 1986, 34(7):3053–7.

Kubo, Isao, et al., "Antimicrobial Activity of Green Tea Flavor Components and Their Combination Effects," *Journal of Agricultural Food Chemistry,* 40:245–248, 1992.

Makimura, M., et al., "Inhibitory Effect of Tea Catechins on Collagenase Activity," *J. Periodontal.* 64(7):630–6, July 1993.

Mukhtar, H., et al., "Green Tea and Skin-anticarcinogenic effects," *J. Invest. Dermatol.* 102(1):3–7, Jan. 1994.

————, et al., "Green Tea Components: Antimugenic and Anticarcinogenic Effects," *Prev. Med.* 21(3):351–60, May 1, 1992.

Nagata, T., et al.; "Differences in Caffeine, Flavonols and Amino Acids Contents in Leaves of Cultivated Species of Camellia," *Jap.J.Breed.* 34(4):459–467, 1984.

Narisawa, T., et al., "A Very Low Dose of Green Tea Polyphenols in Drinking Water Prevents N-methyl-N-nitrosourea-induced Colon Carcinogenesis in F344 Rats," *Jpn. J. Cancer Res.* 84(10):1007–9, Oct. 1993.

Nishida, H., et al., "Inhibitory Effects of (-)-epigallocatechin Gallate on Spontaneous Hepatoma in C3H/HeNCrj Mice and Human Hepatoma-derived PLC/PRF/5 cells," *Jpn. J. Cancer Res.* 85(3):221–5, March 1994.

Shetty, M., et al., "Antibacterial Activity of Tea (*Camillia sinensis*) and Coffee (*Coffee arabica*) With Special Reference to Salmonella Typhimurium," *J. Commun. Dis.* 26(3):147–50, Sept. 1994.

Tao, P., "The Inhibitory Effects of Catechin Derivatives on the Activities of Human Immunodeficiency Virus Reverse Transcriptase and DNA Polymerases," *Chung Kuo I Huo I Hsueh Yuan Hsueh Pao* 14(5):334–8, Oct. 1992.

Tsushida, T., et al., "An enzyme hydrolyzing L-theanine in tea leaves," *Agroc Biol Chem*, 49(10):2913–2917, 1985.

Valstar, E., "Nutrition and Cancer: A Review of Preventive and Therapeutic Abilities of Single Nutrients," *Journal of Nutritional Medicine* 4:176–178, 1994.

Wang, Z. Y., et al., "Inhibitory Effects of Black Tea, Green Tea, Decaffeinated Black Tea, and Decaffeinated Green Tea on Ultraviolet Light-induced Skin Carcinogenesis in 7, 12-dimethylbenz[a]anthracene-initiated SKH-1 Mice," *Cancer Res* 54(13):3428–35, July 1, 1994.

Weisburger, J. H., et al., "Prevention of Heterocyclic Amine Formation by Tea and Tea Polyphenols," *Cancer Lett* 83(1–2):143–7, Aug. 15, 1994.

Yang, Chung S., et al., "Tea and Cancer," *Journal of the National Cancer Institute* 85(13):1038–1049, July 7, 1993.

Yen, Gow-Chin, et al., "Antioxidant Activity of Various Tea Extracts in Relation to Their Antimutagenicity," *Journal of Agricultural and Food Chemistry*, 1995; 43:27–32.

Yin, P., et al., "Experimental Studies of the Inhibitory Effects of Green Tea Catechin on Mice Large Intestinal Cancers Induced by 1,2-Dimethylhydrazine," *Cancer Lett* 79(1):33–8, April 29, 1994.

Yokogoshi, H., et al., "Reduction effect of theanine on blood pressure and brain 5-hydroxyindoles in spontaneously hyptertensive rats," *Bioschi Biotechnol Biochem*, April 1995, 59(4):615–8.

Yoshino, K., et al., "Antioxidative Effects of Black Tea Theaflavins and Thearubigin on Lipid Peroxidation of Rat Liver Homogenates Induced by Tert-butyl Hydroperoxide," *Biol Pharm Bull* 17(1):146–9, Jan. 1994.

CHAPTER 9: DRUGS FOR HEART DISEASE AND THEIR NATURAL ALTERNATIVES

Abbott, Lisa, et al., "Magnesium Deficiency in Alcoholism: Possible Contribution to Osteoporosis and Cardiovascular Disease in Alcoholics," *Alcoholism: Clinical and Experimental Research*, Sept./Oct. 1994;18;(5):1076–1082.

al-Ghamdi, S. M., et al., "Magnesium deficiency: pathophysiologic and clinical overview," *Am J Kidney Dis*, Nov. 1994, 24(5):737–52.

Altura, Burton M., et al., "Role of Magnesium in the Pathogenesis of Hypertension Updated: Relationship to Its Action on Cardiac, Vascular Smooth Muscle and Endothelial Cells," *Hypertension: Pathophysiology, Diagnosis, and Management*, 1995; 72:1213–1242.

Aw, T. Y., et al., "Intestinal absorption and lymphatic transport of peroxidized lipids in rats: effects of exogenous GSH," *Am J Physiol*, Nov. 1992, 263.

Ceconi, C., et al., "The role of glutathione status in the protection against ischaemic and reperfusion damage: effects of N-acetyl cysteine," *J Mol Cell Cardiol*, Jan. 1988, 20(1):5–13.

Classen, U.G., "Influence of high and low dietary magnesium levels on functional, chemical and morphological parameters of 'old' rats," *Magnes Res*, Dec. 1994, 7(3–4):233–43.

Durlach, J., "Primary mitral valve prolapse: a clinical form of primary magnesium deficit," *Magnes Res*, Dec. 1994, 7(3–4):339–40, ISSN 0953-1424.

————————, "Magnesium and therapeutics," *Magnes Res*, Dec. 1994, 7(3–4):313–28.

Elin, R., "Magnesium: The 5th But Forgotten Electrolyte," *American Journal of Clinical Pathology*, 102(5):616–622, 1994.

Flagg, E. W., et al., "Plasma total glutathione in humans and its association with demographic and health-related factors," *Br J Nutr*, Nov. 1993, 70(3):797–808.

"Final report on the aspirin component of the ongoing Physicians' Health Study," *The New England Journal of Medicine*, July 20, 1989, 321(3):129(7).

Giovannucci, Edward, et al., "Alcohol, Low-Methionine-Low Folate Diets and the Risk of Colon Cancer in Men," *Journal of the National Cancer Institute*, Feb. 15, 1995, 87(4):265–273.

Igawa, Akihiko, et al., "Comparison of Frequency of Magnesium Deficiency in Patients with Vasospastic Angina and Fixed Coronary Artery Disease," *American Journal of Cardiology*, April 1, 1995, 75:728–731.

Julius, M., et al., "Glutathione and morbidity in a community-based sample of elderly," *J Clin Epidemiol*, Sept. 1994, 47(9):1021–6.

Kinscherf, R., et al., "Effect of glutathione depletion and oral N-acetyl-cysteine treatment on CD4+ and CD8+ cells," *FASEB J*, April 1, 1994, 8(6):448–51.

Lanza, F. L., "A review of gastric ulcer and gastroduodenal injury in normal volunteers receiving aspirin and other non-steroidal anti-inflammatory drugs," *Scand. J. Gastroenterol. Suppl*, 1989, 24/163 (24–31).

Miura, K., et al., "Cystine uptake and glutathione level in endothelial cells exposed to oxidative stress," *Am J Physiol*, Jan. 1992, 262.

Mizui, T., et al., "Depletion of brain glutathione by buthionine sulfoximine enhances cerebral ischemic injury in rats," *Am J Physiol*, Feb. 1992, 262.

Nozue, Tomio, et al., "Magnesium Status, Serum HDL Cholesterol, and Apolipoprotein A-1 Levels," *Journal of Pediatric Gastroenterology and Nutrition*, 20:316–318, 1995.

Paolisso, G., et al., "Plasma GSH/GSSG affects glucose homeostasis in healthy subjects and non-insulin-dependent diabetics," *Am J Physiol*, Sept. 1992, 263.

Sastre, J., et al., "Exhaustive physical exercise causes oxidation of glutathione status in blood: prevention by antioxidant administration," *Am J Physiol*, Nov. 1992, 263(5Pt2):R992–995.

Toto, K. H., et al., "Magnesium: homeostasis, imbalances, and therapeutic uses," *Crit Care Nurs Clin North A*, Dec. 1994, 6(4):767–83.

Van Zandwijk, Nico, "N-Acetylcysteine for Lung Cancer Prevention," *Chest*, May 1995, 107(5):1437–1441.

High Blood Pressure/Hypertension Drugs

Borok, G., "Nutritional Aspects of Hypertension," *South African Medical Journal*, Aug. 5, 1989, 76:125–126.

Gale, C. R., et al., "Vitamin C and Risk of Death From Stroke and Coronary Heart Disease in Cohorts of Elderly People," *British Medical Journal*, 310:1563–6, 1995.

Kisters, K., et al., "Plasma Magnesium and Total Intracellular Magnesium Ion Content of Lymphocytes in Untreated Normotensive and Hypertensive Patients," *Trace Elements and Electrolytes*, 13(4):163–166, 1996.

Romero-Alvira, D., et al., "High Blood Pressure, Oxygen Radicals and Antioxidants: Etiological Relationships," *Medical Hypotheses*, 1996; 46:414–420.

Sanjuliani, A. F., et al., "Effects of Magnesium on Blood Pressure and Intracellular Ion Levels of Brazilian Hypertensive Patients," *International Journal of Cardiology*, 1996;56:177–183.

Cholesterol-Lowering Drugs

Araghiniknam, Mohsen, et al., "Antioxidant Activity of Dioscorea and Dehydroepiandrosterone (DHEA) in Older Humans," *Life Sciences*, 59(11):147–157, 1996.

Barnard, James R., Ph.D., et al., "Effects of Diet and Exercise on Qualitative and Quantitative Measures of LDL and Its Susceptibility to Oxidation," *Arteriosclerosis, Thrombosis, and Vascular Biology*, Feb. 1996, 16(2):201–207.

Boston, Paul F., et al., "Serum Cholesterol and Treatment-Resistance in Schizophrenia," *Biological Psychiatry*, 40:542–543, 1996.

Brown, Donald, "Hyperlipidemia and Prevention of Coronary Heart Disease," *Quarterly Review of Natural Medicine*, Spring 1997, 61–71.

Chang, et al., "Low Plasma Cholesterol Predicts an Increased Risk of Lung Cancer in Elderly Women," *Preventative Medicine*, 24:557–562, 1995.

Gatto, L. M., et al., "Ascorbic Acid Induces a Favorable Lipoprotein Profile in Women," *Journal of the American College of Nutrition*, 15(2):154–158, 1996.

Harris, William S., "N-3 Fatty Acids and Lipoproteins: Comparison of Results From Human and Animal Studies," *Lipids*, 31(3):243–252, 1996.

Jancin, Bruce, "Psyllium Adds to Diet for Lowering Cholesterol," *Family Practice News*, Nov. 1, 1996, 13.

Kondo, K., et al., "Inhibition of LDL Oxidation by Cocoa," *Lancet*, Nov. 30, 1996, 348:1514.

Kromhout, D., et al., "The Effect of 26 Years of Habitual Fish Consumption on Serum Lipid and Lipoprotein Levels (The Zutphen Study)," *Nutrition, Metabolism and Cardiovascular Disease*, 9h/150:1–7, 1996.

Lien, Wen-Pin, M.D., et al., "Low Serum, High-Density Lipoprotein Cholesterol Concentration Is an Important Coronary Risk Factor in Chinese Patients With Low Serum Levels of Total Cholesterol and Triglyceride," *American Journal of Cardiology*, May 15, 1996, 77:1112–1115.

Malhotra, S. C., Ahuja, M. M. S., Sundarum, K. R., "Long-term clinical studies on the hypolipidemic effect of *Commiphora mukul* (guggul) and clofibrate," *Ind/Med Res* 65:390–95, 1977.

Newman, T. B., et al., "Carcinogenicity of lipid-lowering drugs," *Journal of the American Medical Association*, 275/1(55–60), 1996.

Simons, L. A., et al., "What Dose of Vitamin E Is Required to Reduce Susceptibility of LDL to Oxidation?" *Australian New Zealand Journal of Medicine*, 26:496–503, 1996.

Steiner, Manfred, et al., "A Double-Blind Crossover Study in Moderately Hypercholesterolemic Men That Compared the Effect of Aged Garlic Extract and Placebo Administration on Blood Lipids," *American Journal of Clinical Nutrition*, 1996, 64:866–870.

Temple, N.J., "Dietary Fats and Coronary Heart Disease," *Biomed. and Pharmcother.,* 1996, 50:261–268.

Wander, Rosemary C., et al., "Effects of Interaction of RRR-à-Tocopheryl Acetate and Fish Oil on Low-Density-Lipoprotein Oxidation in Postmenopausal Women With and Without Hormone-Replacement Therapy," *American Journal of Clinical Nutrition,* 1996, 63:194–193.

CHAPTER 10: DRUGS FOR THE DIGESTIVE TRACT AND THEIR NATURAL ALTERNATIVES

Al-Somal, N., Coley, K. E., et al., "Susceptibility of Helicobacter pylori to the antimicrobial activity of manuka honey," *Journal of the Royal Society of Medicine,* Jan. 1994, 87:9–12.

Bachman, A., "Glutamine: Is it a conditionally required nutrient for the human gastrointestinal system?" *Journal of the American College of Nutrition,* 15(3):199–205, 1996.

Batchelder, H. J., Scalzo, R., "Naturopathic Specific Condition Review: Constipation," *Protocol Journal of Botanical Medicine,* vol. 1 no.1, Summer 1995, p. 52–55.

——————, "Allopathic Specific Condition Review: Peptic Ulcer," *Protocol Journal of Botanical Medicine,* vol.1 no.3, Winter 1996, p. 191–196.

Beil, W., Birkholz, C., Sewing, K. F., "Effects of flavonoids on parietal cell acid secretion, gastric mucosal prostaglandin production and Helicobacter pylori growth," *Arzneim-Forsch Drug Research* 45:697–700, 1995.

Buddington, R. K., et al., "Dietary supplement of neosugar alters the fecal flora and decreases activities of some reductive enzymes in human subjects," *American Journal of Clinical Nutrition,* 63:709–16, 1996.

Dunjic, B. S., et al., "Green banana protection of gastric mucosa against experimentally induced injuries in rats," *Scandinavian Journal of Gastroenterology* 28:894–898, 1993.

Goso, Y., et al., "Effects of traditional herbal medicine on gastric mucin against ethanol-induced gastric injury in rats," *Comp. Biochemistry and Physiology,* 113C:17–21, 1996.

Ianoco, G., Carrocio, A., Cavataio, F., et al., "Chronic constipation as a symptom of cow milk allergy," *Journal of Pediatrics,* 126:34–39, 1995.

Liva, R. N.D., "Naturopathic Specific Condition Review: Peptic Ulcer," *The Protocol Journal of Botanical Medicine,* vol.1 no.3, Winter 1996, p.197–202.

Salminen, S., Isolauri, E., Onnela, T., "Gut flora in normal and disordered states," *Chemotherapy* 41(suppl 1):5–15, 1995.

CHAPTER 11: COUGH, COLD, ALLERGY AND ASTHMA DRUGS, AND THEIR NATURAL ALTERNATIVES

Abulhosn, R. A., M.D., et al., "Passive Smoke Exposure Impairs Recovery After Hospitalization for Acute Asthma," *Archives of Pediatric and Adolescent Medicine,* Feb. 1997; 151:135–139.

Baker, Barbara, "Patient History Often Fails to Uncover Allergies," *Skin & Allergy News,* April 1997; 11.

Bogden, J. D., "Micronutrient Nutrition and Immunity," *Nutrition Report,* Feb. 1995;13(2):1.

Broughton, K. S., et al., "Reduced Asthma Symptoms With n-3 Fatty Acid Ingestion Are Related to 5-Series Leukotriene Production," *American Journal of Clinical Nutrition*, 65:1011–1017, 1997.

Cairns, C. B., M.D. and Kraft, M., M.D., "Magnesium Attenuates the Neutrophil Respiratory Burst in Adult Asthmatic Patients," *Academy of Emergency Medicine*, 1996:3:1093–1097.

Carroll, L., "Leukotriene Inhibitors Represent Important Class of Asthma Drugs," *Medical Tribune*, March 6, 1997;4.

The Centers for Disease Control and Prevention: Leads From the Morbidity and Mortality Weekly Report, Atlanta, Ga: Pneumonia and Influenza Death Rates—United States, 1979–1994, *JAMA*, Aug. 16, 1995, 274(7):532.

Donahue, J., D.V.M., Ph.D., "Inhaled Steroids and the Risk of Hospitalization for Asthma," *JAMA*, March 19, 1997:277(11):887–891.

Dowling, C. G. and Hollister, A., "An Epidemic of Sneezing and Wheezing," *Life*, May 1997, p. 76–92.

Eby, G. A., "Zinc Lozenges as Cure for Common Colds," *Annals of Pharmacotherapy*, Nov. 1996;30:1336–1338.

————, "Linearity in Dose-Response From Zinc Lozenges in Treatment of Common Colds," *Journal of Pharmacy Technology*, May/June 1995;22:110–122.

Fantidis, P., et al., "Intracellular (polymorphonuclear) magnesium content in patients with bronchial asthma between attacks," *Journal of the Royal Society of Medicine*, 88(8):441–5, Aug. 1995.

Govaert, T., et al., "The Efficacy of Influenza Vaccination in Elderly Individuals: A Randomized, Double-Blind, Placebo-Controlled Trial," *JAMA*, Dec. 7, 1994; 272:1661–1665.

Hill, D. J., et al., "The Melbourne House Dust Mite Study: Eliminating House Dust Mites in the Domestic Environment," *Journal of Allergy and Clinical Immunology*, March 1997;99:323–329.

Hurst, D. S., M.D., "The Association of Otitis Media With Effusion and Allergy as Demonstrated by Intradermal Skin Testing and Eosinophil Cationic Protein Levels in Both Middle Ear Effusions and Mucosal Biopsies," *Laryngoscope*, Sept.. 1996;106:1128–1137.

————, and Venge, P., M.D., Ph.D., "Levels of Eosinophil Cationic Protein and Myeloperoxidase From Chronic Middle Ear Effusion in Patients With Allergy and/or Acute Infection," *Otalaryngology-Head and Neck Surgery*, 1996;114:531–544.

Knutsen, R., Bohmer, T. and Falch, J., "Intravenous theophylline-induced excretion of calcium, magnesium and sodium in patients with recurrent asthmatic attacks," *Scandinavian Journal of Clinical and Laboratory Investigation*, 54(2):119–25, April 1994.

Majamaa, H., M.D. and Isolauri, E., M.D., "Probiotics: A Novel Approach in the Management of Food Allergy," *Journal of Allergy and Clinical Immunology*, 99:179–185, 1997.

Margolis, K. L., et al., "Frequency of adverse reactions after influenza vaccination," Department of Medicine, University of Minnesota, Minneapolis. *Am J Med*, Jan. 1990, 88(1):27–30.

Mendell, J. J., et al., "Elevated Symptom Prevalence Associated With Ventilation Type in Office Buildings," *Epidemiology*, 7:583–589, 1996.

McCann, J., "Conjugated flu vaccine boosts response in elderly; binding a diphtheria toxoid to the standard influenza vaccine may make flu shots more effective for this group," *Medical World News*, Aug. 8, 1988; 29(15):16(1).

Millqvist, E. and Lowhagen, O., "Placebo-Controlled Challenges With Perfume in Patients with Asthma-Like Symptoms," *Allergy*, 51:434–439, 1996.

Moneret-Vautrin, D. A. and Kanny, G., "Food and Drug Additives: Hypersensitivity and Intolerance," *Human Toxicology*, Chap. 5:259–280, 1996.

Peters, Annette, et al., "Acute Health Effects of Exposure to High Levels of Air Pollution in Eastern Europe," *American Journal of Epidemiology*, 144(6):570–581, 1996.

Scaglione, F., et al., "Efficacy and Safety of the Standardized Ginseng Extract G 115 for Potentiating Vaccination against Common Cold and/or Influenza Syndrome," *Drugs in Experimental and Clinical Research*, 22(2):65–72, 1996.

Seelig, M. S., "Consequences of magnesium deficiency on the enhancement of stress reactions; preventive and therapeutic implications," *J.Am.Coll.Nutr.* 13(5):429–46, Oct. 1994.

Suissa, S., Ph.D and Ernst, P., M.D., "Albuterol in Mild Asthma," *New England Journal of Medicine*, March 6, 1997, 336(10):729.

CHAPTER 12: DRUGS FOR PAIN RELIEF AND THEIR NATURAL ALTERNATIVES

Brown, Scott, J., et al., *Family Practice News*, "Panel OKs Alternative Therapy for Chronic Pain," Dec. 15, 1995;4.

Felson, David T., "Weight and Osteoarthritis," *American Journal of Clinical Nutrition*, 63(suppl.):430S-2S, 1996.

Kjeldsen-Kragh, Jens, "Dietary Treatment of Rheumatoid Arthritis," *Scandinavian Journal of Rheumatology*, 63, 1996.

Kremer, Joel M., M.D., "Effects of Modulation of Inflammatory and Immune Parameters in Patients with Rheumatic and Inflammatory Disease Receiving Dietary Supplementation of N-3 and N-6 Fatty Acids," *Lipids*, (suppl.);31:S-243–S-247, 1996.

McAlindon, Timothy E., et al., "Do Antioxidant Micronutrients Protect Against the Development and Progression of Knee Osteoarthritis?" *Arthritis and Rheumatism*, April 1996, 39(4):648–656.

Peikert, A., et al., "Prophylaxis of Migraine With Oral Magnesium: Results From a Prospective, Multi-Center, Placebo-Controlled and Double-Blind Randomized Study," *Cephalalgia*, 16:257–63, 1996.

Shapiro, Jean A., M.D., et al., "Diet and Rheumatoid Arthritis in Women: A Possible Protective Effect of Fish Consumption," *Epidemiology*, 7:256–263, 1996.

Silman, Alan J., et al., "Cigarette Smoking Increases the Risk of Rheumatoid Arthritis," *Arthritis and Rheumatism*, May 1996;39(5):732–735.

Wilder, Ronald, L., "Adrenal and Gonadal Steroid Hormone Deficiency in the Etiopathogenesis of Rheumatoid Arthritis," *Journal of Rheumatology*, 23(suppl 44):10–12, 1996.

CHAPTER 13: ANTIBIOTICS, ANTIFUNGALS AND THEIR NATURAL ALTERNATIVES

Bergus, George R., M.D., et al., "Antibiotic Use During the First 200 Days of Life," *Archives of Family Medicine*, Oct. 1996; 5:523–526.

Goldman, Erik, et al., "Otitis Accounts for Bulk of Antibiotic Overuse," *Family Practice News*, June 15, 1996;43.

Hansen, B. L. and Andersen, K., "Fungal Arthritis," *Scandinavian Journal of Rheumatology*, 1995;24:248–250.

Hoel, Donna and Williams, David N., "Antibiotics: Past, Present, and Future: Unearthing Nature's Magic Bullets," *Postgraduate Medicine*, Jan. 1997; 101(1):114–122.

Kaiser, Laurent, et al., "Effects of Antibiotic Treatment in the Subset of Common-Cold Patients Who Have Bacteria in Nasopharyngeal Secretions," *Lancet*, June 1, 1996;347:1507–1510.

Mainous, Arch, G., III, Ph.D., et al., "Antibiotics and Upper Respiratory Infection: Do Some Folks Think There Is a Cure for the Common Cold?" *Journal of Family Practice*, April 1996;42(4):357–361.

Nidecker, Anna, "Antibiotic Use Linked to Resistant Organism," *Family Practice News*, Oct. 15, 1996;55.

Norrby, S. Ragnar, "Antibiotic Resistance: A Self-Inflicted Problem," *Journal of Internal Medicine*, 1996;239:373–375.

Saadia, Roger and Lipman, Jeffrey, "Antibiotics and the Gut," *European Journal of Surgery*, 1996; suppl. 576:39–41.

Zajicek, Gershom, M.D., "Antibiotic Resistance and the Intestinal Flora," *Cancer Journal*, Sept.–Oct. 1996;9(5):214.

Zittell, Nicholas K., "Is Antibiotic Use Coming Back to Haunt Us?" *Medical Tribune*, Oct. 24, 1996;18.

CHAPTER 14: DRUGS FOR SLEEPING, ANXIETY AND DEPRESSION AND THEIR NATURAL ALTERNATIVES

Adams, P. B., et al., "Arachidonic acid to eicosapentaenoic acid ratio in blood correlates positively with clinical symptoms of depression," *Lipids*, 1996(suppl.):31:S-157–S-161.

Borok, G., et al., "Atopy: the incidence in chronic recurrent maladies," XVI European Congress of Allergology and Clinical Immunology, June 24–25, 1995.

Corkeron, M. A., "Serotonin syndrome—a potentially fatal complication of antidepressant therapy," *Medical Journal of Australia*, Nov. 6, 1995; 163:481–482.

Cincipirini, P. M., Ph.D., "Depression and cholesterol-lowering chemotherapy: potential influence of smoking cessation, depression history, and dietary change," *Behavioral Medicine*, 85–86, 1996.

Driver, H. S., and Taylor, S. R., "Sleep disturbances and exercise," *Sports Medicine*, Jan. 1996;21(1):1–6.

Herber, K. W., "The influence of kava-special extract WS 1490 on safety-relevant performance alone and in combination with ethylalcohol," *Blutalkohol*, 30:96–105, 1993.

King, A. C., Ph.D., et al., "Moderate-intensity exercise and self-rated quality of sleep in older adults: a randomized controlled trial," *JAMA*, Jan. 1, 1997;277(1):32–37.

Kinzler, E., Kromer, J., and Lehmann, E., "Clinical efficacy of a kava extract in patients with anxiety syndrome: double-blind placebo controlled study over 4 weeks," *Arzneim Forsch* 41:584–8, 1991.

Lebot, V., Merlin, M., Lindstrom, L., *Kava—The Pacific Drug*, Yale University Press, New Haven, 1992.

Lietha, R., M.D., "Neuropsychiatric disorders associated with folate deficiency in the presence of elevated serum and erythrocyte folate: a preliminary report," *Journal of Nutritional Medicine*, 4:441–447, 1994.

Maes, Michael, M.D., Ph.D., et al., "Lower serum L-tryptophan availability in depression as a marker of a more generalized disorder in protein metabolism," *Neuropsychopharmacology*, 1996; 15(3):243–251.

——————, et al., "Fatty acid composition in major depression: decreased omega-3 fractions in cholesterol esters and increased C20:406/C20:503 ratio in cholesterol esters and phospholipids," *Journal of Affective Disorders*, 1996;38:35–46.

Martinez, B., et al., "Hypericum in the treatment of seasonal affective disorders," *Journal of Geriatric Psychiatry and Neurology*, 7(suppl 1):S29–S33, 1994.

Munte, T. F., et al., "Effects of oxazepam and an extract of kava roots on event-related potentials in a word recognition task," *Neuropsychobiol*, 27:46–53, 1993.

Neumeister, Alexander, M.D., et al., "Effects of tryptophan depletion on drug-free patients with seasonal affective disorder during a stable response to bright light therapy," *Archives of General Psychiatry*, 1997;54:133–138.

Pilar, S., M.D., "Amelioration of premenstrual depressive symptomatology with L-tryptophan," *Journal of Psychiatry and Neuroscience*, 1994;19(2):114–119.

Ploeckinger, B., et al., "Rapid decrease of serum cholesterol concentration and post-partum depression," *British Medical Journal*, Sept. 14, 1996;313:664.

Reichert, R. G., N.D., "St. John's wort extract as a tricyclic medication substitute for mild to moderate depression," *Quarterly Review of Natural Medicine*, Winter 1995, p. 275–278.

Reid, Kathryn, et al., "Day-time melatonin administration: effects on core temperature and sleep onset latency," *Journal of Sleep Research*, 1996;5:150–154.

Scholing, W. E., Clausen H. D., "On the effect of d, l-kavain: experience with neuronika," *Med Klin* 72:1301–6, 1977.

Singh, Y. N., "Kava: an overview," *Journal of Ethnopharmacology* 1992; 37:13–45.

Volz, H. P., and Kieser, M., "Kava-kava extract WS 1490 versus placebo in anxiety disorders—a randomized placebo-controlled 25-week outpatient trial," *Pharmacopsychiat*, 1997;30:1–5.

White, H. L., et al., "Extracts of ginkgo biloba leaves inhibit monoamine oxidase," *Life Sciences*, 1996;58(16):1315–1321.

Wright, Kenneth P., Jr., et al., "Caffeine and light effects on nighttime melatonin and temperature levels in sleep-deprived humans," *Brain Research*, 1997;747:78–84.

Zal, H. M., "Seasonal Affective Disorder: How to Lighten the Burden of Winter Depression," *Consultant*, March 1997; 641–649.

CHAPTER 15: DIABETES DRUGS AND THEIR NATURAL ALTERNATIVES

Assan, R., et al., "Dehydroepiandrosterone (DHEA) for Diabetic Patients?" *European Journal of Endocrinology*, 1996;135:37–38.

Basualdo, Carlota G., M.Sc., R.D., et al., "Vitamin A (Retinol) Status of First Nation Adults With Non-Insulin Dependent Diabetes Mellitus," *Journal of the American College of Nutrition*, 1997;16(1):38–45.

Bode, Ann M., "Metabolism of Vitamin C in Health and Disease," *Advances in Pharmacology*, 1997;40:334–44.

Ceriello, Antonio, M.D., et al., "Vitamin E Reduction of Protein Glycosylation in Diabetes: New Prospect for Prevention of Diabetic Complications?" *Diabetes Care*, Jan. 1991;14(1):68–72.

Challem, Jack, "Antioxidants Might Ease Diabetic Complications," *Medical Tribune*, Dec. 12, 1996;18.

Dela, Flemming, "On the Influence of Physical Training on Glucose Homeostasis," *Acta Physiologica Scandinavica*, 1996;5–33.

Jain, Sushil K., Ph.D., et al., "Effect of Modest Vitamin E Supplementation on Blood Glycated Hemoglobin and Triglyceride Levels and Red Cell Indices in Type I Diabetic Patients," *Journal of the American College of Nutrition*, 1996;15(5):458–461.

——————, "Hyperglycemia Can Cause Membrane Lipid Peroxidation and Osmotic Fragility in Human Red Blood Cells," *Journal of Biological Chemistry*, Dec. 15, 1989;264(35):21340–21345.

Kakkar, Rakesh, et al., "Antioxidant Defense System in Diabetic Kidney: A Time Course Study," *Life Sciences*, 60(9):667–679, 1997.

Pick, Mary E., M.Sc., R.D., et al., "Oat Bran Concentrate Bread Products Improve Long-Term Control of Diabetes: A Pilot Study," *Journal of the American Dietetic Association*, Dec. 1996;96(12):1254–1261.

Trehan, Shruti, M.D., et al., "Magnesium Disorders: What To Do When Homeostasis Goes Awry," *Consultant*, Nov. 1996;2485–2497.

Tuominen, J. A., et al. "Exercise Increases Insulin Clearance in Healthy Men and Insulin-Dependent Diabetes Mellitus Patients," *Clinical Physiology*, 17:19–30, 1997.

Osterode, W., et al., "Nutritional Antioxidants, Red Cell Membrane Fluidity and Blood Viscosity in Type I (Insulin Dependent) Diabetes Mellitus," *Diabetic Medicine*, 13:1044–1050, 1996.

Vaccaro, Olga, et al. "Moderate Hyperhomocysteinaemia and Retinopathy in Insulin-Dependent Diabetes," *Lancet*, April 12, 1997, 349:1102–1103.

CHAPTER 16: DRUGS FOR EYE DISEASES AND THEIR NATURAL ALTERNATIVES

Albert, D., M.D., et al., *Principles and Practice of Ophthalmology: Basic Sciences*. W. B. Saunders, 1994.

Baudoin, C., et al., "Expression of inflammatory membrane markers by conjunctival cells in chronically treated patients with glaucoma," *Ophthalmology*, 1994; 101:454–60.

Boulton, M., et al., "Lipofuscin is a photoinducible free radical generator," *Journal of Photochemistry and Photobiology*, B-Biology, Aug. 1993, 19(3):201–4.

Connor, W. E. et al., "Essential Fatty Acids: The Importance of N-3 Fatty Acids in the Retina and Brain," *Nutrition Reviews*, 1992, 50:21–29.

Czernin, J., et al., "Effect of short-term cardiovascular conditioning and low-fat diet on myocardial blood flow and flow reserve," *Circulation*, 92(2):192–204, July 15, 1995.

Ferris, F. L., "Senile macular degeneration: review of epidemiologic features," *Am. J. Epid.* 118:132–50, 1983.

Gottsch, J., et al., "Light-induced deposits in Bruch's membrane of protoporhyric mice," *Archives of Ophthalmology*, Jan. 1993, 111(1):126–9.

Jacob, S., et al., "The antioxidant alpha-lipoic acid enhances insulin-stimulated glucose metabolism in insulin-resistant rat skeletal muscle," *Diabetes*, Aug. 1996, 45(8):1024–9.

Jonas, J., et al., "Parapapillary retinal diameter in normal and glaucomatous eyes," *Investigative Ophthalmology*, 30:1599–1603, 1989.

Kilic, F., et al., "Modelling cortical cataractogenesis 17: in vitro effect of a-lipoic acid on glucose-induced lens membrane damage, a model of diabetic cataractogenesis," *Biochemistry & Molecular Biology International*, Oct. 1995, 37(2):361–70.

Leibowitz, H., Krueger, D., Mauder, L., "The Framingham Eye Study Monograph," *Surv Ophthalmol* 24(suppl):1980.

McDougall, J., et al., "Rapid reduction of serum cholesterol and blood pressure by a twelve-day, very low fat, strictly vegetarian diet," *Journal of the American College of Nutrition*, Oct. 1995, 14(5):491–6.

Nordoy, Arne, "Fish Consumption and Cardiovascular Disease: A Reappraisal," *Nutrition and Metabolism in Cardiovascular Disease*, 6:103–109, 1996.

Rozanowska, M., et al., "Blue light-induced reactivity of retinal age pigment. In vitro generation of oxygen-reactive species," *Journal of Biological Chemistry*, Aug. 11, 1995, 270(32):18825–30.

Sakai, T., Murata, M., Amemiya, T., "Effects of long-term treatment of glaucoma with vitamin B12," *Glaucoma* 14:167–70, 1992.

Seddon, J. M., et al., "Dietary carotenoids, vitamins A, C, and E, and advanced age-related macular degeneration," *JAMA*, 272:1413–1420, 1994.

Snodderly, D. M., "Evidence for protection against age-related macular degeneration by carotenoids and antioxidant vitamins," *Am. J. Clin. Nutr.*, 63(6 suppl):1448S–1461S, Dec. 1995.

Williams, D. E., et al., "Effects of timolol, betaxolol, and levobunolol on human tendon's fibroblasts in tissue culture," *Investigative Ophthalmology and Visual Sciences*, 33:2233–41, 1992.

Ziegler, D., et al., "Treatment of symptomatic diabetic peripheral neuropathy with the antioxidant alpha-lipoic acid. A 3-week multicentre randomized controlled trial (ALADIN study)," *Diabetologica*, Dec. 1995, 38(12):1425–33.

CHAPTER 17: DRUGS FOR THE PROSTATE AND THEIR NATURAL ALTERNATIVES

Giovannucci, Edward, et al., "A Prospective Study of Dietary Fat and the Risk of Prostate Cancer," *Journal of the National Cancer Institute*, Oct. 6, 1993;85(19):1571–1579.

Klein, L. A., Stoff, J. S., "Prostaglandins and the Prostate: An Hypothesis on the Etiology of Benign Prostatic Hyperplasia," *Prostate* 4(3):247–51, 1983.

Milne, David B., Ph.D., and Johnson, Phyllis E., Ph.D., "Effect of Changes in Short-Term Dietary Zinc Intake on Ethanol Metabolism and Zinc Status Indices in Young Men," *Nutrition Research*, 1993; 13:511–521.

Morrison, Howard, et al., "Herbicides and Cancer," *Journal of the National Cancer Institute*, 1992;84:1866–1874.

—————, et al., "Farming and Prostate Cancer Mortality," *American Journal of Epidemiology*, 1993;137(3):270–280.

Rose, David P., "Diet, Hormones and Cancer," *Annual Review of Public Health*, 1993;14:1017.

Talamini, Renato, et al., "Diet and Prostatic Cancer: A Case-Controlled Study in Northern Italy," *Nutrition and Cancer*, 1992;18:277–286.

CHAPTER 18: SYNTHETIC HORMONES AND THEIR NATURAL ALTERNATIVES

Pregnenolone

Akwa, Y. and Young, J., et al., "Neurosteroids: Biosynthesis, metabolism and function of pregnenolone and dehydroepiandrosterone in the brain," *J Steroid Biochem Mol Biol*, 40/1–3:71–81, 1991.

De Wied, D., "Hormone influences on motivation, learning and memory processes," *Hosp Prac*, 11(1):123–131, 1976.

—————, "Pituitary adrenal system hormones and behavior," *Acta Endocrinol*, 85(Suppl 214):9–18, 1977.

Flood, J. F., and Morley, J. E., and Roberts, E., "Memory-enhancing effects in male mice of pregnenolone and steroids metabolically derived from it," *Proc Natl Acad Sci*, 89:1567–1571, 1992.

Morfin, R., and Young, J., et al., "Neurosteroids: Pregnenolone in human sciatic nerves," *Proc Natl Acad Sci USA*, 9/15:6790–6793, 1992.

Paul, S. M., and Purdy, R. H., "Neuroactive steroids," *FASEB J*, 1992;6/6:2311–2322.

Weidenfeld, J., Siegel, R. A. and Chowers, I., "In vitro conversion of pregnenolone to progesterone by discrete brain areas of the male rat," *J Steroid Biochem*, 13/8:961–963, 1980.

Wu, F. S., Gibbs, T. T., et al., "Pregnenolone sulfate: A positive allosteric modulator at the N-methyl-D-aspartate receptor," *Mol Pharmacol*, 40(3):333–336, 1991.

Progesterone

Cundy, T., Evans, M., Roberts, H., et al., "Bone density in women receiving a depot medroxyprogesterone acetate for contraception," *Br Med J* 1991; 303:13–16.

Ellison, P. T., Panter-Brick, C, Lipson, S. F., and O'Rourke, M. T., "The ecological context of human ovarian function," *Human Reprod*, 8:2248–58, 1993.

Hargrove, J. T., Maxson, W. S., et al., "Menopausal hormone replacement therapy with continuous daily oral micronized estradiol and progesterone," *OB&Gyn*, 71:606–612, 1989.

Lee, J. R., M.D., "Osteoporosis reversal: the role of progesterone," *Intern Clin Nutr Rev*, 10:384–391, 1990.

—————, "Osteoporosis reversal with transdermal progesterone," (letter) *Lancet*, 336:1327, 1990.

—————, "Is natural progesterone the missing link in osteoporosis prevention and treatment?" *Medical Hypotheses*, 35:316–318, 1991.

Prior, J. C., Vigna, V. M., "Spinal bone loss and ovulatory disturbances," *N Engl J Med*, 323:1221–1227, 1990.

—————, Vigna, V., Alojado, N., "Progesterone and the prevention of osteoporosis," *Canadian J OB/GYN & Women's Health Care*, 3:178–84, 1991.

—————, "Progesterone as a bone-trophic hormone," *Endocrine Reviews*, 11:386–398, 1990.

Reyes, F. L., Winter, J. S., Paiman, C., "Pituitary ovarian relationships preceding the menopause: A cross-sectional study of serum follicle-stimulating hormone, luteinizing hormone, prolactin, estradiol and progesterone levels," *Am J Obstet Gynecol*, 129:557–564, 1977.

DHEA

Araneo, B., Daynes, R., "Dehydroepiandrosterone functions as more than an antiglucocorticoid in preserving immunocompetence after thermal injury," *Endocrinology*, 136(2):393–401, Feb. 1995.

Assan, R., et al., "Dehydroepiandrosterone (DHEA) for diabetic patients?" *European Journal of Endocrinology*, 1996; 135:37–38.

Barrett-Connor, E., Ferrara, A., "Dehydroepiandrosterone, dehydroepiandrosterone sulfate, obesity, waist-hip ratio, and noninsulin-dependent diabetes in postmenopausal women: the Rancho Bernardo Study," *J Clin Endocrin & Metab*, 81(1):59–64, Jan. 1996.

Baulieu, E. E., "Dehydroepiandrosterone (DHEA): A Fountain of Youth?" *Journal of Clinical Endocrinology and Metabolism*, 1996;81(9):3147–3151.

Beer, N. A., et al., "Dehydroepiandrosterone reduces plasma plasminogen activator inhibitor type 1 and tissue plasminogen activator antigen in man," *Am J of the Med Sci*, 311(5):205–10, May 1996.

Daynes, R. A., Araneo, B. A., "The development of effective vaccine adjuvants employing natural regulators of T-cell lymphokine production in vivo," *Annals of the New York Academy of Sciences* 730:144–61, Aug. 15, 1994.

Eich, D. M., et al., "Inhibition of accelerated coronary atheroslerosis with dehydroepiandrosterone in the heterotropic rabbit model of cardiac transplantation," *Circulation*, 87(1):261–9, Jan. 1993.

Freiss, E. et al., "DHEA administration increases rapid eye movement sleep and EEG power and sigma frequency range," *American Journal of Physiology,* 1995:268:E107–E113.

Haffner, S. M., Valdez, R. A., "Endogenous sex hormones: impact on lipids, lipoproteins, and insulin," *Am J Medicine,* 98(1A):40S–47S, Jan. 16, 1995.

Herbert, J., et al., "The Age of Dehydroepiandrosterone," *Lancet,* May 13, 1995;345:1193–1194.

McLachlan, J. A., Serkin, C. D., Bakouche, O., "Dehydroepiandrosterone modulation of lipopolysaccharide-stimulated monocyte cytotoxicity," *Journal of Immunology,* 156(1):328–35, Jan. 1, 1996.

Morales, A. J., et al., "Effects of replacement dose of dehydroepiandrosterone in men and women of advancing age," *Journal of Clinical Endocrinology and Metabolism,* 1994;78:P1360–1367.

Padgett, D. A., Loria, R. M., "In vitro potentiation of lymphocyte activation by dehydroepiandrosterone, androstenediol, and androstenetriol," *Journal of Immunology,* 153(4):1544–52, Aug. 15, 1994.

Sholnick, Andrew A., "Scientific verdict still out on DHEA," *JAMA,* Nov. 6, 1966, Vol. 276, No. 17.

Toshiyuki, H. M.D., Ph.D., et al., "Effect of Dehydroepiandrosterone Sulfate on Ophthalmic Artery Flow Velocity Wave Forms in Full-Term Pregnant Women," *American Journal of Perinatology,* March 1995; 12(2):135–137.

Watson, D. R., Ph.D., *Exp Opin Invest Drugs,* 1995;4(2):147–154.

Yen, S. S., Morales, A. J., Khorram, O., "Replacement of DHEA in aging men and women, potential remedial effects," *Annual Report of the N.Y. Academy of Sciences,* 1995;774:128–142.

Testosterone

Tenover, J. S., "Effects of testosterone supplementation in the aging male," *Journal of Clinical Endocrinology and Metabolism,* 75(4):1092–8, Oct. 1992.

Growth Hormone

Etherton, T., et al., "Mechanisms by which somatotropin decreases adipose tissue growth," *American Journal of Clinical Nutrition,* 1993; 58(suppl):287S-95S.

Feldman, E., "Aspects of the interrelations of nutrition and aging—1993," *American Journal of Clinical Nutrition,* 58(1):1–3, July 1993.

Hartman, M., et al., "Pulsatile growth hormone secretion in older persons is enhanced by fasting without relationship to sleep stages," *Journal of Clinical Endrocinology and Metabolism,* July 1996, 81(7):2694–701.

Jorgensen, J. O., and Christiansen, J. S., "Brave new senescence: GH in adults," *Lancet,* vol. 341:1247, May 15, 1993.

Kraemer, W. J., et al., "Hormonal and growth factor responses to heavy resistance exercise protocols," *Journal of Applied Physiology,* 1990, 69:1442–1450.

Meling, T., Nylen, E., "Growth hormone deficiency in adults: a review," *American Journal of the Medical Sciences,* 1996; 311(4):153–166.

Rubin, C., M.D., FACP, "Southwestern Internal Medicine Conference: Growth

Hormone-Aging and Osteoporosis," *American Journal of the Medical Sciences,* 1993;305(2):120–129.

Rudman, D., M.D., "Effects of human growth hormone in men over 60 years old," *New England Journal of Medicine,* vol. 323(1):1–6, July 5, 1990.

Schwartz, R., "Trophic factor supplementation: effect on the age-associated changes in body composition," *Journals of Gerontology. Series A,* Biological Sciences and Medical Sciences. 50 Spec No: 151–6, Nov. 1995.

Toogood, A., O'Neill, P., Shalet, S., "Beyond the somatopause: growth hormone deficiency in adults over the age of 60 years," *Journal of Clinical Endocrinology and Metabolism,* Feb. 1996, 81(2):460–5.

Weltman, A., et al., "Endurance training amplifies the pulsatile release of growth hormone: effects of training intensity," *Journal of Applied Physiology* 72(6):2188–2196, 1992.

Wiswell, R., Marcus, R., "Age-dependent effect of resistance exercise on growth hormone secretion in people," *Journal of Clinical Endocrinology and Metabolism,* Aug. 1992, 75(2):404–7.

Yarasheski, K., Zachwieja, J., "Growth hormone for the elderly: the fountain of youth proves toxic [letter]," *JAMA,* Oct. 13, 1993, 270(14):1694.

Melatonin

Reiter, R. J., "Oxygen radical detoxification processes during aging: the functional importance of melatonin," *Aging,* 7(5):340–51, Oct. 1995.

————, "The aging pineal gland and its physiological consequences," *Bioessays,* March 1992, 14(3):169–75.

————, "The role of the neurohormone melatonin as a buffer against macromolecular oxidative damage," *Neurochemistry International,* Dec. 1995, 27(6):453–60.

————, "Functional pleiotropy of the neurohormone melatonin: antioxidant protection and neuroendocrine regulation," *Frontiers in Neuroendocrinology,* Oct. 1995, 16(4):383–415.

CHAPTER 19: DRUGS FOR OSTEOPOROSIS AND THEIR NATURAL ALTERNATIVES

Chilibeck, Philip D., et al., "Exercise and Bone Mineral Density," *Sports Medicine,* 1995;19(2):103–122.

Cooper, C., et al., "Water fluoridation and hip fracture (letter), *JAMA* 1991; 266:513–514.

Danielson, C., Lyon, J. L., Egger, M., Goodenough, G. K., "Hip fractures and fluoridation in Utah's elderly population," *JAMA* 1992; 268:746–747.

Hedlund, L. R., Gallagher, J. C., "Increased incidence of hip fracture in osteoporotic women treated with sodium fluoride," *J Bone & Miner Res* 1989; 4:223–225.

Jacobsen, S. J., Goldenberg, J., Miles, T. P., Brody, J. A., et al., "Regional variation in the incidence of hip fractures; U.S. white women aged 65 years and older," *JAMA* 1990; 264:500–502.

Jacqmin-Gadda, H., Commenges, D., Dartigues, J. F., "Fluorine concentrations in drinking water and fracture in the elderly," *JAMA* 1995;273:775–6.

Kleerekoper, M. E.l, Peterson, E., Phillips, E. Nelson, D., et al., Continuous sodium fluoride therapy does not reduce vertebral fracture rate in postmenopausal osteoporosis [abstract], *J Bone Miner Res* 1989; Res. 4 (suppl. 1):S376.

Lindsay, Robert M.B., Ph.D., "The Burden of Osteoporosis:Cost," *American Journal of Medicine,* Feb. 27, 1995;98(suppl. 2A):2A–9S–2A–11S.

Riggs, B. L., Hodgson, S. F., O'Fallon, W. M., Chao, E. Y. S., et al., "Effect of fluoride treatment on the fracture rate in postmenopausal women with osteoporosis," *N Engl J Med,* 1990; 322:802–809.

Scarbeck, Kathy, "Strength Training May Reduce the Risk of Osteoporotic Fractures," *Family Practice News,* Feb. 15, 1995:10.

Sowers, M. F. R., Clark, M. K., Jannausch, M. L., Wallace, R. B., "A prospective study of bone mineral content and fracture in communities with differential fluoride exposure," *Am J Epidemiol,* 1991; 134:649–660.

REFERENCE BOOKS

Bosker, Gideon, M.D., FACEP, *Pharmatecture: Minimizing Medications to Maximize Results,* Facts & Comparisons, St. Louis, Mo. 1996.

Colvin, Rod, *Prescription Drug Abuse: The Hidden Epidemic,* Omaha, Neb., Addicus Books, 1995.

Dalton, H. R., Grahame-Smith, D. G. and Aronson, J. K., *Oxford Textbook of Clinical Pharmacology and Drug Therapy,* Oxford University Press, Oxford, England, 1992.

Drug Facts & Comparisons, Facts & Comparisons, St. Louis, Mo., 1997.

Ganong, William F., *Review of Medical Physiology,* sixteenth edition, Appleton & Lange, Norwalk, Conn., 1993.

Gradeon, Joel and Teresa, Ph.D., *The People's Guide to Deadly Drug Interactions,* St. Martin's Press, New York, 1995.

——————— and ———————, *The People's Pharmacy,* St. Martin's Griffin, New York, 1996.

Grahame-Smith, D. G. and Aronson, J. K., *Oxford Textbook of Clinical Pharmacology and Drug Therapy,* Oxford University Press, Oxford, England, 1992.

Handbook of Nonprescription Drugs, Eleventh Edition, American Pharmaceutical Association, Washington, D.C., 1996.

Hansten and Horn's Drug Interactions Analysis and Management (Applied Therapeutics, Inc., P.O. Box 5077, Vancouver, WA 98668-5077; (306) 253–7123).

Harness, R. H., *Drug Interactions Guide Book,* Prentice Hall, Englewood Cliffs, N.J., 1991.

Holt, Gary, *Food and Drug Interactions: A Health Care Professional's Guide,* Precept Press, Inc., Chicago, 1992.

The Merck Manual of Diagnosis and Therapy, Merck & Co., Rahway, N.J., 1992.

Physician's Desk Reference, Medical Economics Data Production Company, Montvale, N.J., 1997.

The PDR Family Guide to Prescription Drugs, Crown, New York, 1996.

Thomas, J. H. and Gillham, B., *Wills' Biochemical Basis of Medicine,* Butterworth-Heineman Ltd., Oxford, England, 1992.

INDEX

absorption, 43
acarbose (Precose), 404–405
ACE inhibitors, 135–139
  and kidney damage, 36
acebutolol (Sectral), 130–135
acetaminophen, 285, 286, 287,
    292–293
  and alcohol, 45
  and liver damage, 34
  side effects of, 288
  and surgery, 55–56
  see also Tylenol
acetohexamide (Dymelor), 408–410
acupuncture, and asthma, 272
acyclovir (Zovirax), 503–504
addiction, 28–29, 507
Addison's disease, 482
ADE: see adverse drug events
adenomas, 65
adrenal
  hormones, 473
  insufficiency, and cortisones, 482
adrenaline, 386, 455
adult-onset diabetes, 399–400
  and DHEA, 473–474
adverse drug events, 3, 16–17, 18,
    31, 60, 64, 137
  costs of, 4
  and hospitalization, 50

reporting, 64
aging
  and estrogens, 477
  and hormones, 482–483
  and hypothyroidism, 480
  and melatonin, 390
  see also elderly
agranulocytosis, 65
albuterol, 232–236
alcohol
  and depression, 386
  and drugs, 45–46
  and food allergies, 188
  and heart disease, 91
  and insomnia, 384–385
  and magnesium, 96
  and melatonin, 391
  and mineral absorption, 47
  and osteoporosis, 495
  and surgery, 56
alcoholics, 19, 96
aldosteronism, 126
alendronate (Foxamax), 489–490
alfentanil (Alfenta), 305–308
allergic shiner, 227
allergies, 225–284
  and children, 226
  and DHEA, 474
  and drugs, 31, 62

allergies (*cont.*)
  and eye irritation, 445
  and insomnia, 386, 387
  natural remedies for, 269–271
  prevention of, 266–269
  symptoms of, 226–228
alopecia, 65
alpha-glucosidase inhibitors, 404–405
alpha/beta-adrenergic blockers,
    131–135
alpha lipoic acid, 56
alpha-1 blockers, 152–154
alprazolam (Xanax), 369–372
alternative medicine, 14–16
aluminum
  carbonate gel, 204–208
  hydroxide gel, 204–208, 331
  and osteoporosis, 496
Alzheimer's disease, and estrogens,
    458
amenorrhea, 65
amikacin (Amikin), 349–351
amiloride (Midamor), 125–127
amino acids, 397–399
  and depression, 397
aminoglycosides, 349–351
  and kidney damage, 34
aminophylline, 240–244
amitriptyline (Elavil), 33, 381–384
amlodipine (Norvasc), 139–143
amoxicillin, 336–339
amphotericin B, 352–354
ampicillins, 336–339
amylase, 86, 186
amyl nitrate, 106–108
analgesics, 300–301
anaphylaxis, 65
anemia, 65
angina, 65, 94–95, 104–108
  and natural remedies, 100–102
angiotensin antagonists, 136–139
anorexia, 65
antacids, 185, 204–208, 218, 496

and antibiotics, 329, 331
and calcium, 44, 495
effects of, 217
antazoline (Vascocon-A), 440–441
anti-adrenergic agents
  centrally acting, 144–145
  peripherally acting, 149–150
anti-anxiety drugs, 25–27
antibiotics, 327–332, 333–351, 355
  allergic reactions to, 331
  and antacids, 329, 331
  and birth control pills, 332
  and mineral absorption, 47
  natural remedies as, 356–359
  probiotics, use of, with, 355–356
  resistance to, 328
  see also aminoglycosides;
      cephalosporins;
      fluoroquinolones; macrolides;
      penicillins; tetracyclines
anticoagulants, 108–113
anticonvulsants
  and mineral absorption, 47
  and stroke, 112
antidepressants, 23, 115
  and children, 24
  and insomnia, 386
  natural alternatives to, 365
  see also stimulants
anti-diarrhea drugs, 208–212
antifungals, 352–354
  natural remedies as, 360–362
antihistamines, 251–255
  and allergies, 269
  in eye drops, 440–441
  see also histamine
antihypertensives, 116–142
anti-infectives, 327
antioxidants, 83–86, 97–100
  and cholesterol, 93, 161
  and heart disease, 87, 88
  in preventing infection, 57
  see also free radicals

anxiety, 25, 360–399
  natural remedies for, 383–390
  and sleep, 387
  see also anti-anxiety drugs; stress
appetite suppressants, 23
apraclonidine, 425–428
arginine, 484, 505
arnica, 58
arrhythmia, 65, 96, 104–106
arthralgia, 65
arthritis
  and cortisones, 482
  and dry eye, 425
  and feverfew, 312
  medications, and mineral
      absorption, 47
  natural remedies for, 320–324
  and nightshade family plants, 320
  and overweight, 289
  pain, 288–289
  see also osteoarthritis
ashwagandha, 392
aspartame, 398–399
  and depression, 385
  and dry eye, 425
  and glaucoma, 421
aspirin, 285–288, 294–297
  and heart disease prevention, 89
  and mineral absorption, 47
astemizole, and arrhythmia, 252
asthma, 203, 228–248
  and beta-blockers, 130
  causes of attacks, 270
  drugs aggravating, 230
  and estrogen, 272–273
  natural remedies for, 269–271
  and women, 230
astragalus
  and allergies, 270
  and herpes, 504
atenolol (Tenormin), 130–135
atorvastatin (Lipitor), 171–173
atropine sulfate, 208–210

Ayurvedic medicine, 180, 181, 417
azatadine maleate (Optimine),
      251–255
azelastine (Astelin), 251–255
azithromycin (Zithromax), 346–349

bacampicillin HCI (Spectrobid),
      333–336
back pain, 285, 291
  chronic, 27, 310
bacteria
  friendly: see probiotics
  and high temperature, 355
barbiturates, 27
Barnes basal temperature test,
      480–481
becolomethasone dipropionate
      (Beconase AQ), 260–262
bee pollen, and allergies, 271
Bell's palsy, 502
benazepril (Lotensin), 135–139
bendroflumenthiazide (Naturetin),
      117–121
benign prostatic hypertrophy (BPH),
      448
benzalkonium chloride, 424, 425
benzodiazepines, 25–27, 115,
      369–373
  and diarrhea, 37
  and drug interactions, 49
  and melatonin, 391
  and stroke, 112
  and women, 34
benzthiazide (Exna), 117–121
bepridil (Vascor), 139–143
beta-agonists
  and asthma, 231–243
  and heart disease, 229
beta-blockers, 130–135
  and diarrhea, 37
  in eye drops, 429–431
  and melatonin, 391
  and women, 34

beta-carotene: *see* vitamin A
betaine hydrochloride, 86, 218, 495
betaxolol (Kerlone), 130–135
    eye drops (Betriotic), 429–431
B50 complex, 57
bile, 160, 186
    acid sequestrants (bile-blockers), 165–168
bioflavonoids, 83, 85, 111–112, 280
    and allergies, 268
    and blood flow, 417
    and heart disease, 88
biphosphonates, 489–490
birth control pills, 458, 463–465
    and antibiotics, 332
    and antifungal drugs, 361
    biphasic, 463–465
    and drug interactions, 38
    and mineral absorption, 47
    monophasic, 463–465
bismuth subsalicylate, 211–212
bisoprolol fumarate (Zebeta), 130–135
bladder infections, 359
blood
    circulation, and diabetes, 420
    clots, 92–93, 111–112
    thinners: *see* anticoagulants
blood pressure, 113–116
    and age, 19
    and exercise, 157–158
    and magnesium, 95–96, 158–159
    and potassium, 158–159
    and sodium, 158–159
    and stress, 159
    and sugar, 158–159
    and vitamin E, 84
    and water, 159
    and weight loss, 157–158
blood sugar, 414–419
    and fibrinogen levels, 92
    high, 400, 401
    see also diabetes

bone
    density testing, 500
    and steroid hormones, 472, 477, 487
    see also osteoporosis
boron, 492
bradycardia, 65
breast
    enlargement in men, 36, 137, 448
    feeding, and drugs, 32
brimonidine (Alphagan), 425–428
bromelain, 307
    and arthritis, 320–321
brompheniramine maleate (Dimetapp), 251–255
bronchodilators, 115
    for asthma, 229
bulk-producing laxatives, 213–214, 219
bumetanide (Bumex), 121–125
buprenorphine (Buprenex), 308–309
bupropion (Wellbutrin), 373–375
buspirone (BuSpar), 373
butorphanol (Stadol), 300–309
B vitamins, 395–397
    and diuretics, 117
    and homocysteine, 94
    and inflammation, 311
    and probiotics, 355

cabbage, anti-ulcer effects, 216
caffeine
    drugs containing, 342
    and insomnia, 386
    and melatonin, 391
calcitonin-salmon, 490–491
calcium
    absorption factors, 499
    antacids, 206, 207
    carbonate (Maalox, Mylanta), 204–208
    channel blockers, 139–143
    citrate, 494

and cholesterol, 181
depletion factors, 492, 501
and diuretics, 117
and magnesium, 85–86, 391, 486, 493
and melatonin, 391
and osteoporosis, 486, 491–492, 493–494
and stomach acid, 494
and vitamin D, 494
cancer
    and DHEA, 473, 474, 475–476
    and estrogen, 9
    and growth hormone, 484
    pain, 285
Candida albicans, 189, 357
captopril (Capoten), 135–139, 137
carbachol (Miostat), 431–433
carbamazapine, and folic acid, 94
carbenicillin indanyl, 330–333
carbohydrates, 78
    and diabetes, 414
cardiac glycosides, 104–106
cardiovascular disease: *see* heart disease
carnitine, 101
carpal tunnel syndrome (CTS), 291, 325
    natural remedies for, 325–326
carteolol (Cartrol), 130–135
    eye drops (Ocupress), 429–431
carvedilol (Coreg), 131–134
cataracts, 423–424
    and vitamin E, 84
cat's claw (*Uncaria tomentosa*), 324
cayenne, and cholesterol, 188
cefaclor, 336–339
cefadroxil, 336–339
cefamindole, 336–339
cefazolin, 336–339
cefepime, 336–339
cefizoxime, 336–339
cefmetazole, 336–339

cefonicid, 336–339
cefoperazone, 336–339
cefotaxime, 336–339
cefotetan, 336–339
cefoxitin, 336–339
cefpodoxime proxetil, 336–339
cefprozil, 336–339
ceftazidime, 336–339
ceftibuten, 336–339
ceftriaxone, 336–339
cefuroxime, 336–339
central analgesics, 304–305
cephalexin, 336–339
cephalosporins, 329, 336–339
cephalothin, 336–339
cephapirin, 336–339
cephradine, 336–339
cervical dysplasia, 190
cetirizine, 251–255
children
    and allergies, 226
    cold/flu kit for, 280
    and drug accessibility, 30
Chinese herbs, for colds, 276–278
chlorazepate (Tranxene), 369–373
chlordiazepoxide (Librium), 369–373
    and women, 34
chlorothiazide (Diuril), 117–121
chlorpheniramine (Chlor-Trimeton), 251–255
chlorpropamide (Diabinese), 408–410
chlorthalidone (Thalitone), 117–121
cholesterol, 159–182
    and age, 19
    count, 162–163
    diseases causing rise in, 160
    and estrogen, 179
    and fish oil, 179
    and ginkgo biloba, 97–98
    and hormone production, 455
    and insulin, 405
    and magnesium, 95
    myths about, 160–161

cholesterol (*cont.*)
  natural control of, 178–183
  ratio HDL to total, 163
  and water, 72
cholesterol-blockers, 168–171
cholesterol-lowering
  drugs, 165–168
    and elderly, 164
    and mineral absorption, 47
    natural alternatives to, 177–182
    and women, 163
  supplements, 180–182
cholestipol HCl (Colestid), 165–168
  and folic acid, 94
cholestyramine (Questran), 165–168
  and folic acid, 94
choline salicylate (Arthropan),
  294–297
cholinesterase-inhibiting miotics,
  433–435
chromium
  and blood sugar control, 415–416
  and eye disease, 444
chronic
  fatigue, 482
  illness, and surgery, 51
  infections, 359
  pain, 285, 312–317
    alternative medicine for, 318
    back, 310
    natural remedies for, 310–312,
      315–319
  obstructive pulmonary disease
    (COPD), 241
cimetidine (Tagamet), 44, 195–197
cinnamon, 417–418
ciprofloxacin (Cipro), 339–343
circulation: *see* blood circulation
circumin, 324
  see also turmeric
cisapride (Propulsid), 200–201
clarithromycin (Biaxin), 346–349

clemastine fumarate (Tavist),
  251–255
clofibrate (Atromid-S), 174–175
clonazepam (Klonopin), 369–373
clonidine (Catapres), 146–147
  and stroke, 112
cloxacillin (Cloxapen), 333–336
CNS (central nervous system), 65
codeine, 305–308
  sulfate, 262–265
coenzyme Q10 (*ubiquionone*),
  100–101, 170
coenzymes: *see* digestive enzymes
coffee
  for headache, 319
  and insomnia, 384, 385–386
  and osteoporosis, 496
cold
  liquids, 185
  packs, and pain, 310
  sores, 502, 505
colds, 224–284
  and children, 280
  medications for, 255–265
  and insomnia, 387
  and melatonin, 287, 391
  natural remedies for, 275–281,
    355–357
  symptoms of, 225, 356
  travel kit for, 279
colestipol, 166–169
collagen, 492, 495
  and nonsteroidal anti-
    inflammatory drugs, 289
  and vitamin C, 84
colon cancer, prevention, 189–191
congestive heart failure, 104–106
conjugated estrogen (Premarin),
  458–460
constipation
  drugs causing, 219
  drugs for, 212–215

natural remedies for, 218–220
and water, 72
copper
and cholesterol, 180
and collagen, 492
corn syrup, and chromium
        depletion, 415
corticosteroids, 115
and asthma, 229, 246–249
and melatonin, 391
and mineral absorption, 47
ophthalmic, 439–440
cortisol, 455, 482
and DHEA, 474
excess, 483
and thyroid production, 481
cortisone, 466–468, 481–482
creams, 320
and insomnia, 387
and osteoporosis, 496
cosmetics, and eye irritation, 445
coughs, 224–284
coumarin (Warfarin), 108–111
Crohn's disease, 187
and cortisone, 482
curry, and cholesterol, 180
cyproheptadine (Periactin), 251–255
cysteine, 40
cytochrome P-450 enzymes: see P-
        450 pathways

dairy products, 79, 290
d-alpha tocopherol: see vitamin E
decongestants, 256–260
dehydration, and diuretics, 117
dehydroepiandrosterone (DHEA),
        319–320, 473–476
demecarium (Humorsol), 433–435
demeclocycline (Declomycin),
        343–346
depression, 364–399
drugs causing, 385

and heart disease, 159–160
and low cholesterol, 160
natural remedies for, 384–391
see also antidepressants
dermatitis (defined), 65
DES, 9
dexamethasone (Decadron), 439–440,
        466–468
dexchlorpheniramine maleate
        (Polarmine), 251–255
dexfenfluramine, 9
dextrothyroxine sodium, 172–175
dezocine (Dalgon), 308–309
DHEA: see dehydroepiandrosterone
diabetes, 400–420
drugs for, 404–407, 408–414
foot care in, 420
and heart disease, 400–401
natural remedies for, 414–418
see also blood sugar
diabetic eye diseases, 423–424
natural remedies for, 444
diarrhea
drugs causing, 37
drug treatment for, 208–212
and magnesium, 97
natural remedies for, 215–216
see also anti-diarrhea drugs
diazepam (Valium), 369–372
diclofenac (Voltaren), 297–301
dicloxacillin (Pathocil), 333–336
dicyclomine, 202–204
diet
balanced, 81
and healthy eyes, 442–443
and healthy prostate, 451–453
and heart disease, 162
high fat, and prostate, 448
and infection, 356
vegetarian, and fibrinogen, 93
difenonix with atropine sulfate
        (Motofen), 208–209

diflunisal (Dolobid), 290–293
    and women, 34
digestion, 184–223
    drugs for, 191–216
digestive enzymes, 86
    cofactors of, 186
    and pain, 311
digitalis, and magnesium deficiency,
        96
digitoxin, 104–106
digoxin, 104–106
dihydrotestosterone (DHT), 448, 450
diltiazem (Cardizem), 139–143
dioscorea (yam) creams, 476
diosgenin, 472, 476
diphenhydramine (Benadryl),
        251–255, 368–369
diphenoxylate with atropine sulfate
        (Lomotil), 209–210
dipivefrine (Propine), 425–428
direct-acting miotics, 431–433
dirithromycin (Dynabac), 346–349
diuretics, 117–130
    and melatonin, 390
    and mineral absorption, 47
    and osteoporosis, 497
dl-alpha tocopherol, 100
dl-phenylalanine (DLPA), 311
dorzolamide (Trusopt), 435–43
doxazosin (Cardura), 152–154
doxycycline (Doxychel), 343–346
doxylamine (Unisom Nighttime),
        368–369
drowsiness, and drugs, 41
drug
    abuse: see addiction; drugs, abuse
    companies
        and HMOs, 5, 7, 12–13
        and insurance companies, 12
        physician relations with, 11–13
    information insert, 59–64
    labels, 31, 59–64

drugs
    abuse of, 4–5, 20, 19–35
    accessibility, 30
    and alcohol, 45–46
    and alcoholics, 19
    dangerous, 35
    and diarrhea, 37
    and drowsiness, 41
    effectiveness factors of, 33
    and elderly, 19
    excretion of, 34
    FDA approval of, 8–9, 55, 59
    generic names of, 67
    interactions of, 43–49, 50–53, 61,
        63
    and kidneys, 34, 36
    marketing of, 11–12, 59
    metabolism of, 34
    most abused, 21
    and nutrients, 32, 44–45
    overdosage of, 64
    safe use of, 30–31
    terminology, 65–66
    testing of, 32, 60
    unlabeled uses of, 61–62
    in women, 34
    see also adverse drug events
dry eye, 424–425, 445–446
dyphylline (Dilor), 240–244
dyspepsia (defined), 65
dyspnea (defined), 65
dysuria (defined), 65

ear infections, 359–360
echinacea, 225
    and allergies, 267
    and colds, 274
    and herpes, 504
    and infection, 355
echothiophate, 433–435
edema (defined), 65
eicosapentaenoic acid (EPA), 90

Elavil (amitriptyline), 33, 381–384
elderberry, 281
   and herpes, 505–506
elderly
   and cholesterol-lowering drugs,
      164
   and DHEA, 473
   and drugs, 19, 80
   and medical advice, 50
   and melatonin, 389
   and testosterone, 478
   see also aging
electrolytes, 65, 118
elimination diet, allergen testing,
      222–223
enalapril (Vasitec), 135–139
endocrine system, 455
endorphins, 311
enoxacin (Penetrex), 336–343
enzymes
   digestive, 86
   in small intestine, 186–187
   see also amylase; lactase; lipase;
      protease
ephedra tea, 265–266
ephedrine, 52
   and insomnia, 387
epinephrine, 238–240, 256–260,
      425–428
Epsom salts, 220
erythromycin, 346–349
esmolol (Brevibloc), 130–135
essential fatty acids, 223
   and allergies, 271
   and blood sugar control, 417
   and cholesterol-lowering drugs,
      168
   and depression, 385
   see also gamma linoleic acid
esterified estrogens, 458–460
estradiol, 476–478
estriol, 476–478

estrogen, 476–478
   and arthritis, 321
   and asthma, 231, 272–273
   and cancer, 9, 179
   and carpal tunnel syndrome,
      325–326
   and cholesterol, 179
   and fibrinogen levels, 92–93
   and stroke, 111
   synthetic, 456–457, 458–460
   see also hormone replacement
      therapy (HRT)
estrone, 476–478
estropipate (Ortho-Est), 458–460
ethacrynic acid (Edecrin), 121–125
ethylenediamines, 252
etidronate (Didronel), 115, 488,
      489–490
etodolac (Lodine), 297–301
European black elderberries, 281
evening primrose oil, 223, 417
   and dry eye, 446
excretion, of drugs, 34
exercise, 75–76
   and blood pressure, 157–158
   and cholesterol, 178
   and diabetes, 414, 420
   and fibrinogen levels, 92–93
   and growth hormone, 484
   and headache, 317, 319
   and heart disease, 160
   and menopause, 478
   and osteoporosis, 501
   and pain, 314–315
   and sleep, 386–387
expectorants, 255–256
extremities, blood flow to, 84
eye
   allergies, 445
   diseases, 421–446
      drug treatment for, 425–440
      natural remedies for, 441–446

eye (*cont.*)
  drops
    antihistamine, 440–441
    presevatives in, 424
    use of, 422–423

famciclovir (Famvir), 503–504
famotidine (Pepcid), 193–194
fat, 74, 77
  and GLA oils, 90
  and prostrate enlargement, 448, 449
  and water, 72
fatty acids: *see* essential fatty acids
Federal Drug Administration (FDA),
    8–10
  drug approval, 50, 60
feet, care of, and diabetes, 420
felodipine, 139–143
fenfluramine, 9
fenoprofen (Nalfon), 297–301
fen-phen, 9–10
fentanyl (Duragestic), 305–308
fenugreek, 418
feverfew, 312
  and headache, 319
fexofenadine (Allegra), 251–255
fiber, 56–57, 78, 79–80
  and cholesterol, 179
  and colon health, 190
  and constipation, 219
  and diabetes, 414
fibrinogen, and heart disease, 91–93
fibromyalgia, 286
fibromyositis (defined), 65
filtration system, 72–73
finasteride (Proscar), 448, 449–450
fish, 79
  oil
    and arthritis, 322
    and cholesterol, 179–180, 181
    and depression, 385
    and fibrinogen levels, 92
    and healthy eyes, 442–443

flu
  and children, 280
  natural remedies for preventing,
    358–359
  prevention of, 275–276
  shots for, 225, 277
fluconazole (Diflucan), 352–354
flucytosine (Ancobon), 352–354
fluoride, 497–500
fluorometholone, 439–440
fluoroquinolones, 330
fluoroquinones, 339–343
fluoxetine (Prozac), 377–380
fluoxymesterone (Halotestin),
    465–466
flurbiprofen (Ansaid), 297–301
fluticasone propionate (Flonase),
    260–262
fluvastatin (Lescol), 168–171
folic acid, 82
  and cholesterol-lowering drugs,
    166
  and colon health, 190
  and drug interactions, 44, 94
  and estrogens, 460
  and restless leg syndrome, 394
food
  additives, and allergies, 226, 269
  allergies, 187–188, 220–223
    and arthritis, 285, 321
    elimination diet for, 222–223
    and headache, 286
    tests for, 187–188
  labels, 74–75
foods
  cholesterol-lowering, 182–183
  and drug absorption, 43–44, 47–49
  and drug interactions, 44–45
  for lowering blood pressure, 160
  processed, 73, 226, 270
  vitamin loss in, 80
  whole, 73–75
forskohlhii, 443

FOS: *see* frutooligosacharides
Fosamax (alendronate), 488–490
fosinopril (Monopril), 135–139
free radicals, 83, 97
    and iron, 444
    and sunlight, 441
    see also antioxidants
friendly bacteria: *see* probiotics
fructooligosaccharides (FOS), 189,
    355
fructose, 75
fruits, 74
    sugar in, 75
fungal infections
    internal, 360
    toenail, 361–362
furosemide (Lasix), 121–125
    and insomnia, 387

gamma linoleic acid (GLA), 89–90
ganmaoling, 278
garlic
    and cholesterol, 178
    and fibrinogen levels, 93
    and heart disease, 91
gastrointestinal (defined), 66
gemfibrozil (Lopid), 175–177
genital herpes, 502, 505
gentamicin (Garamycin), 349–351
ginger, 324
ginkgo biloba, 97–98
    and blood flow, 416
    and carpal tunnel syndrome, 326
ginseng, 278, 392
    and diabetes, 416
GLA oils (gamma linoleic acid),
    89–90
glaucoma, 421
    drug treatment for, 425–437
    natural remedies for, 443
glimepiride (Amaryl), 408–410
glipizide (Glucotrol), 408–410
glossitis (defined), 65

glucobalance, 418
glucocorticoids, 466–468, 482
glucosamine
    and carpal tunnel syndrome, 326
    and osteoarthritis, 321–322
glutamine, 223
    in preventing infection, 57
glutathione, 98–99
glyburide, 408–410
glycerin suppositories, 215
goiter, 481
goldenseal, 358
gout, 118
grains, 73–74, 78
grapefruit juice, 37
    and drug interactions, 45
    and drugs, 143
grapeseed extract, 57, 85, 99, 355
    and allergies, 269
    and blood flow, 417
green tea, 85, 99
    and allergies, 269
    and cholesterol, 180
griseofulvin (Fulvicin), 352–354
GSH: *see* glutathione
guaifenesin (Robitussin), 255–256
guanabenz (Wytensin), 148
guanedrel (Hylorel), 150–152
guanethidine (Ismelin), 150–152
guanfacine (Tenex), 147–148
guggul, and cholesterol, 180
guggulipid, 181
gymenma sylvestre, 417

halazepam (Paxipam), 369–372
hawthorn berries, 101
hay fever, 226
headaches, 281
    causes of, 289–291
    chronic, 285
    and feverfew, 312
    natural remedies for, 317–319
    see also migraine headaches

health
  and alternative medicine, 14–16
  and lifestyle, 3
  and modern medicine, 13–14
  principles for optimal, 71–86
  responsibility for, 7–8
heartburn, 185–186
  drugs causing, 218
  natural remedies for, 217–218
heart disease, 87–183
  and antihistamines, 252
  and beta-agonists, 234
  causes of, 87–88, 161
  cost of, 87–88
  and diabetes, 411
  drug treatment for, 104–111
  and estrogens, 458–460
  natural remedies for, 90–102
  and sulfonylureas drugs, 408–410
  and trans fatty acids, 74
  and vitamin E, 84–85
heavy metal poisoning, 157
Helicobacter pylori: see *H. pylori*
hemorrhage (defined), 65
heparins, 108–111
hepatic (defined), 65
hepatoxicity, 34, 36, 62
  and cholesterol-lowering drugs, 166
  drugs causing, 35, 36–38
  and penicillin, 330
  and surgery, 55
herbal teas, 278
  for insomnia, 386
herbicides, and prostate cancer, 449
herbs
  for allergies, 270
  for healthy prostate, 453
  for lowering blood pressure, 157
  for pain, 312, 315–317
  see also herbal teas
herpes, 502–506

  and arginine, 484, 505
  drug treatments for, 503–504
  natural remedies for, 504–506
HGH: *see* human growth hormone
high blood pressure, 113–117, 157–160
  drugs causing, 115
  and insulin, 406
  and kidney disease, 157
  and magnesium, 117, 158
  natural remedies for, 157–159
  see also antihypertensives
high-fat diet: *see* diet
hip fractures, 487
hirsutism (defined), 65
histamine, 84
  in asthma, 269–270
  see also antihistamines
HMG-CoA reductase inhibitors, 168–171
HMOs, and drug companies, 5–7, 12
homeopathic medications, for colds, 275–276
homeostasis, 454–456
homocysteine, 87, 93–94
  and cholesterol-lowering drugs, 165
  and heart disease, 161
hormone
  imbalance
    and carpal tunnel syndrome, 325
    and headache, 286
  replacement therapy (HRT), 180, 272–273, 458–459, 461, 472
    and headache, 286
    and osteoporosis, 486–487
  see also menopause
hormones
  balance of, 454–456
  and carpal tunnel syndrome, 325
  and cholesterol, 455

and headache, 290
natural, 470–484
physiologic vs. pharmacologic
    dosages of, 456
synthetic, 456–470
see also human growth hormone;
    melatonin; steroid hormones;
    thyroid hormones
hospitalization, 16–18
hot packs, and pain, 310–311
H. pylori, 186, 191, 192, 216
H2 blockers, 46, 185, 191–197, 495
human growth hormone (HGH),
    482–484
hydralazine (Apresoline), 154–156
hydrochloride supplement, 218
hydrochlorothiazide, 118–121
hydrocodone (Vicodin), 305–308
hydrocodone combinations, 263–265
hydrocortisone, 481
hydrocortisone/cortisol, 466–468
hydroflumethiazide, 118–121
hydromophone (Dilaudid), 305–308
hyperglycemia, 403
hyperkalemia, 126
hyperkinesia (defined), 66
hypertension: *see* high blood
    pressure
hyperthyroidism, 479
hypocalcemia (defined), 65
hypoglycemia, 402
    defined, 65
    substances causing, 403
    and sulfonylurease drugs, 408
hypokalemia (defined), 66
hypomagnesia (defined), 66
hyponatremia (defined), 66
hypotension (defined), 66
hypothyroidism, 479
    and depression, 364
hysterectomies, and hormone
    imbalance, 456

ibuprofen, 285, 288, 297–301
IGF-1, 483
imipramine, and women, 34
immune system
    and cortisones, 482
    pollution effect on, 82
    and probiotics, 355–356
impotence, drugs causing, 41–42
incontinence, drugs causing, 61
indapamide (Lozol), 118–121
indomethacin (Indocin), 297–301
infection
    bladder, 359
    chronic, 359
    ear, 359–360
    natural remedies for prevention
        of, 355–358
    as result of surgery, 54, 57
    viral, 359
    yeast, 360–361
inflammation
    from allergies, 225–226
    and cortisone, 320, 482
    supplements reducing, 323–324
inositol hexanicotinate, 179, 416
    see also niacin (vitamin B3)
insomnia, 363–399
    drugs causing, 387
    natural remedies for, 384–391
    and stress, 25
insulin, 405–407, 455
    and cholesterol, 406
    excess, 483
    and high blood pressure, 406
    like growth factor 1, 483
    zinc suspension (Humulin U),
        405–407
    zinc suspension lente (Humulin
        L), 405–407
insurance companies, and
    prescription drugs, 11–12
iodine, 481

ipratropium bromide, 250–251
iron, and free radicals, 444
irritable
  bowel syndrome, 187, 189, 202,
    220–222
  colon, 202
isophane insulin suspension
    (Novolin), 405–407
isosorbide
  dinitrate, 106–108
  mononitrate, 107–108
isradipine (DynaCirc), 139–143
itraconazole (Sporanox), 352–354

jaudice (defined), 66
jet lag, and melatonin, 389–390

kanamycin (Kantrex), 349–351
kava (*Piper methysticum*), 316,
    394–395
  and stroke, 112
ketoconazole (Nizoral), 352–354
ketoprofen, 297–301
ketorolac (Toradol), 297–301
kidney
  dialysis, and diabetes, 401
  disease, 34
    and high blood pressure, 157
  and drug damage, 36
  and penicillins, 327
  stones, and water, 72

labels: *see* drug labels; food labels
labetalol, 131–135
lactase, 86
Lactobacillus acidophilus, 356
lactose intolerance, 86, 215
lansoprazole (Prevacid), 197–199
large intestine, and digestion,
    188–189
latanoprost, 436–437
laxatives, 212–215
  and mineral absorption, 47

LDL cholesterol, and fibrinogen
    levels, 92
leaky gut syndrome, 187–188
legumes, 73–74
lemon balm, for herpes, 506
leukopenia, 65
levobunolol (Betagan), 429–431
levomethadyl (ORLAAM), 305–308
levonorgestrel (Progestasert),
    463–465
levorphanol tartate, 305–308
levothyroxine (Synthroid), 468–470
licorice, 216, 482
lifestyle
  and diabetes, 402
  and health, 3
  and heart disease, 88
  and high blood pressure, 113–114
liothyronine (Cytomel), 468–470
liotrix (Euthroid), 468–470
lipase, 86, 186
lisinopril, 135–139
liver damage: *see* hepatoxicity
lomefloxacin (Maxaquin), 339–343
loop diuretics, 121–125
loperamide (Kaopectate), 210–211
loracarbef (Lorabid), 336–339
loratadine (Claritin), 251–255
lorazepam (Ativan), 26, 369–372
lovastatin (Mevacor), 168–171
  and insomnia, 387
low blood sugar: *see* hypoglycemia
lubricants, 214–215
lupus, 482
lutein, 444
lysine, 505

maalox antacid, 204–208
macrolide antibiotics, 329, 346–349
macular degeneration, 421–423
  natural remedies for, 444
magaldrate (Riopan), 204–208
magnesium

and alcohol, 96
aluminum antacids, 207, 208
antacids, 206, 207
and blood pressure, 158–159
and blood sugar control, 416
and calcium, 85–86, 392, 486, 491
calcium supplements, and pain,
    311–312
and cholesterol, 180
and constipation, 220
depletion factors, 96
food sources of, 96
and headache, 319
and heart disease, 89, 94–97, 161
hydroxide (Milk of Magnesia),
    204–208
oxide, 204–208
and osteoporosis, 492, 493
salicylate, 294–297
and vitamin B6, 486
maitake mushrooms, 418
malaise (defined), 66
manganese, 492
and blood sugar control, 416
MAO inhibitors, 53, 115
and reserpine, 149
marshmallow root, 216
meclofenamate sodium (Meclomen),
    297–301
medical terminology, 65–66
medications: see drugs
medicine, 13–16
meditation
    and pain, 313–314
    and stress, 391
medroxyprogesterone acetate
    (Provera), 461–465
medrysone, 439–440
mefenamic acid (Ponstel), 297–301
megestrol acetate (Enovid), 461–463
melatonin, 389–391, 455
    and drugs, 287
memory, and pregnenolone, 470

men, breast enlarging drugs, 36, 448
menopause, 179
    and estrogen, 477
    and exercise, 478
    and hormone replacement
        therapy, 458, 459
    and progesterone, 470
    and sleep, 388
meperidine (Demerol), 305–308
metaformin (Gluophage), 411–412
Metamucil, 80, 214
metformin (Glucophage), 411–412
methacycline (Rondomycin), 343–346
methadone, 305–308
methamphetamine, 21
methicillin (Staphcillin), 333–336
methionine, 93
methotrexate, and folic acid, 94
methychlothiazide, 118–121
methyldopa (Aldomet), 144–146
methyldopate, 144–146
methylprednisolone (Medrol),
    466–468
    and women, 34
methylsulfonylmethane (MSM), 218,
    275, 418
methyltestosterone, 457, 465–466,
    478–479
metipranolol (OptiPranolol), 429–431
metolazone, 118–121
metoprolol (Lopressor), 130–135
Mexican yam (Dioscorea mexicana),
    476
mezlocillin (Mezlin), 333–336
miconazole (Monistat), 352–354
migraine headaches, 140
    drug treatment for, 302–303
    and feverfew, 312
    and milk thistle, 40, 56
minerals
    and bone, 486
    and drug interactions, 44
    imbalance of, 122

minerals (*cont.*)
  and thyroid production, 481
  see also trace minerals
minocycline (Minocin), 343–346
minoxidil (Loniten), 156–157
miotics
  cholinesterase-inhibiting, 433–435
  direct-acting, 431–433
modern medicine, use for, 15–16
moeixpril (Univasc), 135–139
monophasic (Ortho-Novum),
    463–465
monosodium glutamate (MSG), and
    glaucoma, 421
morphine sulphate, 305–308
MSM: *see* methylsulfonylmethane
muscle spasm, and magnesium, 86,
    95
myocardial infarction (defined), 66

nabumetone (Relafen), 297–301
n-acetyl cysteine, 56, 99
  and cholesterol, 180
nadolol (Corgard), 130–135
nafcillin (Nafcil), 333–336
nalbuphine (Nubain), 308–309
naphazoline, 256–260, 437–438
naproxen (Naprosyn), 298–301
narcotic
  agonist-antagonist painkillers,
    308–309
  drugs, 305–309
    withdrawal from, 307
nasal
  congestion, 225
  decongestants, 115
natural healing remedies, 80–81
neomycin, 349–351
  sulfate, 330
nerve pain, 285
netilmicin, 349–351
neuritis (defined), 66

neuropathy (defined), 66
neutropenia (defined), 66
niacin (B3)
  for blood sugar control, 415–416
  and cholesterol, 177–179
nicardipine (Cardene), 139–143
nicotinic acid, 179
nifedipine (Procardia), 139–143
nightshade family plants, and
    arthritis, 285, 317
nimodipine (Nimotop), 139–143
nisoldipine (Sular), 140–143
nitroclycerin, 107–108
nizatidine (Axid), 194
noise, and sleep, 388–389
non-insulin dependent diabetes: *see*
    adult-onset diabetes
non-narcotic painkiller
    combinations, 301–302
nonsteroidal anti-inflammatory
    (NSAID) drugs, 53, 115, 185,
    285
  and arthritis, 320–321
  and collagen, 289
  and melatonin, 287, 389–391
  side effects of, 286–287
  see also acetaminophen; aspirin;
    ibuprofen; ketoprofen;
    naproxen
norethindrone acetate (Aygestin),
    461–463
norfloxacin (Noroxin), 339–343
NSAIDs: *see* nonsteroidal anti-
    inflammatory drugs
nutrients, 44–45
  and drugs, 33, 44–45
  see also diet
nutritional
  deficiencies, 456
  supplements: *see* supplements
nux vomica, 58
nystatin (Mycostatin), 352–354

obesity
 and arthritis, 288
 and fibrinogen levels, 91–92
ofloxacin (Floxin), 339–343
oils: *see* fat
olive oil
 and cholesterol, 178
 and constipation, 220
 and fibrinogen levels, 92–93
omega-3 fish oils
 and healthy eyes, 443
 see also eicosapentaenoic acid
omeprazole (Prilosec), 197–199
ophthalmic
 corticosteroids, 439–440
 vasoconstrictors, 437–438
opium, 305–308
optimal health: *see* Six Core
  Principles of Optimal Health
oral contraceptives: *see* birth control
  pills
ornithine, 484
orthostatic hypotension (defined),
  66
oscillococcinum, 278, 282
osteoarthritis, 289
 and glucosamine, 320–321
osteoporosis, 117, 485–501
 drug treatment for, 488–491
 early signs of, 487
 and estrogens, 458–459, 477
 in men, 478
 natural remedies for, 491–495
 prevention of, 495–500
 and progesterone, 471
 and protein, 76
 symptoms, 487
over-the-counter drugs, and
  prescription drug interactions,
  51–52
oxacillin (Bactocill), 333–336
oxaprozin (Daypro), 298–301

oxazepam (Serax), 369–373
 and women, 34
oxtriphylline (Choledyl), 240–242
oxycodone (Roxicodone), 305–308
oxymetazoline, 256–260, 437–438
oxymorphone (Numorphan),
  305–308
oxytetracycline (Terramysin),
  343–346

pain
 drug treatment for, 285–286
 and kava, 394
 medication abuse, 21–23
 natural remedies for, 310–312
 relief from, 285–326
 see also analgesics; back pain;
  chronic pain; headaches;
  narcotic drugs
pallor (defined), 66
palpitations (defined), 66
panax ginseng, 392
pantothenic acid (B5), 223, 270
parenteral (defined), 66
paresthesia (defined), 66
Parkinson's disease
 drug induced, 366
 and vitamin E, 84
paromomycin (Humatin), 349–351
paroxetine (Paxil), 377–381
PCOs: *see* proanthocyanidins;
  procyanidolic oligomers
penbutolol sulfate (Levatol), 130–135
penciclovir (Denavir), 503–504
penicillin
  G, 333–336
  V, 333–336
penicillins, 329,-330, 333–336
pentazocine (Talwin), 308–309
pesticides, 102–103
P-450 pathways, 36–39
phenindamine (Nolahist), 251–255

pheniramine maleate, 440–441
phen-Pro, 10
phentermine, 9
phentoin, and folic acid, 94
phenylalanine, 398–399
phenylephrine (Neosyndephrine),
       256–260, 437–438
phenylpropanolamine (Propagest),
       256–260
phosphorous, and osteoporosis, 495
photosensitivity, 63
physicians, relations with drug
       companies, 11–12
Physician's Desk Reference, 60
physostigmine, 433–435
pilocarpine, 431–433
pindolol (Visken), 130–135
piperacillin (Pipracil), 333–336
   and tazobactam (Zosyn), 333–336
piroxicam (Feldene), 34, 298–301
pituitary tumors, 483
plantain banana, 216
PMS, 471
pollution
   and allergies, 225
   and antioxidants, 83
   and free radicals, 83, 97
   and hormone imbalance, 455–456
   and immune systems, 82
   see also toxins
polythiazide (Renese), 118–121
Pondimin: *see* fenfluramine
porphyria (defined), 66
postpartum depression, 471
potassium, and blood pressure,
       158–159
   sparing diuretics, 125–130
pravastatin (Pravachol), 168–171
prazepam (Centrax), 369–372
prazosin (Minipress), 152–154
   and stroke, 113
prednisolone, 439–440, 466–468
   and women, 34

prednisone, 466–468, 481
   and osteoporosis, 497
pregnancy
   and DHEA, 475
   and drugs, 32, 63–64
pregnenolone, 455, 470
   and arthritis, 323
Premarin, 457
premenstrual syndrome (PMS), 471
principles for optimal health, 71–86
proanthocyanidins, 85
   and cholesterol, 180
   see also grapeseed extract;
          procyanidolic oligomers (PCOs)
probiotics, 188–189, 216, 355–56
   and constipation, 220
processed foods, 73
prochlorperazine, and stroke, 112
procyanidolic oligomers (PCO), 99
progesterone, 471–473
   cream, 457, 472, 477
   and estrogen balance, 471
   and menopause, 487
   and osteoporosis, 487, 493
   vs. progestin, 457, 472
progestin, 461–463
   and asthma, 231
   vs. progesterone, 457, 472
progestins, 457, 463–465
promethazine (Phenergan), 251–255
Pro-phen, 10
propoxyphene (Darvon), 305–308
propranolol (Inderal), 130–135
   and insomnia, 387
Proscar (finasteride), 448, 449–450
prostaglandins, and aspirin, 89–90
prostate, 447–453
   cancer, and herbicides, 449
   enlarged, 448–449
      drugs for, 450
      natural remedies for, 451–453
      and saw palmetto, 386, 452
protease, 86, 186

protein, 76
  and growth hormone, 484
proton pump inhibitors, 197–199
Prozac (fluoxetine), 10, 24, 59, 62,
    377–380
pruritus, 62
pseudoephedrine, 49, 256–260
psoriasis, and cortisones, 482
psyllium, 80, 219, 220
  and cholesterol, 179, 181
  see also Metamucil
pterygia, 441
pulmonary (defined), 65
  hypertension, and fen-phen, 9–10
pygeum Africanum, 452

qi gong, 313, 420, 501
quercetin, 307
  and allergic inflammation, 445
  and allergies, 267
  for eye disease, 443, 444
quinapril (Accupril), 135–139
quinethazone (Hydromox), 118–121
quinine, 111

ramapril (Altace), 135–139
ranitidine (Zantac), 192–193
red wine
  and cholesterol, 178
  and headaches, 317
Redux: see dexfenfluramin
relaxation, and headache, 316
REM sleep, and DHEA, 474
remifentanil (Ultiva), 305–308
renal (defined), 66
reserpine, 149–150
restless leg syndrome, 396
Reynaud's syndrome, 140
rheumatoid arthritis
  and DHEA, 474
  and pregnenolone, 470
rhinitis, allergic, 226
rimexolone (Vexol), 439–440

SAD: see seasonal affective disorder
St. John's Wort, 313, 394
  and stroke, 112
salicylates, 294–297
salicylsalicyclic acid, 294–297
saline laxatives, 212–213
salmeterol, 235–236
sangchu, 278
saw palmetto (Serena repens),
    387–388, 452, 453
schizophrenia, and low cholesterol,
    161
seasonal affective disorder (SAD),
    364, 395, 399
sedatives
  abuse of, 20
  natural alternatives to, 365
  see also tranquilizers
selective serotonin reuptake
    inhibitors (SSRI), 24, 377–381
selenium, 279
  and blood sugar control, 416
  and colon health, 190
  for herpes, 505–506
  for infection, 357–358
  for prostate enlargement, 451–452
sertraline (Zoloft), 378–381
shingles (herbes zoster), 502, 504
  and arginine, 484, 505
side effects: see adverse drug events
simvastatin (Zocor), 168–171
sinus, remedy, 280, 357
Six Core Principles for Optimal
    Health, 71–86
Sjogren's syndrome, 425
skin, and water, 68
sleep
  and DHEA, 474
  and growth hormone, 483
  see also insomnia
slippery elm, 216
small intestine, and digestion,
    186–187

smoking
  and arthritis, 288
  and depression, 385
  and fibrinogen levels, 92
  and osteoporosis, 496
sodium bicarbonate, 204–208
  and blood pressure, 158
  citrate, 204–208
  salicylate, 294–297
  thiosalicylate (Rexolate), 294–297
somatotropin: *see* human growth
    hormone
sore throat, 281, 356–357
sotalol HCl (Betapace), 130–135
soy, 79
  and osteoporosis, 493
  and phytoestrogens, 478
  and prostate enlargement, 452
sparfloxacin (Zagam), 339–343
spastic colon: *see* irritable colon
spironolactone (Aldactone), 125–128
SSRIs: *see* selective serotonin
    reuptake inhibitors
statins: *see* HMG-CoA reductase
    inhibitors
steroid hormones, 455
  and bone growth, 486
  see also cortisone;
    dehydroepiandrosterone;
    estrogen; progesterone;
    testosterone
steroids, 53
  and glaucoma, 421
  and probiotics, 352
  withdrawal from, 245
  see also corticosteroids
stimulants
  abuse of, 20, 23–24
  and melatonin, 391
  withdrawal from, 23–24
  see also antidepressants; appetite
    suppressants

stinging nettle (*Urtica dioica*), for
  allergies, 270
stomach acid, 185–186, 217–218
  and calcium absorption, 494
  see also antacids
stomatitis (defined), 66
streptomycin, 349–351
stress
  and adrenal function, 482
  and arthritis, 321
  and asthma, 272, 273–274
  and blood pressure, 159
  and DHEA, 474
  and fibrinogen levels, 92
  and food allergies, 188
  and free radicals, 97
  and heart disease, 161
  and insomnia, 25
  natural remedies for, 391–392
  and pain, 310, 313, 315
  and steroid hormones, 455
  see also anxiety
stroke, 108–113
sucralfate (Carafate), 199–200
sufentanil (Sufenta), 305–308
sugar, 75, 78–79
  and blood pressure, 158–159
  and calcium, 492
  and depression, 384–385
  and GLA oils, 90
  see also blood sugar; diabetes;
    hypoglycemia
sulfa, 435
sulfites, 203
sulfonylurea drugs, 408–410
  and hypoglycemia, 408
sulfur, and healthy eyes, 442
sulindac (Clinoril), 298–301
sumatriptan, 115
  succinate (Imitrex), 302–303
sunlight, 441
  and depression, 399

see also vitamin D
supplements, 82–86
  cholesterol-lowering, 180–181
  daily plan for, 82–83
  probiotic, 355
surfactants, 215
surgery, preparing for, 55–57
sympathomimetics (glaucoma),
    425–428
syncope (defined), 65
synthetic hormones, 446–470

tachycardia (defined), 66
Tagamet, 185, 494
tai chi, 313, 501
tartrazine (yellow dye no. 5), 45, 80,
    203, 230–231, 269–270
  and carpal tunnel syndrome, 325
  and vitamin B6, 325
tea: see green tea; herbal teas
temazepam (Restoril), 369–373
terazosin (Hytrin), 152–154, 450
terbinafine (Lamisil), 352–354
terminally ill, and pain, 286
testosterone, 478–479
  and prostate enlargement, 448
  synthetic, 457, 465–466
tetracyclines, 329, 330, 343–346
tetrahydrozoline (Visine), 437–438
thalidomide, 9
theophylline, 51–52, 240–244
  and insomnia, 387
therapy, and stress, 391
thiamine: see vitamin B1
thiazide diuretics, 117–121
thimerosal, 424
thioctic acid: see alpha lipoic acid
thrombophlebitis (defined), 66
thrombosis (defined), 66
thymus extracts, for herpes, 504
thyroglobulin, 468–470
thyroid

hormone, 455, 468–470, 479–481
  natural methods to increase, 481
  testing for, 480
  see also hyperthyroidism;
    hypothyroidism
  medication, and insomnia, 387
  stimulating hormone (TSH), 480
thyroxine, 480
ticarcillin (Ticar), 333–336
  and clavulanate (Timentin),
    333–336
timolol (Timoptic), 429–431
  maleate (Blocadren), 130–135
tobradex, 439–440
tobramin (Nebcin), 349–351
toenail fungus, 361–362
tolazamide (Tolinase), 408–410
tolbutamide (Orinase), 408–410
tolmetin sodium (Tolectin), 298–301
torsemide (Demandex), 121–125
toxins, 103
  and eye irritation, 445
  and food allergies, 188
  and free radicals, 97
  see also heavy metal poisoning;
    pesticides
trace minerals, and calcium
    absorption, 92
tramadol (Ulram), 304–305
trandolapril (Maavik), 135–139
tranquilizers
  abuse of, 20
  Parkinson-like symptoms of, 366
  see also sedatives
trans fatty acids, 74
trazadone, and women, 34
tremor (defined), 66
triamcinolone, 466–468
triamterene (Dyazide), 125–129
trichlormethiazide, 118–121
Tri-Est, 478
triiodothyronine (thyroid T3), 480

tripelennamine (PBZ), 251–255
triphasic (Ortho-Novum), 463–465
troglitazone (Rezulin), 412–414
troleandomycin (Tao), 346–349
tryptophan, and sleep, 396
TSH: see thyroid stimulating
    hormone
turmeric, 324, 417–418
Tylenol (acetaminophen), 285,
    292–293
  effect of, on liver, 34, 40, 55
  side effects of, 288
type II diabetes: see adult-onset
    diabetes
tyramine, 235, 240
tyrosine
  and depression, 398
  and headache, 286
  and thyroid production, 481

ubiquinone: see coenzyme Q10
ulcers, 185–186, 495
  foot, 419
  natural remedies for, 216, 495
ultraviolet rays, and eye disease,
    441
una de gato (Uncaria tomentosa),
    324
uric acid, 118
urtica dioica (stinging nettle), 270
urticaria (defined), 62
USP thyroid, 468–470, 481

vaginal yeast infection, 360–361
valerian, 391
Valium (diazepam), 25, 26, 369–372
vanadium, 416
vanadyl sulfate, 416
vasoconstrictors, ophthalmis,
    437–438
vasodilators, 154–157, 177
vegetables, 74, 80, 219

vegetarian diet, and fibrinogen
    levels, 93
venlafaxine (Effexor), 115, 375–377
ventilation systems, and allergies,
    267–269
verapamil (Verelan), 140–143
vertigo (defined), 66
viral infections, 359
viruses, 281, 283–284
vitamin A
  and collagen, 492, 495
  and diuretics, 125
  and herpes, 504
  and infection, 57, 357
vitamin B1, 124–125
vitamin B3: see niacin
vitamin B5: see pantothenic acid
vitamin B6
  and adrenal function, 482
  and asthma, 272
  and carpal tunnel syndrome,
      325–326
  and cramps, 395–396
  deficiency, 325–326
  and drug interactions, 45
  and estrogens, 460
  and magnesium, 486
  and tartrazine, 325
vitamin B12
  and asthma, 272
  and depression, 396
  and drug interactions, 44
  and glaucoma, 443
vitamin C, 82, 84
  and adrenal function, 482
  and allergic inflammation, 270,
      445
  and anticoagulants, 112
  and arthritis, 323
  and cholesterol, 180
  and colds, 225, 278
  and collagen, 492, 495
  and dry eye, 446

and estrogens, 460
and glucose tolerance, 416
and healthy eyes, 443
and infection, 357
and inflammation, 57, 311
and stroke, 112
vitamin D, 324, 441, 455
and calcium absorption, 494
and diabetes, 416
and osteoarthritis, 324
vitamin E, 4, 84–85
and adrenal function, 482
and anticoagulants, 111
and bloodclots, 460
and cholesterol, 180
and fibrinogen levels, 93
and glucose tolerance, 416
and heart disease prevention, 84–85, 99–100
and inflammation, 311
in preventing infection, 57
synthetic, 100
vitamins
and healthy eyes, 442–443
and inflammation, 311
for lowering blood pressure, 180, 181, 183
see also B vitamins
vitrectomy, 424

walking, 76
warfarin (Coumadin), 50
water, drinking, 71–73
and blood pressure, 159
and constipation, 219
and fluoridation, 497–500
weight
and blood pressure, 157–158
control of, 76–80
and diabetes, 400, 414

gain, drugs causing, 39
and water, 72
white willow bark, 312
whole foods, 73–75
wild yam (Dioscorea villosa), 472, 476
wine, and fibrinogen levels, 92
women
and asthma, 231, 272–273
and cholesterol-lowering drugs, 163–164
and DHEA, 475
and drug metabolism, 34
and headache, 290
wound healing, 57
and vitamin E, 84

yams, 472, 476
yeast infections, 360–361
yellow dye no. 5: see tartrazine
yoga, 271, 313, 420, 501
yogurt, 216

zafirlukast (Accolate), 244–246
Zantac (ranitidine), 185, 192–193, 495
zeaxanthin, 444
zileuton (Zyflo), 244–246
zinc
and blood sugar control, 415–416
and colds, 276
and collagen, 492, 495
and diuretics, 125
and estrogens, 460
and herpes, 505
and infection, 54, 357–358
and prostate enlargement, 451
Zocor (simvastatin), 169–170
Zollinger-Ellison syndrome, 192, 193
Zoloft (sertraline), 24, 377–381
zolpidem tartrate (Ambien), 365–367